a LANGE medical book

CURRENT
ESSENTIALS
of EMERGENCY
MEDICINE

Edited by

C. Keith Stone, MD
Professor and Chairman
Department of Emergency Medicine
Texas A&M University System Health Science ᵒf *Medicine*
Scott & White Memorial Hospital
Temple, Texas

Roger L. Humphrie~
Chairman and Residen
Department of Emerge
University of Kentucky Co
Lexington, Kentucky

Lange Medical Books/McGraw-Hill
Medical Publishing Division

New York   Chicago   San Francisco   Lisbon   London   Madrid   Mexico City
Milan   New Delhi   San Juan   Seoul   Singapore   Sydney   Toronto

The McGraw·Hill Companies

Current Essentials of Emergency Medicine

1 2 3 4 5 6 7 8 9 DOC/DOC 0 1 0 9 8 7 6 5

ISBN: 0-07-144058-5
ISSN: 1553-3085

This book was set in Times Roman by International Typesetting and Composition.
The editors were Andrea Seils, Harriet Lebowitz, and Penny Linskey.
The production supervisor was Catherine H. Saggese.
The cover designer was Elizabeth Pisacreta.
The index was prepared by Patricia Perrier.
RR Donnelley was the printer and binder.

This book is printed on acid-free paper.

Contents

Contributors

Bill Bass, Jr., MD
Assistant Professor of Emergency Medicine
Department of Emergency Medicine
Texas A&M University System Health Science Center College of
 Medicine
Scott & White Memorial Hospital
Temple, Texas
Neurologic Emergencies

Richard Boggs, MD
Medical Director
Department of Emergency Medicine
University of Kentucky College of Medicine
Lexington, Kentucky
Rheumatologic Emergencies; Chest Trauma

Bruce B. Bollinger, MD
Associate Professor of Emergency Medicine
Department of Emergency Medicine
Texas A&M University System Health Science Center College of
 Medicine
Scott & White Memorial Hospital
Temple, Texas
Dermatologic Emergencies

Aleta B. Bonner, MD, DVM
Assistant Professor and Research Director
Department of Emergency Medicine
Texas A&M University System Health Science Center College of
 Medicine
Scott & White Memorial Hospital
Temple, Texas
Pediatric Emergencies

Karina Bush, MD
Resident Physician
Department of Emergency Medicine
University of Kentucky College of Medicine
Lexington, Kentucky
Orthopedic Emergencies

Charles A. Eckerline, Jr., MD, FACEP
Director, Hyperbaric Oxygen Service
Department of Emergency Medicine
University of Kentucky College of Medicine
Lexington, Kentucky
Abdominal Trauma; Vertebral and Spinal Injuries

David A. Fritz, MD
Assistant Professor
Department of Emergency Medicine
Texas A&M University System Health Science Center College of
    Medicine
Scott & White Memorial Hospital
Temple, Texas
Psychiatric Emergencies

Robert D. Greenberg, MD, FACEP
Assistant Professor and Vice-Chair
Department of Emergency Medicine
Texas A&M University System Health Science Center College of
    Medicine
Scott & White Memorial Hospital
Temple, Texas
Eye Emergencies

Kadeer Mohammed Halimi, DO
Resident Physician
Department of Emergency Medicine
Texas A&M University System Health Science Center College of
    Medicine
Scott & White Memorial Hospital
Temple, Texas
Vascular Emergencies

Tom Huhn, MD
Chief Resident
Department of Emergency Medicine
University of Kentucky College of Medicine
Lexington, Kentucky
Abdominal Trauma; Vertebral and Spinal Injuries

Roger L. Humphries, MD
Chairman and Residency Director
Department of Emergency Medicine
University of Kentucky College of Medicine
Lexington, Kentucky
Gastrointestinal Emergencies; Metabolic and Endocrine Emergencies;
  Obstetric and Gynecologic Emergencies; Hand Emergencies

Jon E. Jaffe, MD
Assistant Professor
Department of Emergency Medicine
Texas A&M University System Health Science Center College of
  Medicine
Scott & White Memorial Hospital
Temple, Texas
Hematologic Emergencies; Infectious Disease Emergencies

T. Russell Jones, MD
Assistant Professor
Department of Emergency Medicine
Texas A&M University System Health Science Center College of
  Medicine
Scott & White Memorial Hospital
Temple, Texas
Cardiac Emergencies

Jeremy C. Leslie, MD
Resident Physician
Department of Emergency Medicine
University of Kentucky College of Medicine
Lexington, Kentucky
Gastrointestinal Emergencies

Julia Martin, MD
Director, Air Medical Service
Department of Emergency Medicine
University of Kentucky College of Medicine
Lexington, Kentucky
Head Trauma; Genitourinary Trauma

Charles F. McCuskey, III, MD
Assistant Professor
Department of Emergency Medicine
Texas A&M University System Health Science Center College of
  Medicine
Scott & White Memorial Hospital
Temple, Texas
Genitourinary Emergencies; Vascular Emergencies

David L. Morgan, MD, MS, FACEP
Medical Director, Central Texas Poison Control
Associate Professor
Department of Emergency Medicine
Texas A&M University System Health Science Center College of
    Medicine
Scott & White Memorial Hospital
Temple, Texas
Emergencies Due to Physical & Environmental Agents; Poisoning

Sanjoy Mukerjee, MD
Resident Physician
Department of Emergency Medicine
University of Kentucky College of Medicine
Lexington, Kentucky
Hand Emergencies

Lisa P. Petit, DO
Resident Physician
Department of Emergency Medicine
University of Kentucky College of Medicine
Lexington, Kentucky
Rheumatologic Emergencies; Chest Trauma

Troy Pope, MD
Resident Physician
Department of Emergency Medicine
University of Kentucky College of Medicine
Lexington, Kentucky
Maxillofacial & Neck Trauma

Steve Ragle, MD
Resident Physician
Department of Emergency Medicine
University of Kentucky College of Medicine
Lexington, Kentucky
Orthopedic Emergencies

Troy C. Rock, MD
Medical Director, Kentucky Speedway and UK Athletics
Department of Emergency Medicine
University of Kentucky College of Medicine
Lexington, Kentucky
Maxillofacial & Neck Trauma

David A. Smith, MD
Assistant Professor
Department of Emergency Medicine
Texas A&M University System Health Science Center College of
   Medicine
Scott & White Memorial Hospital
Temple, Texas
Pulmonary Emergencies

Doug Smith, MD
Chief Resident
Department of Emergency Medicine
University of Kentucky College of Medicine
Lexington, Kentucky
Shock; Nuclear, Biologic, & Chemical Agents of Terrorism

Timothy C. Stallard, MD
Assistant Professor and Director, Emergency Medicine Residency
   Program
Department of Emergency Medicine
Texas A&M University System Health Science Center College of
   Medicine
Scott & White Memorial Hospital
Temple, Texas
Electrolyte & Acid-Base Emergencies; ENT Emergencies

William F. Young, MD, FACEP
Education Director
Department of Emergency Medicine
University of Kentucky College of Medicine
Lexington, Kentucky
Shock; Nuclear, Biologic, & Chemical Agents of Terrorism

Preface

We are pleased to present this book as a companion handbook to the *Current Emergency Diagnosis & Treatment*, sixth edition. Our goal was to create a quick reference to common emergency presentations that would assist practitioners of emergency medicine in providing expert care to their patients. The book follows the Current Essentials series format, providing a page for each diagnosis, with bullet points underneath the three headings: Essentials of Diagnosis, Differential Diagnosis, and Treatment. In addition, there is a Pearl included for each condition. The book is presented in twenty-nine sections with conditions covered in each chapter arranged in alphabetical order for easy reference.

We are grateful to the chapter contributors for their commitment to help us create this first edition. In addition we would like to acknowledge Andrea L. Seils and the outstanding team at McGraw-Hill that provided expert guidance and support throughout the project. Lastly, we would like to acknowledge the patience, love, and support of our families for all of our endeavors and in particular for their understanding of the time needed away from them to complete this book.

C. Keith Stone, MD
Roger L. Humphries, MD

1

Shock

Anaphylactic Shock

- **Essentials of Diagnosis**
  - Shock in the presence of massive histamine release
  - Urticaria, soft tissue edema; skin erythematous and warm
  - Wheezing secondary to bronchospasm; stridor secondary to laryngeal edema; hypotension due to vasodilation
  - In severe cases, loss of consciousness, dilation of pupils, incontinence, and convulsions possible

- **Differential Diagnosis**
  - Other distributive shock states: septic or neurogenic shock
  - Reactive airway disease
  - Angioedema

- **Treatment**
  - Supplemental O_2, 5–10 L/min
  - Assisted ventilation; secure airway if necessary
  - Intravenous access; crystalloid infusion
  - Epinephrine, 0.3–0.5 mg IM (children: 0.01 mL/kg/dose of 1:1,000 solution to a maximum of 0.4-mL dose); severe reactions may require intravenous or endotracheal administration (1.0 mL of 1:10,000 solution)
  - Histamine H_2 blockade with diphenhydramine (adults: 50 mg; children: 2 mg/kg IV or IM)
  - Histamine H_1 blockade (eg, ranitidine, 50 mg, or famotidine, 20 mg IV)
  - Hydrocortisone, 100–250 mg, or methylprednisolone, 50–100 mg IV
  - Albuterol or other β-agonist nebulizer
  - Anaphylaxis may recur 12–24 hours after initial episode; admission of patients with severe anaphylaxis for observation

- **Pearl**

If the patient has a severe reaction, prescribe epinephrine for self-administration in response to future events.

Reference

Tang AW: A practical guide to anaphylaxis. Am Fam Physician 2003;68:1325. [PMID: 14567487]

Cardiogenic Shock

- **Essentials of Diagnosis**
  - Shock in the setting of cardiac outflow obstruction (eg, hypertrophic subaortic stenosis) or pump failure (eg, massive myocardial infarction, severe myocardial disease, arrhythmia)
  - Complication of acute myocardial infarction in about 10% of patients; carries grave prognosis (>50% mortality)
  - Hallmark: hypotension accompanied by clinical signs of increased peripheral resistance (weak, thready pulse; cool, clammy skin) and inadequate organ perfusion (altered mental status, decreased urine output)
  - Signs of acute myocardial infarction or preexisting severe cardiac disease typically present
  - CBC, electrolytes, renal function, cardiac enzymes, coagulation studies
  - Electrocardiogram and continuous cardiac monitoring

- **Differential Diagnosis**
  - Hypovolemic shock
  - Hypotension associated with right ventricular infarction (should respond to fluid challenge)

- **Treatment**
  - Oxygenation and ventilation guided by arterial blood gas measurements
  - Intravenous access; crystalloid infusion
  - Identification and vigorous treatment of any potentially correctable myocardial and nonmyocardial factors contributing to or the sole cause of shock in a patient with myocardial infarction (eg, arrhythmias, acidosis, severe valvular disease, ruptured cardiac muscle, cardiac tamponade, pericardial effusion)
  - Dopamine (better if profound hypotension), dobutamine (better in pulmonary edema), and norepinephrine
  - Intra-aortic balloon pump may temporize
  - Percutaneous transarterial coronary angioplasty (PTCA) may improve survival; thrombolytics do not

- **Pearl**

The only therapy shown to improve survival is PTCA in selected cases.

Reference

Yazbek NF, Kleiman NS: Therapeutic strategies for cardiogenic shock. Curr Treat Options Cardiovasc Med 2004;6:29. [PMID: 15023282]

Hypovolemic Shock

- **Essentials of Diagnosis**
  - Decreased intravascular volume resulting from loss of blood or plasma
  - Causes of blood loss: may be due to external trauma or internal hemorrhage (eg, hemothorax, ectopic pregnancy)
  - Causes of plasma loss: may be external (eg, burns, vomiting, diarrhea) or internal (eg, "third spacing" associated with bowel obstruction or pancreatitis)
  - Common but not readily apparent causes: ruptured abdominal aortic aneurysm, aortic dissection, splenic rupture, intestinal obstruction, peritonitis
  - Low central venous pressure; venous and arterial pressures improve rapidly with intravascular volume replacement
  - Early compensatory mechanisms: narrowing of pulse pressure, decreased peripheral blood flow with pallor, tachycardia, agitation, decreased urine output
  - CBC, electrolytes, BUN and creatinine, liver function tests, PT, PTT, blood typing and cross-matching

- **Differential Diagnosis**
  - Cardiogenic, septic, obstructive, or distributive shock

- **Treatment**
  - Close attention to ABCs; stop evident sources of hemorrhage
  - Oxygenation via high-flow O_2
  - Intravenous fluid challenge of 1–2 L isotonic crystalloid
  - Monitoring of urine output, heart rate, blood pressure, mental status, and blood pH to determine effectiveness of resuscitation
  - Identification of possible sources of blood loss: thorax (chest x-ray), abdomen (bedside ultrasound, diagnostic peritoneal lavage, or CT scan), retroperitoneum (CT scan), pelvis, thigh
  - Warmed blood products indicated for shock refractory to 2–3 L of crystalloid infusion

- **Pearl**

Hemoperitoneum associated with ruptured ectopic pregnancy may not manifest tachycardia despite significant hypotension.

Reference

Holmes CL, Walley KR: The evaluation and management of shock. Clin Chest Med 2003;24:775. [PMID: 14710704]

Neurogenic Shock

■ Essentials of Diagnosis
- Hypotension in the presence of spinal cord injury
- Cutaneous and extremity perfusion maintained
- Failure of vasomotor regulation → pooling of blood in dilated capacitance vessels → fall in blood pressure
- Usually due to traumatic quadriplegia or paraplegia but can be induced by high spinal anesthesia and may be seen in severe Guillain-Barré syndrome and other neuropathies
- Hypotension and tachycardia in setting of neurologic disease (eg, traumatic quadriplegia or paraplegia)
- Higher cord lesions associated with greater likelihood of spinal shock (especially lesions above T11; however, disruption of sympathetic output possible with lesions from T1 to L3)

■ Differential Diagnosis
- Vasovagal syncope
- Hypovolemic shock

■ Treatment
- Supine position
- Oxygen
- Fluid replacement with isotonic crystalloids
- If unable to raise mean arterial pressure above 80 mm Hg after adequate fluid resuscitation: intravenous vasopressor agent with α-agonist activity, such as high-dose dopamine, ephedrine, or norepinephrine

■ Pearl

Neurogenic shock should not be confused with spinal shock, which is the loss of cord-mediated reflexes such as anal wink in the acute phase after a spinal cord injury.

Reference

Fehlings MG, Louw D: Initial stabilization and medical management of acute spinal cord injury. Am Fam Physician 1996;54:155. [PMID: 8677831]

Obstructive Shock

- **Essentials of Diagnosis**
  - Hypotension, jugular venous distention (JVD) unless accompanied by severe hypovolemia
  - Impaired filling of the ventricles (decreased preload) causes fall in cardiac output
  - Some causes of obstructive shock difficult to diagnose and treat in the emergency department
  - Causes: cardiac tamponade, tension pneumothorax, massive pulmonary embolism
  - Rare causes: atrial myxoma, mitral thrombus, coarctation of the aorta, obstructive valvular disease, pulmonary hypertension
  - Emergent bedside ultrasound for rapid diagnosis of causes such as pericardial effusion

- **Differential Diagnosis**
  - Hypovolemic, cardiogenic, neurogenic, or anaphylactic shock

- **Treatment**
  - Intravenous fluid resuscitation
  - Oxygenation via high-flow O_2 or endotracheal tube
  - Vasopressors
  - Emergent decompression of tension pneumothorax with needle followed by tube thoracostomy
  - Nontraumatic causes: blind or ultrasound-guided pericardiocentesis of cardiac tamponade; traumatic causes: emergent pericardial window or thoracotomy
  - Thrombolytics for massive pulmonary embolism associated with shock, cardiac arrest, or severe respiratory compromise
  - For stable patients: echocardiography and right heart catheterization may help establish diagnosis

- **Pearl**

The clinical hallmark of pericardial tamponade is the Beck triad (hypotension, decreased heart sounds, JVD).

Reference

Holmes CL, Walley KR: The evaluation and management of shock. Clin Chest Med 2003;24:775. [PMID: 14710704]

Septic Shock

- **Essentials of Diagnosis**
  - Sepsis = systemic inflammatory response syndrome (SIRS) + confirmed infection
  - SIRS = tachypnea: >20 breaths/min, temperature >38°C or <36°C; tachycardia: pulse >90 beats/min, white blood count >12,000 or <4,000
  - Septic shock = sepsis-induced hypotension despite adequate fluid resuscitation or pressor agent support
  - Cause: gram-negative bacteria (most common), other bacteria, fungi, or systemically absorbed toxins (toxic shock syndrome)
  - Clinical features: rigors, fever, petechiae, leukocytosis or leucopenia with a shift to the left, hyperventilation, altered mental status
  - Overt source of infection not always present; consider occult infections in urinary tract, biliary tract, pelvis, retroperitoneum, skin, or perirectal area

- **Differential Diagnosis**
  - Other distributive shock states: anaphylactic or neurogenic shock
  - Hypovolemic or cardiogenic shock
  - Anticholinergic toxidromes

- **Treatment**
  - Initial volume replacement (adults: 1–2 L, children: 10–20 mL/kg) followed by further administration of fluid based on blood pressure, pulse, and urine output response
  - Inotropic agents such as dopamine, norepinephrine, and vasopressin after adequate fluid challenge
  - Broad-spectrum empiric antibiotics based on likely source of infection; tailored later to culture results
  - Identification and drainage of any source of infection requiring surgery (eg, intra-abdominal abscess, biliary obstruction)
  - Potential benefit from inflammatory response attenuation with medications

- **Pearl**

Aggressive resuscitation (early goal-directed therapy) of sepsis patients in the emergency department was associated with lower mortality as compared with patients resuscitated in the ICU.

Reference

Fitch S, Gossage J: Optimal management of septic shock. Postgrad Med 2002;111:53. [PMID: 11912997]

2

Cardiac Emergencies

Acute Coronary Syndrome

- **Essentials of Diagnosis**
  - A spectrum of conditions from unstable angina to acute myocardial infarction due to insufficient myocardial blood flow
  - ST segment elevation or depression on electrocardiogram with chest pain
  - May or may not have elevated myoglobin within 1–3 hours
  - May or may not have elevated troponin T or I within 2–6 hour
  - Cocaine use can induce

- **Differential Diagnosis**
  - Aortic dissection
  - Pericarditis
  - Peptic ulcer disease
  - Pancreatitis
  - Pneumonia
  - Pulmonary embolus

- **Treatment**
  - Depends on whether unstable angina or infarction occurs
  - Aspirin and nitrate therapy
  - Heparin therapy (unfractionated or low-molecular-weight heparin)
  - Intravenous β-blockers
  - Procedural coronary intervention
  - Thrombolytic therapy

- **Pearl**

Electrocardiogram and enzymes may be normal in patients with acute coronary syndrome.

Reference

Diop D, Aghababian RV: Definition, classification, and pathophysiology of acute coronary ischemic syndromes. Emerg Med Clin North Am 2001;19:259. [PMID: 11373977]

Atrial Fibrillation

- ■ Essentials of Diagnosis (Figure 2–1)
  - • Disorganized atrial rate of 400–650 beats/min
  - • Irregularly irregular rhythm with absence of P waves
  - • Most common sustained cardiac arrhythmia in adults
  - • Prevalence increases with age
  - • Can occur in absence of underlying heart disease
  - • Associated with chronic conditions such as hypertension, valvular heart disease, cardiomyopathy, myocardial ischemia, myocarditis or pericarditis, congenital heart disease, and hyperthyroidism
  - • May be associated with acute conditions such as pulmonary embolism, hypoxia, and excess alcohol or caffeine intake
  - • Increased risk of stroke, especially with intermittent atrial fibrillation

- ■ Differential Diagnosis
  - • Multifocal atrial tachycardia
  - • Atrial flutter with a variable atrioventricular block

- ■ Treatment
  - • Unstable patients: immediate synchronized DC cardioversion, starting with 100 J and increasing by 50 J until sinus rhythm restored
  - • Stable patients: rate control with β-blockers, calcium channel blockers, digoxin, or amiodarone
  - • Anticoagulation, especially for intermittent atrial fibrillation and if onset undetermined or symptoms >48 hours
  - • May use antiarrhythmics—class Ia (amiodarone, procainamide, quinidine) or class III (sotalol, ibutilide)—for chemical cardioversion or elective electrical cardioversion after left atrial thrombus has been ruled out by transesophageal echocardiography or the patient has had 3–4 weeks of anticoagulation

- ■ Pearl

Cardiovert only unstable patients or those in whom atrial fibrillation lasts less than 48 hours, to decrease risk of stroke.

Reference

Joglar JA, Kowal RC: Electrical cardioversion of atrial fibrillation. Cardiol Clin 2004;22:101. [PMID: 14994851]

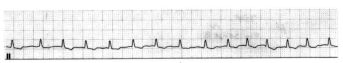

Figure 2–1

Atrial Flutter

- **Essentials of Diagnosis (Figure 2–2)**
  - Characteristic saw tooth flutter waves, particularly in lead II
  - Atrial rate of 25–350 beats/min
  - Typically, a 2:1 atrial to ventricular conduction
  - Can unmask flutter with vagal maneuvers or atrioventricular node blocking agents

- **Differential Diagnosis**
  - Atrial fibrillation
  - Paroxysmal supraventricular tachycardia

- **Treatment**
  - Unstable patients: synchronized DC cardioversion, starting with 50 J and increasing by 50 J until sinus rhythm restored
  - Stable patients: rate control with β-blockers or calcium channel blockers
  - Patients with impaired cardiac function or congestive heart failure: amiodarone is an alternative
  - Anticoagulation is controversial; stroke risk is increased but less than that of atrial fibrillation

- **Pearl**

Consider atrial flutter if the heart rate is a multiple of 75 beats/min (75 beats/min = 3:1 conduction, 150 beats/min = 2:1 conduction, or 300 beats/min = 1:1 conduction).

Reference

Niebauer MJ, Chung MK: Management of atrial flutter. Cardiol Rev 2001;9:253. [PMID: 11520448]

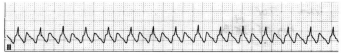

Figure 2–2

Atrioventricular Block, First-Degree

- ■ Essentials of Diagnosis (Figure 2–3)
  - • Characterized by prolongation of the PR interval greater than 0.2 seconds due to myocardial infarction, myocarditis, fibrosis of the SA node, excessive vagal tone, or digoxin toxicity

- ■ Differential Diagnosis
  - • Normal increased vagal tone in athletes
  - • Drug toxicity such as from digoxin
  - • Myocarditis
  - • Inferior wall myocardial infarction with AV node involvement

- ■ Treatment
  - • Treatment directed at underlying cause if indicated

- ■ Pearl

First-degree AV block often is more of an indicator than a problem.

Reference

Barold SS: Atrioventricular block revisited. Compr Ther 2002;28:74. [PMID: 11894446]

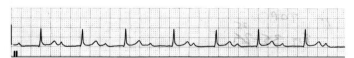

Figure 2–3

Atrioventricular Block, Second-Degree, Type I (Mobitz Type I, Wenckebach)

- ■ Essentials of Diagnosis (Figure 2–4)
  - Progressive lengthening of the PR interval on electrocardiogram followed by a nonconducted P wave leading to a dropped QRS complex
  - Classically, P wave remains constant unless sinus arrhythmia is present
  - Does not commonly progress to complete heart block

- ■ Differential Diagnosis
  - Inferior wall myocardial infarction due to AV nodal ischemia
  - Mobitz II block

- ■ Treatment
  - Observation, but generally does not require pacemaker or other treatment unless patient over age 45 years

- ■ Pearl

Wenckebach *rhymes with* variable interval block. *The Mobitz I (Wenckebach) RR interval is variable (shortens), whereas in the serious Mobitz II block the interval is fixed with a dropped beat.*

Reference

Shaw DB et al: Is Mobitz type I atrioventricular block benign in adults? Heart 2004;90:169. [PMID: 14729789]

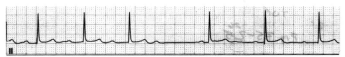

Figure 2–4

Atrioventricular Block, Second-Degree, Type II (Mobitz Type II)

- **Essentials of Diagnosis (Figure 2–5)**
  - Electrocardiogram (ECG) reveals constant PR interval, either normal or prolonged, followed by a nonconducted P wave
  - QRS complex usually wide because this is an infranodal block
  - Test electrolytes and cardiac enzymes

- **Differential Diagnosis**
  - Mobitz type I
  - Anterior myocardial infarction

- **Treatment**
  - ECG monitoring in inpatient setting
  - Strong consideration of cardiac pacing

- **Pearl**

Mobitz II can lead to complete heart block and loss of perfusion, as opposed to Mobitz I, which is far more benign.

Reference

Wogan JM, Lowenstein SR, Gordon GS: Second-degree atrioventricular block: Mobitz type II. J Emerg Med 1993;11:47. [PMID: 8445186]

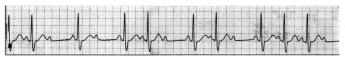

Figure 2–5

Atrioventricular Block, Third-Degree (Complete Heart Block)

- **Essentials of Diagnosis (Figure 2–6)**
  - Independent atrial and ventricular activity
  - No atrial impulses conducted through the atrioventricular (AV) node
  - Atrial rate typically faster than ventricular rate
  - Rate determined by intrinsic escape rhythm
  - AV junctional escape rhythm is 45–60 beats/min
  - Idioventricular escape rhythm is 30–40 beats/min

- **Differential Diagnosis**
  - Digoxin toxicity
  - Calcium channel blocker toxicity
  - β-Blocker toxicity
  - Myocardial infarction or ischemia

- **Treatment**
  - Unstable patients: immediate transcutaneous pacemaker followed by transvenous pacemaker
  - Stable patients: consider atropine or isoproterenol
  - Hospital admission

- **Pearl**

Complete heart block caused by β-blocker or calcium channel blocker overdose may respond to glucagon.

Reference

Brady WJ Jr, Harrigan RA: Diagnosis and management of bradyarrhythmias in the emergency department. Emerg Med Clin North Am 1998;16:361. [PMID: 9621848]

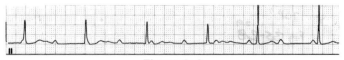

Figure 2–6

Cardiac Tamponade

- ■ **Essentials of Diagnosis**
  - • Tachycardia and hypotension associated with pulsus paradoxus or the Kussmaul sign
  - • Echocardiography: most sensitive and specific test
  - • May observe cardiomegaly on chest x-ray
  - • May note electrical alternans on electrocardiogram

- ■ **Differential Diagnosis**
  - • Pericarditis
  - • Massive pulmonary embolus
  - • Tension pneumothorax
  - • Tension hemothorax

- ■ **Treatment**
  - • Oxygenation
  - • Blood pressure support with crystalloid
  - • Dopamine titrated to support blood pressure
  - • Pericardiocentesis: can be diagnostic and therapeutic

- ■ **Pearl**

Do not administer diuretics, nitrates, or general anesthetics; they may cause severe hypotension in patients with cardiac tamponade.

Reference

Lin CH et al: Spontaneous cardiac rupture. Ann Thorac Surg 2003;76:921. [PMID: 12963231]

Cardiomyopathy

- ■ Essentials of Diagnosis
  - • Three main types: dilated, hypertrophic, restrictive
  - • Myriad causes: ischemic, infectious, immunologic, toxin, muscular dystrophy, metabolic, infiltrative, neoplastic, hypothermic, and pregnancy
  - • Chest x-ray: may be normal or show cardiac enlargement or pulmonary edema
  - • Symptoms associated with congestive heart failure
  - • Electrocardiogram: may reveal left ventricular hypertrophy and intraventricular conduction defects
  - • Echocardiography: often diagnostic
  - • Endomyocardial biopsy: can be diagnostic

- ■ Differential Diagnosis
  - • Myocardial infarction
  - • Acute coronary syndrome
  - • Pulmonary embolus
  - • Pericarditis
  - • Myocarditis

- ■ Treatment
  - • Therapy directed for specific cause
  - • Treat complications such as arrhythmias, embolization, and heart failure

- ■ Pearl

Progressive dyspnea can indicate that the patient is developing cardiomyopathy.

Reference

Cruickshank S: Cardiomyopathy. Nurs Stand 2004;18:46. [PMID: 15017816]

Congestive Heart Failure

- **Essentials of Diagnosis**
  - Caused by extensive myocardial infarction, volume overload, arrhythmia, acute mitral regurgitation, or ventricular septal rupture
  - In right heart failure: elevated central venous pressure, hepatomegaly, peripheral edema, or right ventricular gallop
  - In left heart failure: dyspnea, rales or rhonchi, pulmonary congestion on chest x-ray
  - B-type natriuretic peptide (BNP) levels: can be diagnostic
  - Echocardiography: can help differentiate among causes

- **Differential Diagnosis**
  - Pulmonary embolus
  - Reactive airway disease or chronic obstructive pulmonary disease
  - Myocarditis
  - Cardiomyopathy
  - Massive myocardial infarction
  - Acute respiratory distress syndrome

- **Treatment**
  - Airway management
  - Diuretics unless right ventricular infarct suspected
  - Nitrates unless inferior or right ventricular infarct suspected; may precipitate hypotension
  - Morphine sulfate
  - Natrecor BNP

- **Pearl**

Use of atrial peptides such as Natrecor will falsely elevate BNP levels, which will preclude following these levels to assess the effectiveness of therapy.

Reference

Murcoch DR, McMurray JJ: Acute heart failure: a practical guide to management. Hosp Med 2000;61:725. [PMID: 11103286]

Hypertensive Crisis

- **Essentials of Diagnosis**
  - Evidence of elevated blood pressure with end-organ dysfunction such as of the brain, heart, and kidneys
  - Mental status changes
  - Cardiac ischemia or congestive heart failure
  - Acute renal failure

- **Differential Diagnosis**
  - Chronically elevated blood pressure with no end-organ effects
  - Hypertensive urgency
  - Intracerebral bleed with autoregulation

- **Treatment**
  - Rapid but controlled reduction of blood pressure using intravenous medications
  - Goal is 25% reduction in mean pressure over 1 hour as tolerated by patient; remaining reduction over 24 hours to patient's baseline
  - Nitroprusside
  - Labetalol
  - Nitroglycerin
  - Hydralazine
  - Fenoldopam

- **Pearl**

Make certain that the patient does not have an intracerebral bleed because blood pressure elevations may be a secondary and not a primary phenomenon.

Reference

Cherney D, Straus S: Management of patients with hypertensive urgencies and emergencies. J Gen Intern Med 2002;17:937. [PMID: 12472930]

Idioventricular Rhythm

- **Essentials of Diagnosis (Figure 2–7)**
    - Six or more consecutive ventricular escape beats
    - Rate usually 30–40 beats/min
    - Duration of QRS complex often exceeds 0.16 seconds
    - May develop as a response to severe bradycardia or advanced atrioventricular (AV) block
    - If rate is 40–100 beats/min, the term accelerated idioventricular rhythm (AIVR) is applied
    - AIVR occurs with thrombolytic therapy

- **Differential Diagnosis**
    - Preventricular contractions
    - Ventricular tachycardia

- **Treatment**
    - Directed at treating underlying AV block
    - AIVR associated with thrombolytic treatment of myocardial infarction: no treatment may be necessary as this may be associated with reperfusion

- **Pearl**

Treat the patient, not the rhythm.

Reference

Wehrens XH et al: A comparison of electrocardiographic changes during reperfusion of acute myocardial infarction by thrombolysis of percutaneous transluminal coronary angioplasty. Am Heart J 2000;139:430. [PMID: 10689257]

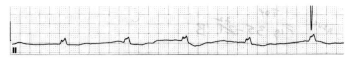

Figure 2–7

Junctional Rhythm

- **Essentials of Diagnosis (Figure 2–8)**
  - Escape rhythm with six or more consecutive junctional beats; ventricular rate of 45–60 beats/min with a narrow QRS complex
  - If junctional escape rhythm is greater than 60 beats/min, the term atrioventricular junctional tachycardia is applied

- **Differential Diagnosis**
  - Sinus bradycardia
  - Idioventricular bradycardia
  - Junctional bradycardia

- **Treatment**
  - Depends on underlying cause

- **Pearl**

Evaluate patient for digoxin toxicity if the junctional rate is greater than 60 beats/min.

Reference

Swart G et al: Acute myocardial infarction complicated by hemodynamically unstable bradyarrhythmia: prehospital and ED treatment with atropine. Am J Emerg Med 1999;17:647. [PMID: 10597081]

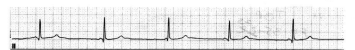

Figure 2–8

Mitral Regurgitation, Acute

- **Essentials of Diagnosis**
  - Associated with myocardial infarction
  - Abrupt severe congestive heart failure
  - Pansystolic regurgitation murmur
  - Echocardiography to detect mitral regurgitation

- **Differential Diagnosis**
  - Preexisting murmur
  - Congestive heart failure
  - Bacterial endocarditis

- **Treatment**
  - Treatment of congestive heart failure
  - Urgent cardiologic consultation
  - Urgent cardiac surgical consultation
  - Intra-aortic balloon pump may temporize

- **Pearl**

Rule out acute mitral regurgitation in the setting of an acute myocardial infarction with a new murmur.

Reference

Yoshida S, Sakuma K, Ueda O: Acute mitral regurgitation due to total rupture in the anterior papillary muscle after acute myocardial infarction successfully treated by emergency surgery. Jpn J Thorac Cardiovasc Surg 2003;51:208. [PMID: 12776954]

Multifocal Atrial Tachycardia

- ■ Essentials of Diagnosis (Figure 2–9)
  - • At least three different P wave morphologies; heart rate typically 100–130 beats/min
  - • May have varying PR intervals
  - • Unless aberrancy is present, the QRS complex is narrow
  - • Associated with severe underlying chronic obstructive pulmonary disease (COPD) in 60–85% of cases
  - • Also associated with congestive heart failure, hypokalemia, hypomagnesemia, pulmonary hypertension, hypoxia, hypercapnia, and methylxanthine toxicity

- ■ Differential Diagnosis
  - • Atrial fibrillation

- ■ Treatment
  - • Achieve heart rate control (metoprolol, esmolol, amiodarone, digoxin, diltiazem)
  - • Treatment of underlying cause (eg, correct magnesium or potassium)
  - • Does not respond to electrical cardioversion
  - • Consider hospitalization depending on cause and on patient's response to therapy

- ■ Pearl

Patients with COPD, who most commonly have multifocal atrial tachycardia (MAT), are also most commonly taking methylxanthines, which are etiologic agents of MAT.

Reference

Pierce WJ, McGroary K: Multifocal atrial tachycardia and ibutilide. Am J Geriatr Cardiol 2001;10:193. [PMID: 11455238]

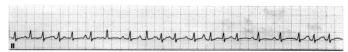

Figure 2–9

Myocardial Infarction, Acute

- **■ Essentials of Diagnosis**
  - Due to atherosclerotic coronary artery disease
  - ST segment elevation on electrocardiogram (ECG) with chest pain
  - ST segment elevation on serial ECGs
  - Myoglobin elevation within 1–3 hours
  - Elevated troponin T or I within 2–6 hours
  - Elevated CK-MB isoenzyme in 4–6 hours
  - S4 or S3 gallop may be associated
  - Ventricular dysfunction on echocardiogram
  - Cocaine use can induce

- **■ Differential Diagnosis**
  - Aortic dissection
  - Pericarditis
  - Peptic ulcer disease
  - Pancreatitis
  - Pneumonia
  - Pulmonary embolus

- **■ Treatment**
  - Procedural coronary intervention
  - Thrombolytic therapy
  - Aspirin and nitrate therapy
  - Intravenous β-blockers
  - Heparin therapy

- **■ Pearl**

Hypotension is common in right ventricular myocardial infarction and should be treated with fluid resuscitation.

Reference

Cheng JW: Recognition, pathophysiology, and management of acute myocardial infarction. Am J Health Syst Pharm 2001;58:1709. [PMID: 11571813]

Myocardial Rupture

- **Essentials of Diagnosis**
  - Associated with myocardial infarction
  - Abrupt hypotension with increased venous pressure (cardiac tamponade)

- **Differential Diagnosis**
  - Massive pulmonary embolus
  - Tension hemothorax
  - Tension pneumothorax
  - Tension pneumopericardium

- **Treatment**
  - Pericardiocentesis: may be life saving
  - Urgent cardiac surgical consultation

- **Pearl**

Ultrasound is the diagnostic test of choice and can help guide life-saving pericardiocentesis.

Reference

Davis N, Sistino JJ: Review of ventricular rupture: key concepts and diagnostic tools for success. Perfusion 2002;17:63. [PMID: 11817532]

Myocarditis

- **Essentials of Diagnosis**
  - Myocarditis can result from myriad causes: infectious, immunologic, toxin, muscular dystrophy, metabolic, infiltrative, neoplastic, hypothermic, and pregnancy
  - Chest x-ray: may be normal or show cardiac enlargement or pulmonary edema
  - Chest pain with associated congestive heart failure, arrhythmias, and systemic embolization
  - May see intraventricular conduction defects
  - Echocardiography: may detect wall motion abnormalities or pericardial effusion
  - May see elevated cardiac enzymes
  - Endomyocardial biopsy: may be diagnostic

- **Differential Diagnosis**
  - Myocardial infarction
  - Acute coronary syndrome
  - Pulmonary embolus
  - Pericarditis
  - Ischemic cardiomyopathy

- **Treatment**
  - Therapy for specific cause
  - Bed rest
  - Treat complications such as arrhythmias, embolization, and heart failure

- **Pearl**

Early consultation with a cardiologist can ensure that the appropriate studies are done to help make the diagnosis.

Reference

Calabrese F, Thiene G: Myocarditis and inflammatory cardiomyopathy; microbiological and molecular biological aspects. Cardiovasc Res 2003;60:11. [PMID: 14522403]

Paroxysmal Supraventricular Tachycardia

- ■ Essentials of Diagnosis (Figure 2–10)
  - • Heart rate usually 180–200 beats/min
  - • 90% associated with a reentrant mechanism, atrioventricular nodal reentrant tachycardia (AVNRT), or atrioventricular reciprocating tachycardia (AVRT); remainder a result of increased automaticity
  - • Can be classified as atrioventricular (AV) nodal dependent or independent; classification useful in formulating treatment
  - • Both AVNRT and AVRT are AV nodal dependent

- ■ Differential Diagnosis
  - • Atrial fibrillation with rapid ventricular response
  - • Atrial flutter

- ■ Treatment
  - • Unstable patients: synchronized DC cardioversion, starting with 50 J and increasing by 50 J until sinus rhythm restored
  - • Stable patients: can try vagal maneuvers (Valsalva or Mueller), cold water facial immersion, gagging, or carotid sinus massage (in younger patients without bruits)
  - • First-line therapy: adenosine
  - • β-Blockers, calcium channel blockers, and digoxin in AV-nodal-dependent tachycardia
  - • Procainamide and amiodarone in AV-nodal-independent tachycardia
  - • Admit patients with serious signs or symptoms

- ■ Pearl

When you are administering adenosine and the patient has a prolonged block, cough CPR can maintain blood flow temporarily.

Reference

Chauhan VS et al: Supraventricular tachycardia. Med Clin North Am 2001;85:193. [PMID: 11233946]

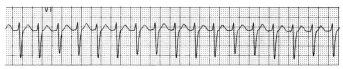

Figure 2–10

Pericardial Effusion

- **Essentials of Diagnosis**
    - Suspected on physical exam by pericardial friction rub
    - Suspected on chest x-ray with enlarged cardiac silhouette
    - Dullness to percussion below the left scapula (Ewart sign)
    - Electrocardiogram: may show findings of pericarditis or electrical alternans
    - Diagnosis by echocardiography

- **Differential Diagnosis**
    - Pulmonary friction rub
    - Pericardial tamponade

- **Treatment**
    - Pericardiocentesis: may be diagnostic for cause
    - Pericardiocentesis in emergency department only for decompensation suggesting tamponade

- **Pearl**

Physical exam and all studies may be normal, except echocardiography.

Reference

Soler-Soler J, Sagrista-Sauleda J, Permanyer-Miralda G: Management of pericardial effusion. Heart 2001;86:235. [PMID: 11454853]

Pericarditis

- ■ Essentials of Diagnosis
  - • Chest pain that worsens when patient lies down and improves when he or she sits up and leans forward
  - • Pericardial friction rub
  - • Electrocardiogram (ECG): may have diffuse ST segment elevation, be normal, or have diffuse ST segment depression
  - • Echocardiography: most sensitive and specific noninvasive test

- ■ Differential Diagnosis
  - • Infection
  - • Collagen vascular diseases
  - • Uremia
  - • Trauma
  - • Myocardial infarction
  - • Surgery
  - • Neoplasm
  - • Irradiation
  - • Drugs or toxins

- ■ Treatment
  - • Treatment of underlying cause
  - • Nonsteroidal anti-inflammatory agents
  - • Monitor ECG
  - • Pain control
  - • Cardiology consultation

- ■ Pearl

Patients classically report feeling as though they have a hot iron on their chest when they lay back; the sensation improves when they sit up, as if the hot iron fell off.

Reference

Groyle KK, Walling AD: Diagnosing pericarditis. Am Fam Physician 2002;66:1695. [PMID: 12449268]

Sick Sinus Syndrome

- **Essentials of Diagnosis**
  - Sinus node dysfunction leading to bradyarrhythmias
  - Comprises numerous arrhythmias, including sinus bradycardia, sinus pause, sinus arrest, and sinoatrial block
  - Dizziness, weakness, confusion, or syncope possible

- **Differential Diagnosis**
  - Sinus bradycardia

- **Treatment**
  - Admission required for symptomatic patients
  - Atropine for symptomatic bradycardia
  - Pacemaker may be required on a permanent basis

- **Pearl**

During emergency department evaluation of the patient, the monitor may manifest a series of bradycardic and tachycardic rhythms or no dysrhythmia at all.

Reference

Adan V, Crown LA: Diagnosis and treatment of sick sinus syndrome. Am Fam Physician 2003;67:1725. [PMID: 12725451]

Sinus Arrest

- ■ Essentials of Diagnosis
  - • Failure of sinus node impulse formation
  - • Electrocardiogram: random periods of absent cardiac activity with lengthy pauses unless escape beats occur
  - • Pauses greater than 2.5 seconds: may progress to asystole

- ■ Differential Diagnosis
  - • Sick sinus syndrome
  - • Digoxin toxicity
  - • β-Blocker toxicity

- ■ Treatment
  - • Cardiac pacing may be required

- ■ Pearl

Atrial or dual-chamber pacemakers are superior to ventricular pacemakers for sinus node dysfunction.

Reference

Adan V, Crown LA: Diagnosis and treatment of sick sinus syndrome. Am Fam Physician 2003;67:1725. [PMID: 12725451]

Sinus Bradycardia

- ■ **Essentials of Diagnosis (Figure 2–11)**
  - • Sinus rate slower than 60 beats/min
  - • Usually 45–59 beats/min
  - • Occasionally as slow as 35 beats/min
  - • Often seen in young, healthy, or athletic patients
  - • Pathologic when associated with end-organ dysfunction
  - • Associated with hypothermia, hypothyroidism, or increased intracranial pressure
  - • Associated with medications such as β-blockers, calcium channel blockers, clonidine, digoxin, and lithium

- ■ **Differential Diagnosis**
  - • Normal in young, healthy, or athletic patients
  - • Drug induced (see above)
  - • Cardiac ischemia
  - • Vagus mediated
  - • Increased intracranial pressure

- ■ **Treatment**
  - • Symptomatic patients: use atropine first; consider pacing if atropine produces no response
  - • Permanent pacemaker if patient has recurrent symptoms
  - • Treatment of drug toxicity if drug induced
  - • Treat underlying condition

- ■ **Pearl**

Base treatment decision on how well the patient is tolerating the sinus bradycardia.

Reference

Mangrum JM, DiMarco JP: The evaluation and management of bradycardia. N Engl J Med 2000;342:703. [PMID: 10706901]

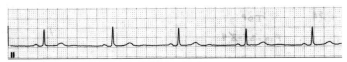

Figure 2–11

Sinus Tachycardia

- **Essentials of Diagnosis (Figure 2–12)**
  - Sinus rate faster than 100 beats/min
  - Usually 101–160 beats/min
  - Young, healthy patients: rate can be 180–200 beats/min during exercise
  - Often a response to other illness or condition

- **Differential Diagnosis**
  - Pain
  - Fever
  - Stress
  - Hyperadrenergic states
  - Anemia
  - Hypovolemia
  - Myocardial ischemia
  - Pulmonary edema
  - Shock
  - Hypothyroidism
  - Toxins, drugs, and medications
  - Hypoxia

- **Treatment**
  - Treatment of underlying cause
  - Vagal maneuvers may help differentiate from paroxysmal supraventricular tachycardia (PSVT)
  - Adenosine may help differentiate from PSVT

- **Pearl**

Many patients use cocaine who you might not suspect of doing so, including the elderly; consider the possibility of cocaine use when a patient presents with an unexplained tachycardia.

Reference

Cossu SF, Steinberg JS: Supraventricular tachyarrhythmias involving the sinus node: clinical and electrophysiologic characteristics. Prog Cardiovasc Dis 1998;41:51. [PMID: 9717859]

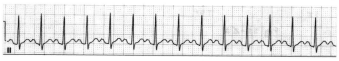

Figure 2–12

Torsades de Pointes

- **Essentials of Diagnosis (Figure 2–13)**
    - Means "twisting of the points"
    - A form of polymorphic ventricular tachycardia
    - Heart rate 200–250 beats/min
    - Prolonged QT interval
    - Paroxysmal or sustained
    - Can degenerate to ventricular fibrillation
    - Medications can induce

- **Differential Diagnosis**
    - Ventricular tachycardia

- **Treatment**
    - Magnesium, 2 g IV slow push over 5 minutes
    - Maintenance infusion of magnesium, 1–2 g/h
    - Isoproterenol to increase heart rate while preparing for a ventricular pacemaker
    - Consider supplemental potassium to keep serum potassium in high normal range

- **Pearl**

Consider a diagnosis of torsades de pointes when the monitor shows a wide complex tachycardia.

Reference

Passman R, Kadish A: Polymorphic ventricular tachycardia, long Q-T syndrome and torsades de pointes. Med Clin North Am 2001;85:321. [PMID: 11233951]

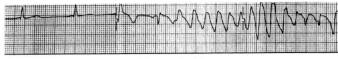

Figure 2–13

Ventricular Fibrillation

- **Essentials of Diagnosis** (Figure 2–14)
  - Irregular ventricular rhythm
  - No distinction between the QRS complex, ST segment, and T wave
  - Common cause of sudden cardiac death
  - A nonperfusing rhythm

- **Differential Diagnosis**
  - Polymorphic ventricular tachycardia
  - Torsades de pointes

- **Treatment**
  - Asynchronous defibrillation starting with 200 J
  - Progressive defibrillation with 200–300 J, followed by 360 J
  - Vasopressin or epinephrine
  - Antiarrhythmics: amiodarone or lidocaine

- **Pearl**

Start a drip of an antiarrhythmic agent that is successful in converting fibrillation.

Reference

Flinders DC, Roberts SD: Ventricular arrhythmias. Prim Care 2000;27:709. [PMID: 10918676]

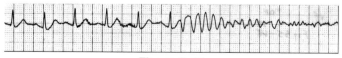

Figure 2–14

Ventricular Septal Rupture

■ Essentials of Diagnosis
- Associated with myocardial infarction
- Abrupt severe congestive heart failure
- Pansystolic regurgitation murmur
- Echocardiography to detect abnormal velocity jet of a ventricular septal defect

■ Differential Diagnosis
- Preexisting murmur
- Congestive heart failure
- Bacterial endocarditis

■ Treatment
- Treatment of congestive heart failure
- Urgent cardiologic consultation
- Urgent cardiac surgical consultation
- Intra-aortic balloon pump may temporize

■ Pearl

Ventricular septal rupture should be considered and ruled out in the setting of an acute myocardial infarction with a new systolic murmur.

Reference

Rhydwen GR, Charman S, Schofield PM: Influence of thrombolytic therapy on the patterns of ventricular septal rupture after acute myocardial infarction. Postgrad Med J 2002;78:408. [PMID: 12151656]

Ventricular Tachycardia

- ■ Essentials of Diagnosis (Figure 2–15)
  - • Ventricular rate usually 180–250 beats/min
  - • Can occur at rates slower than 160 beats/min
  - • Six or more consecutive ventricular beats together
  - • Sustained ventricular tachycardia characterized by an episode longer than 30 seconds and hemodynamic compromise
  - • Wide complex has QRS complex greater than 120 ms in duration

- ■ Differential Diagnosis
  - • Supraventricular tachycardia with aberrancy
  - • Atrioventricular reciprocating tachycardia

- ■ Treatment
  - • Unstable patients: synchronized DC cardioversion, starting with 50–100 J and increasing by 50 Joules until sinus rhythm restored
  - • Stable patients: antiarrhythmics such as amiodarone, lidocaine, or procainamide; if unsuccessful, consider cardioversion

- ■ Pearl

Among patients with a wide complex tachycardia, 80% will have ventricular tachycardia, whereas only 20% will have SVT with aberrancy.

Reference

Talwar KK, Naik N: Etiology and management of sustained ventricular tachycardia. Am J Cardiovasc Drugs 2001;1:179. [PMID: 14728033]

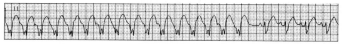

Figure 2–15

Wolff-Parkinson-White Syndrome

■ Essentials of Diagnosis

- Most common form of ventricular preexcitation
- Short PR interval and presence of a delta wave
- Most common arrhythmia is orthodromic atrioventricular reciprocating tachycardia (AVRT)
- Second most common arrhythmia is atrial fibrillation
- Rarely antidromic AVRT occurs that masquerades as ventricular tachycardia

■ Differential Diagnosis

- Ventricular tachycardia
- Atrial fibrillation with rapid ventricular response (RVR)
- Lown-Ganong-Levine syndrome

■ Treatment

- Unstable orthodromic AVRT patients: DC cardioversion, starting with 50 J and increasing by 50 J until sinus rhythm is restored
- Stable orthodromic AVRT patients: adenosine, β-blockers, or calcium channel blockers
- Unstable patient with atrial fibrillation with ventricular preexcitation: synchronized DC cardioversion, starting with 100 J; atrioventricular nodal blocking agents (β-blockers, calcium channel blockers, digoxin) are contraindicated because they can result in ventricular fibrillation
- Procainamide: drug of choice for Wolff-Parkinson-White-associated atrial fibrillation with RVR
- Amiodarone: alternative for atrial fibrillation with ventricular preexcitation and congestive heart failure

■ Pearl

Ibutilide may offer a new way to terminate atrial fibrillation in Wolff-Parkinson-White syndrome.

Reference

Varriale P, Sedighi A, Mirzaietehrane M: Ibutilide for termination of atrial fibrillation in the Wolff-Parkinson-White syndrome. Pacing Clin Electrophysiol 1999;22:1267. [PMID: 10461309]

3

Pulmonary Emergencies

Acute Respiratory Distress Syndrome (ARDS)

- Essentials of Diagnosis
  - Acute onset of diffuse lung injury
  - Bilateral infiltrates on chest x-ray
  - Hypoxemia (PaO_2/FiO_2 ratio ≤ 200 mm Hg)
  - Absence of pulmonary vascular congestion (PCWP <18 mm Hg)
  - Causes of lung injury: pneumonia (bacterial or viral), major trauma with multiple transfusions, toxic inhalation, pulmonary contusion, burns, sepsis, fat embolism, or near drowning

- Differential Diagnosis
  - Pulmonary edema (PCWP >18 mm Hg)
  - Pulmonary embolus
  - Right-to-left intra- or extracardiac shunting of blood
  - Pneumothorax
  - Respiratory failure

- Treatment
  - Intubation and ventilation with low tidal volumes (6–7 mL/kg) in support of oxygenation and to prevent barotrauma
  - Positive end-expiratory pressure (PEEP)
  - Appropriate antibiotics for pneumonia or systemic infection
  - Optimization of supportive therapy in sepsis and shock
  - Limit further lung injury from high concentrations of oxygen

- Pearl

Noninvasive positive-pressure ventilation may be useful temporarily, but virtually all patients with ARDS will ultimately need invasive positive-pressure ventilation.

Reference

Rivers E et al: Early goal-directed therapy in the treatment of severe sepsis and septic shock. N Engl J Med 2001;345:1368. [PMID: 11794169]

Aspiration Pneumonia

- **Essentials of Diagnosis**
  - Fever, cough, rales, and hypoxemia following an observed episode of aspiration indicates chemical pneumonitis
  - Suctioning of particulate or liquid foreign material from the lungs
  - Infiltrates following aspiration typically in dependent areas of the lungs
  - Depressed mentation or ineffective cough and clearing of secretions due to muscle weakness or neurologic impairment predispose to aspiration pneumonia

- **Differential Diagnosis**
  - Community- or hospital-acquired bacterial or viral pneumonia
  - Lung abscess
  - Pleural effusion
  - Empyema
  - Primary or metastatic tumors of the lung or pleura

- **Treatment**
  - Antibiotics not required; they do not prevent subsequent infectious pneumonia and may select for resistant organisms
  - Immediate suctioning of aspirated material and positioning to prevent additional aspiration
  - If antibiotics are given, provide empiric coverage: levofloxacin, 500 mg/d, or ceftriaxone, 1–2 g/d; piperacillin/tazobactam, 3.375 g every 6 hours, or imipenem, 500 mg to 1 g every 6–8 hours, if severe periodontal disease exists
  - Protection from additional aspiration: semi-erect positioning and use of small-bore feeding tubes into the small bowel

- **Pearl**

The posterior segments of the upper lobes and the superior segments of the lower lobes are most often affected when patients aspirate in the supine position. The basilar segments of the lower lobes are most often affected when patients aspirate when upright or semierect.

Reference

Marik PE: Aspiration pneumonitis and aspiration pneumonia. N Engl J Med 2001;344:665. [PMID: 11228282]

Asthma

■ Essentials of Diagnosis
  • Wheezing, cough, and dyspnea with chest tightness
  • Severely ill patients: wheezing may be absent when they tire and airflow becomes severely limited
  • Episodic in nature, sometimes seasonal; attacks may be precipitated by infection, inhaled allergens, or exercise
  • Chest x-ray usually normal but may show hyperinflation

■ Differential Diagnosis
  • Chronic obstructive pulmonary disease (COPD)
  • Congestive heart failure
  • Upper respiratory tract infection
  • Bronchitis
  • Pneumonia
  • Interstitial lung diseases
  • Croup and other causes of upper airway obstruction
  • Aspirated foreign bodies such as peanuts

■ Treatment
  • Inhaled short-acting bronchodilators (albuterol, levalbuterol): first-line therapy for acute asthma
  • Ipratropium: labeled for use in COPD but also effective in combination with β-agonists for acute asthma
  • Oral or parenteral steroids: added for severe attacks
  • Inhaled corticosteroids: effective for persistent asthma

■ Pearl

Long-acting β-agonists may blunt the response to short-acting rescue medications.

Reference

National Asthma Education and Prevention Program: Expert panel report: guidelines for the diagnosis and management of asthma update on selected topics—2002. J Allergy Clin Immunol 2002;110:S141. [PMID: 12542074]

Bronchitis

- **Essentials of Diagnosis**
  - Acute onset of productive cough
  - Lack of clinical evidence for pneumonia, including tachycardia, tachypnea, hypoxia, and high fever
  - Chest x-ray usually not indicated but should not demonstrate an infiltrate
  - Rhonchi sometimes with wheezing, but rales indicating parenchymal involvement are lacking
  - Cannot differentiate between viral and bacterial causes based on color or amount of purulent sputum
  - Patients with asthma and chronic obstructive pulmonary disease: productive cough frequently present during exacerbations of chronic illness

- **Differential Diagnosis**
  - Pneumonia
  - Viral upper respiratory tract infection
  - Asthma
  - Hypersensitivity pneumonitis
  - Bacterial trachitis

- **Treatment**
  - Viral cause in approximately 90% of episodes
  - Antibiotic therapy: little effect or only marginal benefit in uncomplicated acute bronchitis
  - Antibiotic treatment directed to *Haemophilus influenza* and pneumococci (trimethoprim-sulfamethoxazole, amoxicillin, or a macrolide): may hasten resolution of symptoms
  - Bronchodilators (eg, albuterol) decrease cough by 50%

- **Pearl**

Troublesome cough and bronchial inflammation may persist for weeks or months following the initial infection.

Reference

Edmonds ML: Evidence-based emergency medicine. Antibiotic treatment for acute bronchitis. Ann Emerg Med 2002;40:110. [PMID: 12085081]

Chronic Obstructive Pulmonary Disease (COPD)

- ■ Essentials of Diagnosis
  - • Cough, dyspnea, and wheezing caused by exacerbations
  - • History of smoking present in most patients
  - • Hyperinflation and flattened diaphragms with increased anterior-posterior diameter seen on chest x-ray in emphysematous patients
  - • Spirometry: mild disease, FEV_1/FVC <70%, FEV_1 >80% predicted
  - • Peak flows also reduced
  - • Patients with chronic bronchitis: frequently obese, hypoxic, and have signs of right heart failure; patients predominately with emphysema: usually very thin and mildly hypoxic

- ■ Differential Diagnosis
  - • Congestive heart failure
  - • Pneumonia (may be present in patients with acute exacerbations)
  - • Pulmonary embolus
  - • Pneumothorax

- ■ Treatment
  - • Inhaled bronchodilators: albuterol, levalbuterol
  - • Inhaled ipratropium bromide
  - • Oral steroids for acute exacerbations
  - • Bilevel positive airway pressure is effective; may prevent morbidity associated with intubation, but patients must be able to cooperate and protect their airway

- ■ Pearl

A serum B-type natriuretic peptide test is useful to detect associated congestive heart failure in patients presenting with symptoms suggesting an exacerbation of COPD.

Reference

Sin DD et al: Contemporary management of chronic obstructive pulmonary disease: scientific review. JAMA 2003;290:2301. [PMID: 14600189]

Cystic Fibrosis

- **Essentials of Diagnosis**
  - Cough, frequently loose and productive of purulent sputum
  - Recurrent wheezing and hyperinflation of lungs
  - Recurrent pneumonia
  - Chest x-ray: often demonstrates increased lung markings; areas of focal pneumonia may be present in acute disease
  - Maldigestion and failure to thrive
  - Endocrine pancreatic insufficiency with hyperglycemia
  - Dehydration and salt depletion in warm weather
  - Positive quantitative sweat test ($[Cl^-] \geq 60$ mEq/L)
  - Positive family history

- **Differential Diagnosis**
  - Asthma
  - Chronic bronchitis
  - IgA deficiency
  - Bronchiectasis

- **Treatment**
  - Chest physical therapy and postural drainage frequently used to clear secretions from airways
  - Maintenance of hydration, to help clear mucous secretions
  - Antibiotic therapy, oral or aerosolized and guided wherever possible by sensitivities of isolated pathogens
  - Immunoprophylaxis specifically against rubeola, pertussis, and influenza

- **Pearl**

Because the development of drug-resistant infection is the most significant obstacle to long-term control of symptoms, make every effort to use antibiotic therapy appropriately.

Reference

Aitken ML: Cystic fibrosis. Curr Opin Pulm Med 1995;1:425. [PMID: 9363078]

Interstitial Pulmonary Disease

■ Essentials of Diagnosis
- May be acute pneumonitis or chronic from fibrosis or pneumoconiosis
- Acute pneumonitis: nonproductive cough, fever, dyspnea, and sometimes chest pain
- Chronic interstitial disease: dyspnea and progressive decline in pulmonary function with hypoxia and decreased exercise tolerance
- Pneumoconiosis, which includes asbestosis, silicosis, and kaolinosis (white clay): caused by exposure to inorganic dusts
- Hypersensitivity pneumonitis: caused by exposure to inhaled organic antigens such as molds, organic dusts, and pollens
- Acute or chronic interstitial lung disease possible from amiodarone, nitrofurantoin, bleomycin, and other chemotherapeutic agents
- Characteristic chest x-ray finding: interstitial pattern of reticular or reticulonodular infiltrates diffusely affecting both lungs
- Diffuse fibrotic changes interspersed with cystic changes may produce honeycomb appearance on chest x-ray
- Characteristic and etiologically specific changes within the interstitial lung tissue seen on biopsy

■ Differential Diagnosis
- Viral or atypical (eg, *Pneumocystis carinii* pneumonia)
- Congestive heart failure
- Noncardiogenic pulmonary edema
- Lymphangitic carcinomatosis of the lungs

■ Treatment
- Therapy directed at specific cause, the diagnosis of which may require lung biopsy
- Therapy often primarily preventive, by avoiding offending stimulus (eg, pneumoconiosis), or supportive (eg, supplemental oxygen)
- Hypersensitivity pneumonitis or drug-induced parenchymal lung disease if present long enough will lead to irreversible pulmonary fibrosis

■ Pearl

Amiodarone is now the most frequent cause of drug-induced interstitial lung disease.

Reference

Drent M, du Bois RM, Poletti V: Recent advances in the diagnosis and management of nonspecific interstitial pneumonia. Curr Opin Pulm Med 2003;9:411. [PMID: 12904713]

Pleural Effusion

- **Essentials of Diagnosis**
    - Dyspnea from compressing and shifting lung position
    - Pleuritic pain if cause is inflammatory
    - Dullness to percussion and diminished breath sounds
    - Hypoxia and tachypnea if effusion is large
    - Opacity visible at lung bases on upright chest x-ray
    - Pleural effusions produce curved meniscus
    - Decubitus views or echocardiography may be helpful prior to thoracentesis
    - Diagnostic thoracentesis necessary to demonstrate presence of hemorrhage, infection, or an empyema
    - Complicated parapneumonic effusions are culture negative, but the LDH is >1,000 IU/L, pH is <7.2, or glucose is <40 mg/dL

- **Differential Diagnosis**
    - Pneumonia
    - Atelectasis
    - Tumors
    - Pulmonary edema
    - Pleural thickening from fibrosis or malignancy

- **Treatment**
    - Treatment of underlying cause (eg, congestive heart failure, cirrhosis, pulmonary embolus, pneumonia, cancer, rheumatoid arthritis, systemic lupus erythematosus, pancreatitis)
    - Symptomatic thoracentesis usually indicated when large malignant effusions compromise respiration causing tachypnea
    - Chest tube thoracostomy connected to a drainage system may be necessary, especially if hemothorax or infection suspected
    - Effusions that are complicated, gram stain or culture positive, or frankly purulent require chest tube drainage
    - Pleurodesis through a catheter or chest tube with bleomycin, or talc for palliation of recurrent malignant effusions
    - Thoracoscopy to break up adhesions may be required

- **Pearl**

A marked decrease in pleural liquid pressure from thoracentesis may cause unilateral pulmonary edema, especially if a large volume is removed.

Reference

Jones JS: The pleura in health and disease. Lung 2001;179:397. [PMID: 12040428]

Pneumonia

- ■ **Essentials of Diagnosis**
  - Fever, frequently high; cough almost universal (may produce bloody or rust-colored sputum)
  - Rigors may herald onset of pneumococcal pneumonia
  - Pleuritic pain with involvement of pleural surface
  - Dyspnea and hypoxia may occur with extensive involvement of pulmonary parenchyma or in patients already compromised by preexisting lung disease such as asthma, congestive heart failure, or chronic obstructive pulmonary disease
  - Rales over involved area with fremitus and bronchial breathing where dense consolidation exists
  - Alveolar infiltrates seen on chest x-ray in bacterial pneumonia; interstitial infiltrates in viral and atypical pneumonias (chlamydia, mycoplasma, *Pneumocystis carinii* pneumonia)
  - Extrapulmonary manifestations: may be prominent in some pneumonias, especially legionnaires disease, which may produce an altered mental status, diarrhea, abnormal liver function tests, hyponatremia, and impairment of renal function

- ■ **Differential Diagnosis**
  - Bronchitis
  - Pulmonary embolus
  - Congestive heart failure
  - Primary or metastatic lung tumor
  - Inflammatory or aspiration pneumonitis
  - Pleural effusions loculated in the fissures of the lung

- ■ **Treatment**
  - Antibiotics given empirically based on setting
  - Community-acquired disease: quinolones, macrolides, or third-generation cephalosporins
  - Staphylococcal pneumonia: vancomycin may be necessary
  - Nosocomial- and ventilator-associated pneumonias: gram-negative coverage frequently necessary
  - Supportive care: supplemental oxygen, bronchodilators, and judicious rehydration to prevent fluid overload

- ■ **Pearl**

All patients with pneumonia should receive antibiotics before leaving the emergency department.

Reference

American College of Emergency Physicians: Clinical policy for the management and risk stratification of community-acquired pneumonia in adults in the emergency department. Ann Emerg Med 2001;38:107. [PMID: 11859897]

Pneumothorax, Spontaneous

- **Essentials of Diagnosis**
  - More frequent in young males who are smokers, especially those who are tall and thin
  - Pleuritic chest pain most frequent complaint
  - Dyspnea and hypoxia may occur with a large pneumothorax or if presence of tension displaces mediastinum
  - Absent or diminished breath sounds over affected lung
  - Chest x-ray demonstrates curved line representing edge of lung with lack of lung markings between this and chest wall
  - May occur adjacent to base of lung if adhesions prevent typical location at the apex
  - When both fluid and air are present in pleural space, fluid does not track up between lung and chest in a curved meniscus but appears as horizontal air fluid level in the hemithorax on upright chest x-rays

- **Differential Diagnosis**
  - Emphysema associated blebs
  - Viral pleurisy
  - Pneumonia
  - Pulmonary embolus
  - Cardiac ischemia
  - Aortic dissection
  - Pericarditis

- **Treatment**
  - Less than 15% pneumothorax: observation in hospital or 6 hours of emergency department observation on O_2 (without progression), discharge with close follow-up
  - More than 15% pneumothorax or progression of smaller pneumothorax: catheter placement with aspiration, observation as above; tube thoracostomy and hospitalization

- **Pearl**

Patients with Pneumocystis carinii *pneumonia may present with a spontaneous pneumothorax.*

Reference

Sahn SA, Heffner JE: Spontaneous pneumothorax. N Engl J Med 2000;342:868. [PMID: 10727592]

Pulmonary Embolus

■ Essentials of Diagnosis

- Dyspnea, tachypnea, tachycardia, chest pain
- Risk factors: immobilization, recent surgery, trauma, malignancy, estrogen
- Chest x-ray usually normal but occasionally shows signs of pulmonary infarction (ie, pleural effusions, infiltrates sometimes pleural based, elevation of the hemidiaphragm)
- Hypoxia common (85% of patients), but 15% have normal PaO_2
- Electrocardiographic (ECG) findings: tachycardia, T wave inversion in the anterior chest leads, right bundle branch block, right axis deviation, and new-onset atrial fibrillation or flutter
- D-Dimer to exclude only cases of low probability
- Helical CT scan or ventilation/perfusion for imaging

■ Differential Diagnosis

- Pneumonia
- Pneumothorax
- Myocardial ischemia and infarction
- Congestive heart failure
- Exacerbations of asthma and chronic obstructive pulmonary disease

■ Treatment

- Anticoagulation: unfractionated heparin, 80 IU/kg intravenous bolus followed by 18 IU/kg/h; low-molecular-weight heparin (Enoxaparin, 1 mg/kg subcutaneously twice daily)
- Bedrest, supplemental O_2, ECG monitoring, pulse oximetry
- Vena cava filter when anticoagulation is contraindicated
- Evaluation of possible precipitating causes: antiphospholipid antibodies, lupus anticoagulants, protein C or S deficiency, unrecognized malignancies

■ Pearl

Spiral CT scanning with intravenous contrast has essentially replaced ventilation perfusion scanning as an imaging study.

Reference

Sadosty AT, Boie ET, Stead LG: Pulmonary embolism. Emerg Med Clin North Am 2003;21:363. [PMID: 12793619]

Pulmonary Tuberculosis

■ **Essentials of Diagnosis**

- Cough, sputum production, hemoptysis, chest pain
- Weight loss, anorexia, fatigue, low-grade fever, night sweats
- Infiltrates on chest x-ray nonspecific in primary infection; may affect lower and upper lobes
- Reactivation tuberculosis: usually involves apical and posterior segments of upper lobes
- Adenopathy, pleural effusions, calcified granulomas or nodes
- Cavities, nodules, or scarring of lungs
- Positive tuberculin skin test (PPD) documents infection with tuberculosis but not active infection
- Positive acid-fast bacilli in sputum, washings, or biopsy
- Nontuberculous mycobacteria retain acid-fast stains and may cause confusion between tuberculosis and atypical mycobacteria
- Culture from sputum or tissue may require up to 6 weeks

■ **Differential Diagnosis**

- Pneumonia
- Aspiration pneumonia
- Lung cancer
- Lung abscess
- Bronchiectasis
- Pulmonary embolus

■ **Treatment**

- Combination therapy with isoniazid, rifampin, pyrazinamide, and ethambutol recommended
- Compliance important to prevent emergence of drug-resistant organisms; may require supervised enforcement
- Isoniazid used alone for 9 months in close contacts and persons recently converted to positive PPD

■ **Pearl**

Children with pneumonia should be skin tested with PPD if they reside in endemic areas or are exposed to immigrant populations.

Reference

Blumberg HM et al: American Thoracic Society/Centers for Disease Control and Prevention/Infectious Diseases Society of America: Treatment of tuberculosis. Am J Respir Crit Care Med 2003;167:603. [PMID: 12588714]

4

Gastrointestinal Emergencies

Appendicitis

- **Essentials of Diagnosis**
  - Abdominal symptoms classically begin as a vague poorly localized, diffuse, periumbilical or epigastric pain that, over 12–24 hours, becomes sharper and more well localized usually to the right lower quadrant (McBurney point)
  - Typically pain symptoms begin before anorexia, nausea, or vomiting
  - Fever (usually low grade) often occurs
  - Abdominal tenderness is localized to the right lower quadrant; in later stages, peritoneal signs (rebound tenderness, Rovsing sign [pain in the right lower quadrant when the left lower quadrant is palpated] or involuntary guarding) are present
  - Abdominal pain may improve if appendiceal rupture occurs; when diffuse peritonitis develops, symptoms worsen
  - Urinalysis, CBC with differential (although not very helpful)
  - Abdominal CT with oral and intravenous contrast has become a popular study in the evaluation of suspected appendicitis (90–100% sensitivity, 91–99% specificity); ultrasound is helpful if the appendix is well visualized

- **Differential Diagnosis**
  - Ureterolithiasis
  - Testicular or ovarian torsion
  - Ruptured ovarian cyst
  - Other intra-abdominal infections such as diverticulitis or pelvic inflammatory disease
  - Inflammatory bowel disease (ie, Crohn disease)

- **Treatment**
  - Intravenous fluids and broad-spectrum antibiotics
  - Definitive treatment: appendectomy

- **Pearl**

The astute clinician will be careful not to ascribe abdominal pain and vomiting symptoms to gastroenteritis without carefully considering appendicitis (especially in the absence of diarrhea).

Reference

Paulson EK, Kalady MF, Pappas TN: Clinical practice. Suspected appendicitis. N Engl J Med 2003;348:236. [PMID: 12529465]

Ascites

- **Essentials of Diagnosis**
  - Abnormal accumulation of fluid in peritoneal cavity
  - Exam may reveal signs of liver disease (palmar erythema, spider angiomata, caput medusa), bulging flanks, shifting dullness, or fluid wave
  - Causes include portal hypertension, low albumin, or peritoneal disease
  - SAAG (difference between serum and ascitic fluid albumin) >1.1 mg/dL highly suggestive of portal hypertension
  - New-onset ascites should receive diagnostic paracentesis with fluid sent for cell count, albumin, culture, cytology, protein, and Gram stain
  - Neutrophil count >250 cells/µL suggests bacterial peritonitis
  - Ascites usually easily seen by ultrasound

- **Differential Diagnosis**
  - Portal hypertensive (SAAG >1.1): hepatic failure, cirrhosis, congestive heart failure, Budd-Chiari syndrome
  - Hypoalbuminemic (SAAG <1.1): nephrotic syndrome, protein malnutrition
  - Peritoneal (SAAG <1.1): tuberculous peritonitis, bacterial peritonitis, peritoneal carcinomatosis (often painful)

- **Treatment**
  - Sodium restriction
  - Diuretic therapy (spironolactone, loop diuretics, thiazide diuretics)
  - Transjugular intrahepatic portacaval shunt (TIPS) for refractory ascites
  - Therapeutic paracentesis for tense ascites

- **Pearl**

Acute ascites in a previously stable cirrhotic patient may be secondary to hepatocellular carcinoma.

Reference

Garcia-Tsao G: Current management of the complications of cirrhosis and portal hypertension: variceal hemorrhage, ascites, and spontaneous bacterial peritonitis. Gastroenterology 2001;120:726. [PMID: 11179247]

Biliary Colic

■ Essentials of Diagnosis

- Pain thought to arise from the passage of small stones through the gallbladder or impaction of stones in the neck of the gallbladder
- Presentation with pain typically in the right upper quadrant and radiating to the scapula; associated with nausea and emesis and lasting 2–6 hours
- Association with fatty food ingestion likely in other disorders; thus not clinically useful
- Frequently occurs at night
- Risk factors for gallstones: cholesterol stones—age, female gender, obesity, weight loss, cystic fibrosis, family history, malabsorption; black stones—sickle cell disease, spherocytosis; brown stones—Asian descent, parasitic infection, bacterial infection
- CBC, electrolytes, BUN, creatinine, liver enzymes, lipase, urinalysis, urine pregnancy test
- Most lab studies will be normal; evaluate for common duct obstruction, pancreatitis, hepatitis
- Ultrasound: 98% sensitive and specific for cholelithiasis and 95% sensitive for cholecystitis
- Fever, leukocytosis, or elevated liver enzymes may suggest cholecystitis

■ Differential Diagnosis

- Cholecystitis
- Cholangitis
- Hepatitis
- Myocardial ischemia
- Peptic ulcer disease
- Nonulcer dyspepsia
- Abdominal aortic aneurysm

■ Treatment

- Fluid and electrolyte replacement
- Pain control with ketorolac, antispasmodics, or opiates
- Referral for surgical management

■ Pearl

Risk factors are the F's: Forty, Fat, Female, Fertile.

Reference

Ahmed A, Cheung RC, Keeffe EB: Management of gallstones and their complications. Am Fam Physician 2000;61:1673. [PMID: 10750875]

Boerhaave Syndrome

- ■ **Essentials of Diagnosis**
  - Rupture of the esophagus (not secondary to iatrogenic complication, foreign body, or trauma)
  - Most commonly distal esophagus on the left side
  - Commonly follows episode of emesis followed by chest pain, which may radiate to left shoulder
  - Mackler triad (vomiting, chest pain, subcutaneous emphysema) characteristic but uncommon
  - Other symptoms: fever, abdominal pain, odynophagia, tachypnea, dyspnea; cyanosis and shock often present
  - Physical exam may reveal decreased breath sounds over one hemithorax, Hamman sign (crackling sound over the heart during systole), or subcutaneous emphysema
  - Chest x-ray may show pneumomediastinum, pleural effusion (90%), pneumothorax or hydropneumothorax, or pneumoperitoneum; chest x-ray abnormal in 97% of cases but diagnostic in only 25%
  - Gastrografin can confirm diagnosis; false negatives are common (~10%); confirm negative study with barium swallow
  - High mortality rate (worse with delayed diagnosis)

- ■ **Differential Diagnosis**
  - Acute myocardial infarction
  - Spontaneous pneumothorax
  - Pericarditis
  - Gastroesophageal reflux disease
  - Spontaneous pneumomediastinum

- ■ **Treatment**
  - Nothing by mouth
  - Broad-spectrum antibiotics
  - Chest tube drainage may be required
  - Admit to ICU; surgical consult

- ■ **Pearl**

Always consider Boerhaave syndrome in any patient with chest, back, or abdominal pain.

Reference

Janjua KJ: Boerhaave's syndrome. Postgrad Med J 1997;73:265. [PMID: 9196697]

Cholangitis

- ■ Essentials of Diagnosis
  - • Infection of biliary tree caused by obstruction
  - • Obstruction most commonly by choledocholithiasis but may be due to stricture, tumor, or endoscopic retrograde cholangiopancreatography (ERCP)
  - • Charcot triad (right upper quadrant pain, fever, jaundice): present in 70% of patients
  - • Reynold pentad = Charcot triad + mental status changes and sepsis
  - • Common organisms: *Escherichia coli, Klebsiella, Enterobacter,* enterococci
  - • In 79% of cases, WBC >10,000, mean bilirubin = 6.6, elevated AST, ALT, and alkaline phosphatase
  - • Ultrasound sensitive for gallstones but not common duct stones; moderately sensitive for biliary dilation
  - • CT insensitive for stones but may show biliary dilation; also can evaluate for other conditions in differential diagnosis
  - • HIDA may show nonvisualization of small intestine consistent with obstruction but loses sensitivity at high bilirubin levels

- ■ Differential Diagnosis
  - • Hepatitis
  - • Hepatic abscess
  - • Pancreatitis
  - • Biliary colic
  - • Acute cholecystitis

- ■ Treatment
  - • Depends on severity
  - • Mild cholangitis: volume resuscitation, intravenous antibiotics, close observation; 70–85% of mild cases respond to medical therapy
  - • Severe cholangitis and patients failing medical therapy: immediate decompression via surgery or ERCP

- ■ Pearl

Consider cholangitis in elderly patient who has sepsis syndrome, because they may not be able to localize discomfort to the right upper quadrant.

Reference

Hanau LH, Steigbigel NH: Acute (ascending) cholangitis. Infect Dis Clin North Am 2000;14:521. [PMID: 10987108]

Cholecystitis, Acute

■ **Essentials of Diagnosis**

- Inflammation of the gallbladder due to chemical, mechanical, or infectious causes
- Bacterial agents contribute in 50–80% of cases (mainly *Escherichia coli* and *Klebsiella*)
- More than 90% of cases caused by cholelithiasis with stone impacted in cystic duct
- Acalculous cholecystitis in elderly due to trauma, burns, diabetes mellitus
- Pain in right upper quadrant or epigastrium similar to biliary colic but >6 hours duration; nausea and vomiting, low-grade fevers common
- Murphy sign: inspiratory arrest during right subcostal firm palpation (97% sensitive)
- Ultrasound: may show cholelithiasis, distended gallbladder, gallbladder wall thickening, ductal dilatation, pericholecystic fluid, or sonographic Murphy sign (95% sensitive)
- Usually WBC = 10,000–15,000 with left shift; bilirubin may be mildly elevated (~5) in the absence of common duct stone
- HIDA scan reliable if bilirubin <5; nonvisualization of gallbladder 98% sensitive, 81% specific

■ **Differential Diagnosis**

- Biliary colic
- Pancreatitis
- Peptic ulcer disease
- Hepatitis
- Ascending cholangitis
- Appendicitis
- Pneumonia

■ **Treatment**

- Nothing by mouth; intravenous hydration
- Antibiotics; analgesics (meperidine causes less spasm of sphincter of Oddi)
- Surgery

■ **Pearl**

When only clinical criteria are used, 20% of patients with acute cholecystitis will be missed; HIDA or ultrasound is required for diagnosis.

Reference

Trowbridge RL et al: Does this patient have acute cholecystitis? JAMA 2003;289:80. [PMID: 12503981]

Cirrhosis

- ■ Essentials of Diagnosis
  - • Replacement of normal hepatic tissue by fibrotic tissue and abnormal nodules
  - • Ninth leading cause of death
  - • Caused typically by hepatitis B, hepatitis C, and alcohol but may be caused by a variety of diseases including Wilson disease, hemochromatosis, autoimmune hepatitis, primary biliary cirrhosis, sclerosing cholangitis, drug-induced liver disease, and Budd-Chiari syndrome
  - • Presents with complications including ascites, variceal bleeding, or encephalopathy
  - • Physical exam may reveal spider angiomata, palmar erythema, jaundice, ascites, caput medusae, muscle wasting, gynecomastia
  - • Liver is enlarged in 70% of cases
  - • Lab studies are normal or minimally abnormal until late in disease when PT prolongation, hypoalbuminemia, and hyperbilirubinemia develop
  - • Ascites: SAAG (difference between serum and ascitic fluid albumin) >1.1 mg/dL highly diagnostic for portal hypertension (99% sensitivity)
  - • Hepatorenal syndrome manifested by oliguria; azotemia in the absence of shock suggests poor prognosis

- ■ Differential Diagnosis
  - • Noncirrhotic portal hypertension may be due to portal vein thrombosis, splenic vein thrombosis, or schistosomiasis
  - • Ascites may be caused by nephrotic syndrome, protein malnutrition, tuberculous peritonitis, or bacterial peritonitis
  - • Congestive heart failure or constrictive pericarditis may result in secondary "cardiac" cirrhosis

- ■ Treatment
  - • Stop alcohol use
  - • Diuretics for ascites
  - • Paracentesis for tense ascites or respiratory difficulty
  - • Mild protein restriction
  - • β-Blockers to prevent variceal bleeding
  - • Liver transplantation

- ■ Pearl

Vitamin K therapy is ineffective in end-stage liver disease; fresh frozen plasma may be used for procedures.

Reference

Menon KV et al: Managing the complications of cirrhosis. Mayo Clin Proc 2000;75:501. [PMID: 10807079]

Colitis, Ischemic

- **Essentials of Diagnosis**
  - Disease most commonly affecting the elderly
  - Abdominal pain often in the left lower quadrant; bloody diarrhea
  - Almost always a nonocclusive disease; infarction is rare
  - Plain x-rays may reveal thumbprinting indicative of submucosal edema
  - CT may show thickening of the bowel wall in a segmental pattern or, in more advanced cases, pneumatosis and gas in the mesenteric veins
  - Barium enema contraindicated due to risk of perforation
  - May result in stricture formation
  - Colonoscopy reveals segmental distribution and rectal sparing, distinguishing ischemic colitis from ulcerative colitis
  - Serum markers of ischemia not useful

- **Differential Diagnosis**
  - Infectious colitis
  - Inflammatory bowel disease
  - Colon cancer
  - Pseudomembranous colitis

- **Treatment**
  - Without evidence of peritonitis or perforation: supportive treatment; disease often self-limited
  - If infarction or perforation is present: immediate surgical consult
  - Avoid vasopressors

- **Pearl**

Always consider ischemic colitis when an elderly patient presents with what seems to be inflammatory bowel disease.

Reference

MacDonald PH: Ischaemic colitis. Best Pract Res Clin Gastroenterol 2002;16:51. [PMID: 11977928]

Colitis, Ulcerative

- **■ Essentials of Diagnosis**
  - Idiopathic inflammatory disorder involving the submucosa of the rectum and spreading proximally without skip areas
  - Mucosa granular and friable; may have pseudopolyps
  - Chronic recurrent abdominal pain, bloody diarrhea, tenesmus, vomiting, fever
  - May have extraintestinal manifestations: sacroiliitis, peripheral arthritis, uveitis, episcleritis, pyoderma gangrenosum, erythema nodosum, sclerosing cholangitis
  - May have leukocytosis, anemia, elevated erythrocyte sedimentation rate
  - Send stool for leukocytes, ova and parasites, bacterial culture, *Clostridium difficile* toxin
  - Rule out amebiasis by serologic testing
  - Most useful diagnostic study is endoscopy with biopsy; procedures should not be performed on acutely ill patients
  - Toxic megacolon: severe colitis manifested by continuous air-filled loop of colon (>6 cm) that may have thumbprinting or loss of haustra

- **■ Differential Diagnosis**
  - Crohn colitis
  - Ischemic colitis
  - Infectious colitis
  - Pseudomembranous colitis

- **■ Treatment**
  - 5-Amino salicylic acid (ASA) agents (sulfasalazine, mesalamine)
  - Corticosteroid or 5-ASA enemas
  - Intravenous steroids for severe acute colitis
  - Immunosuppressive agents
  - Surgery is curative
  - Patients with toxic megacolon: administer intravenous fluids, steroids, and antibiotics; surgery if not improved in 24–48 hours

- **■ Pearl**

Patients with ulcerative colitis have a 10- to 30-fold increased risk for colon cancer.

Reference

Roy MA: Inflammatory bowel disease. Surg Clin North Am 1997;77:1419. [PMID: 9431347]

Crohn Disease

- **Essentials of Diagnosis**
  - Segmental granulomatous inflammation that can affect any portion of the gastrointestinal tract but characteristically affects the terminal ileum
  - In contrast to ulcerative colitis, inflammation is through all layers of bowel wall and may result in fissures, fistulas, or abscesses
  - May have extraintestinal manifestations including sacroiliitis, peripheral arthritis, uveitis, episcleritis, pyoderma gangrenosum, erythema nodosum, sclerosing cholangitis
  - Presentation generally includes low-grade fevers, fatigue, and intermittent nonbloody diarrhea
  - Diagnosis usually confirmed months to years after symptom onset
  - Diagnosis by upper GI with small bowel follow-through, air-contrast enema, or colonoscopy
  - Lab evaluation may reveal mild leukocytosis; marked elevations suggest complication
  - Erythrocyte sedimentation rate may be used to monitor disease activity
  - Evaluate stool for leukocytes, ova and parasites, bacterial culture, *Clostridium difficile* toxin

- **Differential Diagnosis**
  - Ulcerative colitis
  - Appendicitis or diverticulitis
  - Amebiasis
  - Ileocecal tuberculosis
  - *Yersinia* enterocolitis

- **Treatment**
  - Bowel rest, nasogastric suction, intravenous hydration, and admission if evidence of obstruction or peritonitis
  - 5-Amino salicylic acid agents (sulfasalazine, mesalamine)
  - Glucocorticoids useful in acute exacerbation but should not be used for maintenance
  - Immunosuppressives (6-mercaptopurine or azathioprine)
  - Metronidazole for colitis, perianal disease, and fistulas

- **Pearl**

Patients with Yersinia *enterocolitis may present with terminal ileitis and erythema nodosum, closely mimicking Crohn disease.*

Reference

Fiocchi C: Inflammatory bowel disease: etiology and pathogenesis. Gastroenterology 1998;115:182. [PMID: 9649475]

Diverticulitis

- ■ Essentials of Diagnosis
  - • Inflammation of a colonic diverticulum caused by fecalith formation in the neck followed by bacterial proliferation
  - • May perforate limited to serosa (peridiverticulitis) or form a pericolic abscess or generalized peritonitis
  - • Presentation often with left lower quadrant abdominal pain, fever, nausea, emesis
  - • May have dysuria, pyuria, or frequency if adjacent ureter inflamed or secondary to colovesical fistula
  - • Physical exam reveals abdominal tenderness and may demonstrate mass in left lower quadrant
  - • Stool positive for occult blood in 25–50% of patients; gross bleeding rare
  - • Leukocytosis common but may be absent in immunocompromised or elderly
  - • Plain abdominal x-rays may show evidence of free air
  - • CT is test of choice for suspected diverticulitis
  - • Contrast enema studies should not be performed due to risk of perforation

- ■ Differential Diagnosis
  - • Ischemic colitis
  - • Infectious colitis
  - • Inflammatory bowel disease
  - • Pelvic infection
  - • Colon cancer
  - • Cecal diverticulitis (may mimic appendicitis)

- ■ Treatment
  - • Bowel rest, intravenous fluids, analgesics, intravenous antibiotics (ie, gentamycin and metronidazole)
  - • Mild cases: outpatient treatment with nonopioid analgesics and oral antibiotics (ie, ciprofloxacin and metronidazole)
  - • Surgical consult for peritonitis, perforation, or abscess formation
  - • Abscess often drained percutaneously

- ■ Pearl

The risk of perforation is high in immunocompromised patients (43%, compared with 14% for the nonimmunocompromised).

Reference

Stollman N, Raskin JB: Diverticular disease of the colon. Lancet 2004;363:631. [PMID: 14987890]

Diverticulosis

- **Essentials of Diagnosis**
    - Outpouching of the mucosa and submucosa through the muscularis, most commonly affecting the sigmoid colon (right sided in Asians)
    - Acquired disorder linked closely to western low-fiber diet
    - Very common; increases to two-thirds prevalence by age 85; rare before age 40
    - Only 10–20% of patients become symptomatic
    - May result in pain, diverticulitis, lower gastrointestinal bleeding, perforation, or fistula formation
    - Uncomplicated diverticular pain is transient left lower quadrant abdominal pain often associated with flatulence without signs of acute diverticulitis (fever, tenderness, elevated white count)
    - Diverticulitis: inflammation of diverticulum secondary to impacted fecal material; may result in perforation, fistula, or abscess
    - Bleeding secondary to diverticular disease is secondary to erosion of the dome into a colonic artery with acute painless hematochezia or bright red blood per rectum
    - Most common cause of significant lower gastrointestinal bleeding

- **Differential Diagnosis**
    - Pain: appendicitis, ischemic colitis, colitis, ulcerative colitis, cancer
    - Bleeding: angiodysplasia, upper gastrointestinal bleed, colitis, cancer, rectal bleeding (fissure, hemorrhoid)

- **Treatment**
    - Uncomplicated pain: high-fiber diet, antispasmodic
    - Diverticulitis: antibiotics, possible admission
    - Diverticular bleeding: 75–90% of cases stop spontaneously; those with continued bleeding will require transfusion and angiography, surgery, or endoscopy
    - Recurrent diverticulitis or patient age <40 years: refer for elective surgical resection

- **Pearl**

Diverticular bleeding is the most common cause of significant painless lower gastrointestinal bleeding.

Reference

Stollman N, Raskin JB: Diverticular disease of the colon. Lancet 2004;363:631. [PMID: 14987890]

Gastritis

- ■ Essentials of Diagnosis
  - • Inflammatory changes in gastric mucosa due to a variety of insults; diagnosed histologically
  - • Presentation with epigastric pain, nausea, emesis, or gastrointestinal bleeding
  - • Categorized as erosive/hemorrhagic, nonerosive, or specific
  - • Erosive disease: may be secondary to nonsteroidal anti-inflammatory drugs (NSAIDs), alcohol, stress from severe medical or surgical disease, or portal hypertension; may be asymptomatic, or presentation with abdominal pain or upper gastrointestinal bleeding; gastrointestinal bleeding usually clinically insignificant
  - • Nonerosive disease: often due to *Helicobacter pylori* or pernicious anemia; serologic testing for *H pylori* sensitive and specific but may not indicate active infection; urea breath tests, biopsy, or fecal antigen indicate active infection but not usually available; no evidence that *H pylori* is associated with nonulcer dyspepsia
  - • Specific causes include cytomegalovirus gastritis in immunocompromised, anisakiasis from raw fish or sushi, candida, disseminated histoplasmosis, or phlegmonous gastritis from bacterial infection

- ■ Differential Diagnosis
  - • Peptic ulcer disease or functional dyspepsia
  - • Biliary tract disease or pancreatitis
  - • Variceal bleeding
  - • Vascular disease (ruptured abdominal aortic aneurysm, myocardial infarction, or intestinal ischemia)

- ■ Treatment
  - • Patients with abdominal pain and presumptive diagnosis of gastritis: histamine blockers, antacids; primary care referral
  - • Patients with upper gastrointestinal bleeding: hemodynamic monitoring, histamine blockers or proton pump inhibitors, intravenous fluids, possible blood transfusion, endoscopy
  - • Discontinuation of NSAIDs and aspirin, or take only with meals

- ■ Pearl

Obtain an electrocardiogram for patients over age 40 who present with epigastric pain.

Reference

Tally NJ, Hunt RH: What role does Helicobacter pylori play in dyspepsia and nonulcer dyspepsia? Arguments for and against H. pylori being associated with dyspeptic symptoms. Gastroenterology 1997;113(6 Suppl):S67. [PMID: 9394764]

Gastroenteritis

- **Essentials of Diagnosis**
  - Nonspecific term referring to acute diarrhea secondary to a variety of toxins or bacterial, parasitic, or viral infections
  - Manifests as diarrhea, often with nausea and emesis, with or without abdominal pain
  - 50–70% of cases are viral in origin; most common agents are Norwalk virus in adults and rotavirus in children
  - Patients with viral gastroenteritis tend to have low-grade fever or are afebrile and do not have bloody stools
  - ~20% secondary to bacteria may be invasive or toxigenic
  - Parasitic infections, preformed toxins
  - Invasive diarrhea associated with fever, leukocytes in stool and blood in stool due to infection with *Shigella,* enteroinvasive *Escherichia coli, Salmonella, Campylobacter, Yersinia, Clostridium difficile*
  - Short incubation period suggests preformed toxin (*Staphylococcus aureus, Bacillus cereus*)
  - Stool for leukocytes and RBCs if invasive disease suspected
  - Stool cultures for patients who are immunocompromised, ill appearing, febrile, or at extremes of age
  - *C difficile* toxin if recent antibiotic usage
  - Stool for ova and parasites if persistent diarrhea, travel to endemic area, or immunocompromised

- **Differential Diagnosis**
  - Appendicitis or inflammatory bowel disease
  - Bowel obstruction
  - Toxin (cholinergic toxidrome, withdrawal)

- **Treatment**
  - In otherwise uncomplicated cases: history and physical followed by intravenous or oral hydration therapy
  - Antibiotics useful if bacterial infection suspected (trimethoprim-sulfamethoxazole or a fluoroquinolone)
  - Use antimotility agents with caution

- **Pearl**

Vomiting without diarrhea must always prompt a search for noninfectious causes and cannot be referred to as gastroenteritis.

Reference

DuPont HL: Guidelines on acute infectious diarrhea in adults. The Practice Parameters Committee of the American College of Gastroenterology. Am J Gastroenterol 1997;92:1962. [PMID: 9362174]

Gastroesophageal Reflux Disease

■ Essentials of Diagnosis

- Most common symptom: heartburn after meals and during recumbency
- May report reflux of bitter contents into oropharynx
- May also manifest as asthma, chronic cough, sore throat, chest pain
- Often diagnosed clinically
- Endoscopy shows mucosal changes in 50% of patients
- pH probe useful to document temporal relationship between reflux and chest pain or asthma

■ Differential Diagnosis

- Angina
- Peptic ulcer disease
- Nonulcer dyspepsia
- Infectious esophagitis
- Pancreatitis

■ Treatment

- Elevate head of bed
- Avoid eating 3 hours prior to sleep
- Avoid acidic foods, alcohol, chocolate, and smoking
- Antacids
- Promotility agents (metoclopramide)
- Histamine antagonists effective in most patients
- Proton pump inhibitors: for patients unresponsive to histamine antagonists or for severe or extraesophageal symptoms

■ Pearl

Response of chest pain to gastrointestinal anesthetics (the common "GI cocktail") has no diagnostic utility and should not be used to rule out ischemic cardiac causes.

Reference

Heidelbaugh JJ et al: Management of gastroesophageal reflux disease. Am Fam Physician 2003;68:1311. [PMID: 14567485]

Hemorrhoids

- ■ Essentials of Diagnosis
    - • Dilated arteriovenous complexes
    - • Most common cause of hematochezia in adults
    - • Internal hemorrhoids are from above the dentate line, covered in anal mucosa, and free from sensory innervation; may cause painless bleeding or painful prolapse
    - • First-degree: internal protrude into lumen
    - • Second-degree: protrude out of anal canal during defecation but reduce spontaneously
    - • Third-degree: must be reduced manually
    - • Fourth-degree: cannot be reduced
    - • External hemorrhoids originate from below the dentate line, appear like surrounding skin, and have sensory innervation; may become thrombosed and acutely painful
    - • Patients with either type may present with painless bright red bleeding

- ■ Differential Diagnosis
    - • Anal cancer
    - • Anal fissure
    - • Perianal abscess
    - • Rectal prolapse
    - • Condylomata acuminata
    - • Pruritus ani

- ■ Treatment
    - • WASH regimen: warm water, analgesia, stool softeners, high-fiber diet
    - • Acutely thrombosed external hemorrhoids: excision
    - • Second- and third-degree internal: referral to surgeon
    - • Fourth-degree internal: requires surgical consult

- ■ Pearl

Lower gastrointestinal bleeding should not be attributed to hemorrhoids without careful consideration of a more proximal (and serious) cause.

Reference

Madoff RD, Fleshman JW: American Gastroenterological Association technical review on the diagnosis and treatment of hemorrhoids. Gastroenterology 2004;126:1463. [PMID: 15131807]

Hepatic Abscess

■ Essentials of Diagnosis
- Abdominal pain, fevers, chills, anorexia, nausea and vomiting, weight loss, weakness, and malaise
- Categorized as amebic or pyogenic
- Amebic abscess: amebiasis in 10% of world population, 2% of U.S. population; *Entamoeba histolytica* ascends portal vein; one-third of patients have concurrent diarrhea, more may recall recent diarrheal illness; pulmonary symptoms in 20% of patients secondary to rupture of abscess into pleural cavity—classically with anchovy-paste sputum; stool studies 30% sensitive, serologic testing more sensitive
- Pyogenic abscess: commonly associated with biliary obstruction or cholangitis, although other intra-abdominal processes (such as ruptured appendicitis) can be causes
- Ultrasound sensitive for abscess
- Technetium scanning is useful for differentiating an amebic liver abscess from a pyogenic abscess

■ Differential Diagnosis
- Biliary disease
- Hepatitis
- Pneumonia

■ Treatment
- Amebic abscess: metronidazole is treatment of choice with drainage reserved for refractory cases; mild cases may be treated on outpatient basis
- Pyogenic abscess: broad-spectrum antibiotics (some recommend gentamicin and metronidazole) until specific cultures are available, drainage (usually percutaneously), and admission

■ Pearl

Only one-third of patients with amebic abscess will have concurrent intestinal amebiasis.

Reference

Hoffner RJ, Kilaghbian T, Esekogwu VI: Common presentations of amebic liver abscess. Ann Emerg Med 1999;34:351. [PMID: 10459092]

Hepatic Encephalopathy

- **Essentials of Diagnosis**
  - Syndrome of altered mental status ranging from confusion to coma secondary to hepatocellular dysfunction or portal systemic shunting
  - Ammonia is a commonly used marker for the disease; 10% of patients have normal ammonia and many patients with elevated levels do not have symptoms
  - Pathophysiology incompletely understood but may be secondary to false neurotransmitters and neurotoxins passing through a dysfunctional blood-brain barrier
  - Physical exam may show evidence of cirrhosis: spider angiomata, palmar erythema, ascites, or asterixis
  - May have fetor hepaticus (sweet pungent smell of the breath) due to mercaptans (dimethylsulfide)
  - Lab studies often reveal evidence of decreased synthetic function with low albumin, elevated PT
  - Characteristic changes evident on electroencephalogram

- **Differential Diagnosis**
  - Hypoglycemia
  - Alcohol withdrawal or ingestion
  - Seizure or postictal state
  - Intracranial bleed or structural disorder
  - CNS infection
  - Toxin ingestion

- **Treatment**
  - Lactulose or neomycin
  - Avoid medications with CNS effects (benzodiazepines)
  - Admission for severe cases
  - Lower protein diet

- **Pearl**

Gastrointestinal bleeding is a common cause of worsening hepatic encephalopathy.

Reference

Lizardi-Cervera J et al: Hepatic encephalopathy: a review. Ann Hepatol 2003;2:122. [PMID: 15115963]

Hepatitis, Alcoholic

- **Essentials of Diagnosis**
  - Inflammatory liver injury caused by heavy alcohol consumption
  - Risk of injury increases for greater than 80 g of alcohol (about a 6 pack of beer) per day for men, 20 g for women
  - Ranges in severity from asymptomatic to liver failure
  - Fever, hepatomegaly, right upper quadrant tenderness, encephalopathy, jaundice, or bleeding
  - AST/ALT elevated usually <10 times normal
  - Alkaline phosphatase may be elevated mildly (larger elevations suggest common duct obstruction), GGT often elevated
  - Conjugated hyperbilirubinemia, bilirubinuria, hypoalbuminemia
  - Coagulopathy noted by prolonged PT, which usually is not responsive to vitamin K
  - Discriminant function (DF) for prognosis = $4.6 \times$ PT prolongation + bilirubin (>32 suggests severe disease with 50% 30-day mortality)

- **Differential Diagnosis**
  - Viral hepatitis
  - Drug-induced hepatitis
  - Choledocholithiasis
  - Hepatic abscess
  - Nonalcoholic fatty liver
  - Hemochromatosis

- **Treatment**
  - With cessation of alcohol, hepatitis improves over months
  - Intravenous hydration with replacement of thiamine, magnesium
  - In severe hepatitis (DF >32), corticosteroids are sometimes used
  - Vitamin K may be given for coagulopathy but improvement unlikely as the cells are nonfunctional
  - Fresh frozen plasma for bleeding

- **Pearl**

In alcoholic hepatitis, AST is usually greater than ALT: the ratio is often reversed in other causes of hepatitis.

Reference

McCullough AJ, O'Connor JF: Alcoholic liver disease: proposed recommendations for the American College of Gastroenterology. Am J Gastroenterol 1998;93:2022. [PMID: 9820369]

Hepatitis, Viral

- **Essentials of Diagnosis**
  - Hepatitis A: fecal oral transmission, associated with poor hygiene, crowded environment; usually a mild self-limited disease
  - Hepatitis B: transmitted parentally or sexually; associated with intravenous drug use, blood transfusion, occupational exposure; may cause chronic active hepatitis or acute hepatic failure
  - Hepatitis C: transmitted perinatally, sexually, or parentally; associated with intravenous drug use, blood transfusion, occupational exposure; 80% progress to chronic active hepatitis, 80% of patients are nonicteric during acute infection
  - Hepatitis D: incomplete virus that requires hepatitis B to replicate, transmitted similarly to hepatitis B; increased incidence of chronic hepatitis in patients with hepatitis D compared with patients with hepatitis B alone
  - Nausea, emesis, scleral icterus (visible if bili >2.5), jaundice, hepatomegaly, abdominal tenderness
  - AST/ALT 10–100 times normal; ALT >AST (in contrast to alcoholic hepatitis)
  - Alkaline phosphatase may be up to 2 times normal; greater elevations suggest abscess or biliary obstruction
  - Bilirubin elevated; conjugated and unconjugated in nearly equal amounts
  - Elevated PT suggests severe disease

- **Differential Diagnosis**
  - Cholecystitis
  - Cholangitis
  - Hepatic abscess
  - Autoimmune hepatitis
  - Drug-induced hepatitis
  - Alcoholic hepatitis

- **Treatment**
  - Supportive care
  - Admission for patients with encephalopathy, PT prolongation, bilirubin >30, intractable emesis

- **Pearl**

Hepatitis A is not associated with chronic infection.

Reference

Vail BA: Management of chronic viral hepatitis. Am Fam Physician 1997; 55:2749. [PMID: 9191459]

Incarcerated Hernia

- **Essentials of Diagnosis**
    - Abdominal pain usually with palpable abdominal mass sometimes associated with erythema of the overlying skin
    - Gastrointestinal symptoms include anorexia, nausea or vomiting, and occasionally gastrointestinal bleeding
    - Hernias can occur congenitally or postsurgically or can develop from inherent abdominal wall weakness
    - Incarceration denotes a nonreducible mass that is at significant risk of becoming ischemic (strangulated); fever, leukocytosis, or gastrointestinal bleeding suggest ischemia
    - Diagnosis usually made on clinical grounds; for unclear cases, abdominal CT with oral and intravenous contrast can be diagnostic

- **Differential Diagnosis**
    - Nonincarcerated hernia
    - Intra-abdominal palpable mass with no abdominal wall defect
    - Inguinal adenopathy

- **Treatment**
    - Urgent reduction of the hernia (often using procedural sedation to facilitate abdominal musculature relaxation) unless signs and symptoms already suggest strangulation
    - Emergent surgical consult if reduction is not easily accomplished in the emergency department
    - Broad-spectrum antibiotics if associated ischemic bowel is suspected
    - If reduction is possible in emergency department, outpatient follow-up with a surgeon is recommended for definitive repair

- **Pearl**

Search carefully for hernia in any patient with small bowel obstruction.

Reference

McCollough M, Sharieff GQ: Abdominal surgical emergencies in infants and young children. Emerg Med Clin North Am 2003;21:909. [PMID: 14708813]

Intestinal Obstruction

- ■ Essentials of Diagnosis
  - • Symptoms include intermittent colicky abdominal pain of sudden onset that rises to a peak and then subsides
  - • Vomiting usually occurs and may be feculent if obstruction is distal and long-standing
  - • Tachycardia and oliguria indicate severe dehydration
  - • Fever may indicate strangulation and bowel infarction
  - • Abdominal findings: distension, tenderness, and tinkling bowel sounds; look carefully for incarcerated umbilical or inguinal hernias
  - • Abdominal x-rays show dilated loops of bowel with air fluid levels and can confirm the diagnosis; differentiation of small vs. large bowel obstruction is possible by identifying valvulae conniventes that cross the entire lumen of the small bowel and haustra in the large bowel that do not cross the entire lumen
  - • When plain x-rays are nondiagnostic, abdominal CT with oral and intravenous contrast can confirm diagnosis
  - • Renal and hepatic function studies, serum glucose and lipase, urinalysis

- ■ Differential Diagnosis
  - • Paralytic ileus
  - • Colonic pseudoobstruction (Ogilvie syndrome)

- ■ Treatment
  - • Intravenous fluid therapy for dehydration
  - • Nasogastric suction
  - • Surgical consult for possible operative therapy

- ■ Pearl

It is difficult to distinguish on clinical grounds alone between a simple and a strangulated obstruction.

Reference

Bass KN, Jones B, Bulkley GB: Current management of small-bowel obstruction. Adv Surg 1997;31:1. [PMID: 9408486]

Irritable Bowel Syndrome

- ■ Essentials of Diagnosis
  - • Functional disorder characterized by abdominal pain and altered bowel habits without structural or biochemical abnormalities
  - • Rome criteria: chronic abdominal discomfort with 2 out of 3 criteria: (1) relieved by defecation, (2) onset associated with a change in frequency of stool, (3) onset associated with change in form of stool
  - • Other symptoms: abnormal stool frequency, abnormal stool form, abnormal stool passage, mucorrhea, or distension
  - • Acute symptoms (it is a chronic disease), nocturnal diarrhea, gastrointestinal bleeding, weight loss, or fever suggest other disorder
  - • CBC, erythrocyte sedimentation rate, serum albumin, hemoccult should be negative
  - • Up to 20% of population has symptoms consistent with diagnosis; most do not seek medical attention
  - • More than 50% of patients who seek medical attention for this disorder have depression, anxiety, or somatization

- ■ Differential Diagnosis
  - • Inflammatory bowel disease (Crohn disease, ulcerative colitis)
  - • Colon cancer
  - • Celiac sprue
  - • Lactose intolerance
  - • Biliary colic
  - • Peptic ulcer disease
  - • Porphyria

- ■ Treatment
  - • High-fiber diet recommended; stop caffeine intake
  - • Drug therapy controversial; placebo resulted in improvement in up to 70% of cases
  - • Anticholinergic for postprandial pain; loperamide or diphenoxylate with atropine for diarrhea; fiber for constipation; antidepressants

- ■ Pearl

The development of symptoms in patients older than 40 years does not exclude irritable bowel syndrome but should prompt a closer search for an underlying organic cause.

Reference

Maxwell PR, Mendall MA, Kumar D: Irritable bowel syndrome. Lancet 1997;350:1691. [PMID: 9400529]

Mallory-Weiss Syndrome

- **Essentials of Diagnosis**
  - Arterial bleeding from tears in distal esophagus or proximal stomach
  - Believed to arise from large pressure gradient between chest and stomach
  - Causes 10% of upper gastrointestinal bleeding
  - Patients usually present with acute hematemesis but can present with melena, hematochezia, abdominal pain, or syncope
  - History of vomiting prior to hematemesis in 50% of patients
  - Diagnosis confirmed at endoscopy

- **Differential Diagnosis**
  - Peptic ulcer disease
  - Gastritis
  - Esophagitis
  - Esophageal or gastric varices

- **Treatment**
  - Usually supportive—most bleeding stops spontaneously
  - Intravenous access, CBC, blood type and cross-match, electrolytes, liver studies, PT, PTT
  - Nasogastric lavage with normal saline (room temperature) until clear
  - Crystalloid infusion/packed RBCs if systolic blood pressure <90 mm Hg despite 2 L of crystalloid
  - Endoscopy for diagnosis or treatment
  - Sclerotherapy or coagulation usually effective; surgery or embolization if necessary
  - Gastroenterology or surgery consult

- **Pearl**

Some 50% of patients do not report a preceding event (eg, retching).

Reference

Kortas DY et al: Mallory-Weiss tear: predisposing factors and predictors of a complicated course. Am J Gastroenterol 2001;96:2863. [PMID: 11693318]

Meckel Diverticulum

- ■ Essentials of Diagnosis
  - • Remnant of omphalomesenteric duct
  - • Patients may present with gastrointestinal bleeding, intestinal obstruction, or diverticulitis
  - • Most commonly discovered incidentally at laparotomy
  - • 60% contain heterotopic tissue including pancreatic, duodenal, and gastric mucosa
  - • Classic presentation is males age <5 years with painless gastrointestinal bleeding
  - • Diagnosis by Meckel scan (technetium scan): 90% sensitive when gastric mucosa present; sensitivity may be increased by pentagastrin, histamine blockers; less sensitive in adults

- ■ Differential Diagnosis
  - • Anal fissures
  - • Hemorrhoids
  - • Vascular malformation
  - • Swallowed maternal blood (differentiate by Apt test)

- ■ Treatment
  - • Symptomatic patients: surgical treatment

- ■ Pearl

Rule of 2's: Occurs in 2% of population, 2 inches in length, 2 feet proximal to ileocecal valve, and 2% are symptomatic.

Reference

Martin JP et al: Meckel's diverticulum. Am Fam Physician 2000;61:1037. [PMID: 10706156]

Pancreatitis, Acute

■ Essentials of Diagnosis

- Gallstones and alcohol cause 60–80% of cases
- Usually abrupt onset of severe, unrelenting epigastric pain with nausea and emesis
- May have fever, paralytic ileus, or signs of shock or multiple organ dysfunction syndrome
- Epigastric tenderness may have signs of retroperitoneal hemorrhage such as Grey-Turner (flanks) or Cullen sign (periumbilical area)
- Ranson criteria: if 3 or more are present on admission, severe course with necrosis predicted (60–80% sensitivity): (1) age >55 years; (2) WBC >16,000; (3) glucose >200 mg/dL; (4) LDH >350 IU/L; (5) AST >250 IU/L
- Plain x-rays may show sentinel loop or "colon cut-off sign"
- Serum amylase and lipase (more specific) >3 times normal in 90% of cases
- CT with contrast useful in uncertain diagnosis or to detect complication such as abscess, necrosis, or pseudocyst formation

■ Differential Diagnosis

- Peptic ulcer disease
- Cholecystitis
- Aortic aneurysm
- Small bowel obstruction
- Gastritis
- Cholangitis
- Myocardial ischemia

■ Treatment

- Nothing by mouth; consider nasogastric suction
- Intravenous fluids; monitor urine output closely
- Analgesics (meperidine causes less spasm of sphincter of Oddi)
- Imipenem if necrosis is present
- Ranson criteria 0–2: admit to floor; 3–5: admit to ICU
- Surgical consult for severe pancreatitis, hemorrhagic pancreatitis, or abscess

■ Pearl

Patients with pancreatitis may develop hypocalcemia due to saponification.

Reference

Powell JJ et al: Diagnosis and early management of acute pancreatitis. Hosp Med 2003;64:150. [PMID: 12669481]

Peptic Ulcer Disease

- ■ Essentials of Diagnosis
  - • Diagnosed in 10% of patients who present to emergency department with abdominal pain
  - • Epigastric pain typically described as burning; may be relieved by foods or antacids
  - • Main cause (>95% of cases): nonsteroidal anti-inflammatory drugs (NSAIDs) or *Helicobacter pylori* infection
  - • Serologic tests for *H pylori* IgG antibodies widely available with good sensitivity and specificity but does not confirm active infection; antibodies remain for several years
  - • Physical exam usually reveals only mild epigastric tenderness but may show peritonitis if perforation is present
  - • Rectal exam mandatory to evaluate for bleeding
  - • Consider CBC, electrolytes, BUN, creatinine, liver enzymes, bilirubin, lipase, and blood type and cross-match if gastrointestinal bleeding is present; upright abdominal x-ray to evaluate for perforation; consider electrocardiogram in older population
  - • Definitive diagnosis by endoscopy or upper GI
  - • Accounts for half of all upper gastrointestinal bleeding
  - • Complications include gastrointestinal bleeding, gastric outlet obstruction, and perforation

- ■ Differential Diagnosis
  - • Gastritis or gastroesophageal reflux disease
  - • Gallbladder disease, cholangitis, pancreatitis
  - • Vascular disease: abdominal aortic aneurysm, myocardial infarction, mesenteric ischemia
  - • Functional dyspepsia

- ■ Treatment
  - • Stop NSAIDs and aspirin
  - • Treat *H pylori* infection
  - • Patients presenting with dyspepsia: trial of histamine blocker, antacids, with or without test for *H pylori*
  - • Patients with gastrointestinal bleeding: obtain large-bore intravenous access, start proton pump inhibitor, nasogastric lavage (to monitor bleeding and clear for endoscopy), gastroenterology consult for endoscopy or surgical consult

- ■ Pearl

Dyspepsia will have an identifiable cause in only 50% of patients.

Reference

Chan FK, Leung WK: Peptic-ulcer disease. Lancet 2002;360:933. [PMID: 12354485]

Perforated Peptic Ulcer

- **Essentials of Diagnosis**
  - Usually sudden severe upper abdominal pain accompanied by shallow breathing and drawing of the knees toward the chest; shoulder pain may occur from diaphragmatic irritation
  - Epigastric abdominal tenderness accompanied by a rigid abdomen (involuntary guarding)
  - Upright abdominal or chest x-ray may be diagnostic of gastric or bowel perforation demonstrating pneumoperitoneum
  - When abdominal or chest x-rays are nondiagnostic, abdominal CT with intravenous and water-soluble oral contrast may demonstrate a perforation
  - Renal and hepatic function studies, serum glucose and lipase, urinalysis

- **Differential Diagnosis**
  - Gastritis
  - Pancreatitis
  - Cholelithiasis or cholecystitis

- **Treatment**
  - Careful attention to the ABCs and continuous cardiac monitoring
  - Resuscitation with intravenous isotonic fluids for tachycardia, hypotension, or signs of shock
  - Intravenous isotonic fluids for dehydration
  - Nasogastric suction
  - Surgical consult for operative therapy
  - Broad-spectrum intravenous antibiotics

- **Pearl**

Posterior ulcer perforation may result in elevations of amylase and lipase secondary to pancreatic involvement.

Reference

Espinoza R, Rodriguez A: Traumatic and nontraumatic perforation of hollow viscera. Surg Clin North Am 1997;77:1291. [PMID: 9431340]

Variceal Bleeding

- ■ Essentials of Diagnosis
  - • Dilated submucosal veins in the distal esophagus secondary to portal hypertension and collateral blood flow
  - • Cause of 10% of upper gastrointestinal bleeding
  - • 50% of cirrhotic patients have varices; one-third of them develop bleeding
  - • 70% chance of rebleeding; one-third are fatal
  - • Obtain intravenous access; blood for type and cross-match; CBC, PT, PTT, electrolytes, BUN, creatinine, liver studies
  - • Bleeding varices: place nasogastric tube and lavage to prepare for endoscopy
  - • Urgent endoscopy indicated in any cirrhotic patient with suspected gastrointestinal bleeding

- ■ Differential Diagnosis
  - • Erosive gastritis
  - • Peptic ulcer disease
  - • Mallory-Weiss tear
  - • Gastric cancer

- ■ Treatment
  - • Patients with varices without bleeding have been treated with β-blockers to decrease risk of bleeding
  - • Fresh frozen plasma or platelet transfusion for INR >1.5 or platelet count less than 50,000, respectively
  - • Octreotide, 50 μg bolus followed by 50 μg/h by intravenous infusion, controls bleeding in 80% of patients (vasopressin has been used in the past but with no improvement in mortality rate)
  - • Sclerotherapy or banding by endoscopy
  - • Balloon tamponade as temporizing measure; associated with significant complications and requires intubation of the patient
  - • Transjugular intrahepatic portosystemic shunt (TIPS) or surgical shunting if bleeding not controlled by endoscopy

- ■ Pearl

Patients with bleeding from esophageal varices have higher morbidity and mortality rates than do patients with bleeding from any other source of upper gastrointestinal bleeding.

Reference

Peter DJ et al: Evaluation of the patient with gastrointestinal bleeding: an evidence-based approach. Emerg Med Clin North Am 1999;17:239. [PMID: 10101349]

5

Neurologic Emergencies

Bell's Palsy

- **Essentials of Diagnosis**
    - Dysfunction of the peripheral 7th cranial nerve
    - Unilateral (less than 1% bilateral) paralysis of facial muscles including the forehead without sensory deficit
    - Hyperacusis on the affected side due to chordae tympani dysfunction
    - Impaired ability to close the eye due to orbicularis oculi paralysis resulting in a danger of corneal ulceration
    - Loss of taste in the anterior part of the tongue
    - No associated tinnitus, vertigo, or signs of increased intracranial pressure
    - Postauricular pain is common
    - May be a symptom of Lyme disease

- **Differential Diagnosis**
    - Stroke
    - Multiple sclerosis
    - Cerebropontine angle tumor
    - Mastoiditis or other basal skull infections

- **Treatment**
    - Prednisone, 40–60 mg/d for 10 days, with acyclovir, 400 mg 5 times a day for 10 days
    - Careful protection of the cornea with taping of the eyelid after instillation of a bland ophthalmic ointment when sleeping and methylcellulose drops when awake
    - Physical therapy and nerve stimulation sometimes beneficial in keeping the facial muscle strong while awaiting nerve function return

- **Pearl**

Numbness of the interior portion of the external auditory canal suggests pressure on the nervus intermedius, which can be associated with acoustic neuroma.

Reference

Grogan PM, Gronseth GS: Practice parameter: steroids, acyclovir, and surgery for Bell's palsy (an evidence-based review): report of the Quality Standards Subcommittee of the American Academy of Neurology. Neurology 2001;56:830. [PMID: 11294918]

Brain Abscess

- **Essentials of Diagnosis**
  - Caused by spread from intravenous drug use, endocarditis, or other source of septic emboli; localized spread from sinuses, face, mastoid air cells, or penetrating injury
  - Classically, fever, headache (often unilateral and constant in nature), and localized neurologic deficit
  - Suspect brain abscess in all patients with headache and fever
  - Frequently associated with increased intracranial pressure; even small abscesses are surrounded by a considerable area of cerebral edema
  - Significant elevation in intracranial pressure associated with abscess is one of the indications for CT scan preceding lumbar puncture
  - Most brain abscesses are seen on CT scan before lumbar puncture is performed; cerebrospinal fluid exam may be normal in the face of significant abscess

- **Differential Diagnosis**
  - Stroke
  - Toxoplasmosis
  - Echinococcosis
  - Cysticercosis
  - Nocardia
  - Subdural empyema
  - Epidural abscess
  - Metastatic or primary brain tumors
  - Vasculitis or giant cell arteritis

- **Treatment**
  - Urgent neurosurgical consult for diagnostic and therapeutic intervention
  - Start antibiotics after blood cultures are obtained; selection based on suspected source of infection: penicillin for odontogenic abscess, vancomycin for endocarditis, and antistaphylococcal antibiotics for direct penetrating injury
  - Control intracranial pressure with hyperventilation, mannitol, and steroids if necessary

- **Pearl**

Always listen carefully for a heart murmur in patients presenting with fever and headache and keep a high index of suspicion for this relatively rare but devastating condition.

Reference

Calfee DP, Wispelwey B: Brain abscess. Semin Neurol 2000;20:353. [PMID: 11051299]

Brain Tumor

- **Essentials of Diagnosis**
  - Patients with primary brain tumor usually present before fifth decade; after age 50 years, metastatic lesions from lung, breast, and kidney are far more common
  - Presenting symptoms are usually headache (about 50%) associated with lateralizing neurologic dysfunction or seizure
  - Headache is usually worse at night and associated with Valsalva, cough, and exertion
  - Symptoms generally have been present for some time but worsen suddenly in association with increased intracranial pressure and frequently papilledema
  - Vomiting may develop with significantly increased intracranial pressure
  - Metastatic tumors have significant associated cerebral edema; best imaged with a contrast CT or MRI scan
  - Meningiomas can be very slow growing and develop into very large tumors with little symptomology
  - Patients with temporal lobe tumors may present with personality changes; frontal lobe tumors are manifested as cognitive disorders

- **Differential Diagnosis**
  - Brain abscess
  - Chronic subdural hematoma
  - Stroke
  - Subarachnoid or intracerebral hemorrhage

- **Treatment**
  - Control increased intracranial pressure with glucocorticoids (dexamethasone, 10 mg IV, followed by 4 mg IV every 6 hours), hyperventilation, and mannitol as needed
  - Seizures: lorazepam and phenytoin as needed

- **Pearl**

Meningiomas can grow through the suture lines and appear as a tumor of the scalp, the so-called dumbbell meningioma.

Reference

Purdy R, Kirby S: Headaches and brain tumors. Neurol Clin 2004;22:39. [PMID: 15062527]

Guillain-Barré Syndrome

- **Essentials of Diagnosis**
  - Classically described as an acute inflammatory demyelinating polyneuropathy associated with an antecedent viral infectious process; now recognized to have multifactorial cause
  - Appears to be an autoimmune disease caused by a misdirected immune response against components of peripheral nerve
  - Classic manifestations: symmetric weakness; may involve the cranial nerves causing difficulty swallowing and speaking, paraesthesias, and hyporeflexia
  - Gradual onset of weakness usually beginning in the lower extremities and progressively involving more of the CNS; 25% of cases involve respiratory failure and require mechanical ventilation
  - Elevated cerebrospinal protein (up to 400 mg/dL) without leukocytosis is common

- **Differential Diagnosis**
  - Hysteria or conversion reaction
  - Poliomyelitis
  - Rabies
  - Transverse myelitis
  - Epidural abscess or cauda equina syndrome
  - Vitamin B_{12} or folate deficiency
  - Tick paralysis
  - Lyme disease
  - Botulism

- **Treatment**
  - Admission for monitoring of respiratory status, which can decline precipitously
  - Severe cases: plasmapheresis started within 10 days
  - No benefit demonstrated with corticosteroid use

- **Pearl**

Guillain-Barré syndrome may be associated with immunizations; if so, further immunizations should be avoided.

Reference

Kuwabara S: Guillain-Barré syndrome: epidemiology, pathophysiology, and management. Drugs 2004;64:597. [PMID: 15018590]

Headache, Cluster

- **Essentials of Diagnosis**
  - Acute, unilateral, sharp, stabbing pain around the eye and in the distribution of the trigeminal nerve
  - Occurs in clusters, with several attacks a day for several weeks, followed by a period of time without headache
  - Associated autonomic symptoms essential for acute diagnosis: lacrimation, ptosis, nasal congestion, and facial sweating
  - Onset is frequently during sleep
  - Many patients have a chronic partial Horner syndrome
  - Episodes precipitated by alcohol, vasodilators, and nitroglycerin

- **Differential Diagnosis**
  - Trigeminal neuralgia
  - Ramsay-Hunt syndrome of geniculate ganglion herpes
  - Migraine
  - Intracranial mass lesion
  - Posterior pharyngeal tumor
  - Cracked tooth syndrome or severe dental caries
  - Drug-seeking behavior

- **Treatment**
  - High-flow O_2, 7–10 L/min, effective in up to 70% of cases
  - Sumatriptan, 6 mg, subcutaneously
  - Intranasal lidocaine has been effective; cocaine has been tried, but abuse potential limits its use
  - Prophylaxis: verapamil, up to 480 mg/d; lithium to maintain therapeutic levels; and methysergide
  - Avoidance of alcohol and tobacco recommended
  - Treatment of last resort: partial or complete section of the trigeminal nerve

- **Pearl**

The diagnosis of cluster headache is suspect without demonstrable autonomic symptoms.

Reference

Jarrar RG et al: Outcome of trigeminal nerve section in the treatment of chronic cluster headache. Neurology 2003;60:1360. [PMID: 12707445]

Headache, Migraine

■ Essentials of Diagnosis

- Classified as with aura or without aura
- Migraine with aura preceded by a transient neurologic deficit that may include scintillations, scotomas, visual field cuts that fade; headache then begins
- Classic description: unilateral throbbing-type pain exacerbated by lights and loud noises; up to half of migraines are bilateral
- May be precipitated by alcohol, tobacco, monosodium glutamate, and tyramine-containing foods
- Usually associated with nausea and vomiting
- Estrogens, especially birth control pills, seem to increase frequency of migraine attacks
- Incidence greater in females than in males (3:1)
- Look for spontaneous retinal venous pulsations that seem to be common in migraine and help rule out increased intracranial pressure
- Carefully evaluate for the presence of meningeal irritation (nuchal rigidity, positive Kernig and Brudzinski signs) to help rule out subarachnoid hemorrhage and meningitis

■ Differential Diagnosis

- Glaucoma
- Temporal arteritis
- Tumors
- Brain abscess
- Meningitis
- Subarachnoid hemorrhage

■ Treatment

- Oral administration of a nonsteroidal anti-inflammatory drug and metoclopramide at the first sign of headache may abort or markedly decrease severity
- Triptans: specific serotonin 5-HT receptor antagonists that are effective in many cases; very expensive and generally no more effective than intravenous metoclopramide or prochlorperazine

■ Pearl

Scalp tenderness, though frequently present, should suggest an investigation for temporal arteritis in patients over age 50 years.

Reference

Goadsby PJ, Lipton RB, Ferrari MD: Migraine—current understanding and treatment. N Engl J Med 2002;346:257. [PMID: 11807151]

Headache, Tension

- **Essentials of Diagnosis**
    - Common recurrent pain syndrome affecting a large percentage of the population; may be a continuum of the headache syndrome with migraine
    - Gradual onset of headache described as a bandlike syndrome without nausea, photophobia, or neurologic symptoms
    - Occasionally associated with muscle tension and tight neck muscles; headache can exist without this finding
    - Usually not disabling but may be a symptom of emotional stress or depression
    - Normal neurologic exam and vital signs
    - Frequently a diagnosis of exclusion after normal neuroimaging and cerebrospinal fluid analysis

- **Differential Diagnosis**
    - Pseudotumor cerebri (idiopathic intracranial hypertension)
    - Temporomandibular dysfunction
    - Cervical spondylosis
    - Sinusitis
    - Intracranial masses
    - Glaucoma

- **Treatment**
    - Nonsteroidal analgesics usually sufficient
    - Patients occasionally benefit from combination products with butalbital, caffeine, and aspirin or acetaminophen
    - Refractory headaches may improve with diazepam or treatment for depression

- **Pearl**

Bruxism and poor dental occlusion can lead to recurrent headache.

Reference

Ashina S, Ashina M: Current and potential future drug therapies for tension-type headache. Curr Pain Headache Rep 2003;7:466. [PMID: 14604506]

Myasthenia Gravis

- **Essentials of Diagnosis**
  - Autoimmune disease caused by autoantibodies directed at the neuromuscular junction acetylcholine receptor
  - Typical presentation: weakness of bulbar muscles causing symptoms of ptosis, blurred vision, difficulty swallowing, and dysarthria
  - Essential finding: muscle fatigability (worsening of weakness with repeated use)
  - No sensory abnormalities
  - Pain may occur in fatigued muscles; strength improves with muscle rest
  - Administration of edrophonium with unequivocal improvement: thought to be diagnostic and therapeutic
  - Avoid neuromuscular blockers if intubation required
  - Aminoglycoside antibiotics, tetracycline, and class I antiarrhythmics may worsen myasthenia

- **Differential Diagnosis**
  - Multiple sclerosis
  - Botulism
  - Pernicious anemia
  - Poliomyelitis
  - Hyperthyroidism

- **Treatment**
  - Pyridostigmine, 60 mg tabs, 1–4 every 4–6 hours
  - Prednisone, 40–60 mg/d
  - Thymectomy if thymoma present; less effective if thymoma not present
  - Plasmapheresis or intravenous immunoglobulin
  - Hospitalization for myasthenic crisis

- **Pearl**

Botulism affects the pupillary light reflex; it is spared in myasthenia gravis.

Reference

Graves M, Katz JS: Myasthenia gravis. Curr Treat Options Neurol 2004;6:163. [PMID: 14759348]

Poliomyelitis

- **Essentials of Diagnosis**
    - Enteroviral infection that attacks the anterior horn cell resulting in paralysis
    - Viral syndrome of headache, fever, sore throat, myalgias, and vomiting may precede paralysis
    - Severe muscle pain with spasm precedes weakness
    - Generally affects lower limbs more than upper limbs
    - Paraesthesias common, but no sensory deficit can be demonstrated
    - Bulbar form associated with dysphagia, dysphasia, diaphragmatic paralysis, and autonomic dysfunction
    - Respiratory failure develops in severe cases
    - Most cases in the United States currently caused by an immuno-compromised patient being exposed to a live, attenuated virus in the oral polio vaccine

- **Differential Diagnosis**
    - Botulism
    - Guillain-Barré syndrome
    - Myasthenia gravis
    - Spinal epidural abscess

- **Treatment**
    - Preventable with adequate immunization
    - Only supportive care is recommended; no antiviral specific agent is available

- **Pearl**

Suspect polio in an immunocompromised patient exposed to an oral polio vaccine recipient.

Reference

Marx A, Glass JD, Sutter RW: Differential diagnosis of acute flaccid paralysis and its role in poliomyelitis surveillance. Epidemiol Rev 2000;22:298. [PMID: 11218380]

Pseudotumor Cerebri

- **Essentials of Diagnosis**
  - Also known as idiopathic intracranial hypertension
  - Markedly more common in middle-aged, obese females
  - Typical manifestations: headache, elevated cerebrospinal pressure (>20 cm H_2O), and visual blurring and field cuts
  - Neuroimaging is normal or may show small ventricles
  - Thought to be produced by diminished absorption of cerebrospinal fluid (CSF)
  - Symptoms exacerbated similarly to other causes of increased intracranial pressure such as the Valsalva maneuver and the recumbent position
  - Visual disturbance, 6th nerve palsy, or papilledema may be seen

- **Differential Diagnosis**
  - Tumor
  - Posttraumatic hydrocephalus
  - Brain abscess
  - Chronic subdural hematoma
  - Chronic fungal meningitis

- **Treatment**
  - Acetazolamide
  - Corticosteroids, although rebound common with discontinuation
  - Thiazide diuretics
  - Weight loss in obese patients and stopping of estrogens
  - Repetitive lumbar puncture
  - Neurosurgical CSF shunting procedure in refractory cases

- **Pearl**

Measure CSF pressure with patient in the lateral decubitus position, and be sure that the height of the column of fluid varies with respiration to ensure accurate measurement.

Reference

Binder DK et al: Idiopathic intracranial hypertension. Neurosurgery 2004;54:538. [PMID: 15028127]

Seizure

- **Essentials of Diagnosis**
  - Manifested by an uncontrollable motion or behavior caused by unregulated cerebral neuronal discharge
  - Classic grand mal epilepsy described as having the order of aura, incontinence, tonic, clonic, and postictal phases
  - Temporal lobe epilepsy: may manifest itself as behavioral aberrations only; partial simple or complex seizures: any portion of the seizure complex may be present
  - Suspect pseudoseizure in any patients with tonic-clonic movements who do not bite their tongue or become incontinent
  - New-onset seizures in the fourth decade are symptomatic of tumor until proved otherwise
  - Focal seizures in the febrile patient suggest brain abscess
  - Consider and correct hypoglycemia, hypocalcemia, and hypomagnesemia as initial evaluation step
  - Patients with significant seizure activity can develop leukocytosis, fever, and lactic acidosis, all of which resolve with control of the seizures

- **Differential Diagnosis**
  - Tetany from hypocalcemia, strychnine, or tetanus
  - Pseudoseizure
  - Occasional brief tonic-clonic activity that follows a period of simple syncope in an otherwise normal patient

- **Treatment**
  - Maintain airway; a nasal trumpet is sometimes effective, rather than trying to work around clenched teeth
  - Evaluate and treat for hypoglycemia if needed
  - Lorazepam, 0.1 mg/kg IV, up to 10 mg slowly to control seizure activity
  - Phenytoin, 15–18 mg/kg, or fosphenytoin in equivalent doses
  - Protect patient from injury and aspiration

- **Pearl**

An elevated prolactin level suggests an actual seizure rather than pseudoseizure.

Reference

Ahmed SN, Spencer SS: An approach to the evaluation of a patient for seizures and epilepsy. West Med J 2004;103:49. [PMID: 15101468]

Status Epilepticus

■ Essentials of Diagnosis
- Seizure activity that continues without remission for more than 5–10 minutes (classically, 30 minutes) or that recurs without an intervening period of consciousness
- May be manifested by nonconvulsive states, with behavior such as lip smacking, nystagmus, or unresponsiveness
- Electroencephalogram (EEG): essential for the diagnosis of nonconvulsive status epilepticus
- Focal seizures suggest irritative cortical lesion such as abscess, tumor, or old scar from trauma or stroke
- Overdose of stimulants such as cocaine or methamphetamine can cause status epilepticus
- Evaluation and treatment of hypoglycemia and hypocalcemia are essential

■ Differential Diagnosis
- Tetanus
- Pseudoseizure
- Strychnine-induced tetany

■ Treatment
- Establish and maintain airway and ventilation
- Lorazepam, 0.1 mg/kg, up to 8 mg
- Phenytoin, 15–18 mg/kg, or fosphenytoin in equivalent doses
- Phenobarbital, 10 mg/kg IV
- Consider paraldehyde, 0.1–0.5 cc/kg of a 4% solution
- Consider lidocaine, 50 mg IV, followed by a 1–2 mg/min drip if effective
- General anesthesia: pentobarbital, 15 mg/kg IV, then 0.5–1.0 mg/kg/h, with EEG monitoring to ensure that seizures are controlled

■ Pearl

As for any unconscious patient, give thiamine, 100 mg, due to the relatively high incidence of alcoholism in status epilepticus patients.

Reference

Lowenstein DH, Alldredge BK: Status epilepticus. N Engl J Med 1998;338:970. [PMID: 9521986]

Stroke, Hemorrhagic (Intracerebral Hemorrhage)

- ■ Essentials of Diagnosis
  - • Clinical findings depend on hemorrhage site
  - • Common presentation: headache and vomiting with associated focal neurologic deficit
  - • Hypertension is causative and complicating in most cases
  - • Diagnosis by CT scan

- ■ Differential Diagnosis
  - • Meningitis
  - • Migraine
  - • Pseudotumor
  - • Subarachnoid hemorrhage

- ■ Treatment
  - • Maintain airway and ventilation
  - • Control blood pressure to mean arterial pressure below 130 mm Hg; do not lower more than 25%
  - • Consider seizure prophylaxis with fosphenytoin or phenytoin
  - • Surgical treatment can be life saving but is controversial owing to associated mortality and morbidity

- ■ Pearl

No specific clinical signs or symptoms reliably differentiate between hemorrhagic and ischemic stroke; a CT scan is required.

Reference

O'Rourke F et al: Current and future concepts in stroke prevention. Can Med Assoc J 2004;170:1123. [PMID: 15051698]

Stroke, Ischemic

- **Essentials of Diagnosis**
  - Abrupt onset of hemiparesis, monoparesis, visual or visual field loss, dysarthria, ataxia, or vertigo
  - May be associated with numbness, tingling, or a generally uncomfortable sensation only
  - Can be either thrombotic or embolic from atrial fibrillation or other sources
  - May be associated with significant hypertension
  - Initial CT scan is usually normal for first 12 or more hours

- **Differential Diagnosis**
  - Tumor
  - Brain abscess
  - Chronic subdural hematoma
  - Hemorrhagic stroke
  - Migraine
  - Transient ischemic attack

- **Treatment**
  - Thrombolytic therapy with tissue plasminogen activator if patient is older than 18 years; patient has a measurable deficit on the NIH stroke scale; CT scan is negative for hemorrhage; time since onset of symptoms is less than 3 hours (if patient wakes up with symptoms, time of onset is when he or she went to sleep); blood pressure <185 mm Hg systolic and 110 mm Hg diastolic; and if patient has no history of intracranial hemorrhage, head injury, or previous stroke in the past 3 months
  - Other contraindications to thrombolysis: clinical suspicion of subarachnoid hemorrhage despite negative CT scan, known arteriovenous malformation or aneurysm, active internal bleeding, prior intracranial hemorrhage, known bleeding diathesis, major surgery in past 14 days, pregnancy, or post–myocardial infarction pericarditis
  - Control blood pressure to mean arterial pressure <130 mm Hg
  - Elevate the head of the bed to reduce cerebral edema
  - Consider antiplatelet agents after hemorrhage ruled out

- **Pearl**

If intracerebral bleeding is suspected due to an acute change in condition during thrombolytic therapy, stop the infusion and obtain another CT scan immediately.

Reference

O'Rourke F et al: Current and future concepts in stroke prevention. Can Med Assoc J 2004;170:1123. [PMID: 15051698]

Subarachnoid Hemorrhage

- **Essentials of Diagnosis**
    - Sudden, severe (thunderclap) headache usually described as "the worst headache of my life"
    - Usually associated with nausea and occasionally back or leg pain
    - Nuchal rigidity eventually present but may not develop immediately
    - In small, sentinel bleeds, nuchal rigidity may be subtle and develop up to 4 hours after the event
    - Gradation varies from a slight headache (grade I) to profound obtundation and paralysis (grade V)
    - May be associated with trauma, coagulopathy, intracranial neoplasm, adrenergic stimulant use, or atrioventricular malformation
    - Usual cause is a saccular aneurysm of the circle of Willis
    - CT scan misses 5% of subarachnoid hemorrhages; must be followed by lumbar puncture to exclude the diagnosis completely
    - Major problem in patients with a sentinel bleed is rebleeding when the clot undergoes fibrinolysis and catastrophic subarachnoid hemorrhage develops

- **Differential Diagnosis**
    - Migraine
    - Meningitis
    - Brain abscess
    - Brain tumor
    - Encephalitis

- **Treatment**
    - Vasospasm prevention: nimodipine, 60 mg orally every 4 hours
    - Blood pressure control: to decrease rebleeding and maintain cerebral perfusion pressure; labetalol is agent of choice if antihypertensive effects of nimodipine are inadequate
    - Seizure prevention is important; give phenytoin or fosphenytoin
    - Correction of coagulopathies
    - Urgent neurosurgical consult is essential

- **Pearl**

Assume any headache associated with syncope is a subarachnoid hemorrhage.

Reference

Edlow JA: Diagnosis of subarachnoid hemorrhage in the emergency department. Emerg Med Clin North Am 2003;21:73. [PMID: 12630732]

Syncope

- **Essentials of Diagnosis**
  - Sudden, transient loss of awareness and CNS function associated with postural collapse
  - Majority of cases are related to loss of cerebral and brain stem function due to inadequate perfusion pressure or deficient glucose and oxygen delivery
  - First seek extracranial causes for syncope
  - Direct attention initially to hypoperfusion caused by dysrhythmia, volume loss, or medications
  - Institute electrocardiographic and cardiac monitoring as soon as possible
  - Syncope occurring while patient is recumbent or sitting suggests dysrhythmia or seizure
  - Orthostatic testing to evaluate for hypovolemia
  - Vasovagal syncope: can be associated with events that trigger the emotions, exposure to sight of blood or other procedures, prolonged motionless standing, micturition, and migraine
  - A few tonic-clonic movements may be present with syncope, but there is never a postictal period

- **Differential Diagnosis**
  - Seizures
  - Drug and alcohol intoxication
  - Hysteria
  - Pseudoseizure
  - Hypotension caused by vasodilator drugs
  - Fixed-output syncope caused by aortic stenosis, subclavian steal, idiopathic hypertrophic subaortic stenosis, or the like

- **Treatment**
  - Target workup at finding underlying cause
  - Younger healthy patients without structural heart disease and a good history for vasovagal, hypovolemia, or medication-induced syncope can be discharged with follow-up
  - Consider admission for all other patients

- **Pearl**

In over one half of the patients presenting with syncope, a definitive etiology will not be found.

Reference

Maisel WH, Stevenson WG: Syncope—getting to the heart of the matter. N Engl J Med 2002;347:931. [PMID: 12239264]

Temporal Arteritis (Giant Cell Arteritis)

- ■ Essentials of Diagnosis
  - Multinucleated giant cell infiltration of the branches of the carotid artery
  - Age over 50 years and erythrocyte sedimentation rate above 50 in a patient with a headache or pain in the upper face suggests temporal arteritis
  - Pain may be in the posterior part of the scalp or occasionally in the occiput
  - Temporal artery tenderness is a common finding, although its absence does not rule out temporal arteritis
  - Temporal arteritis is associated with aortic aneurysm; chest x-ray should be part of annual follow-up
  - Twice as common in women compared with men
  - May cause sudden catastrophic blindness if not recognized and treated promptly
  - An elevated platelet count may be risk factor for permanent visual loss in patients with temporal arteritis

- ■ Differential Diagnosis
  - Glaucoma
  - Temporomandibular joint syndrome
  - Migraine headache
  - Amaurosis fugax

- ■ Treatment
  - Patients without visual manifestations: prednisone, 40–60 mg/d
  - Patients with visual manifestations: methylprednisolone, 250–500 mg/d IV
  - Expeditious referral for biopsy of the temporal artery for definitive diagnosis

- ■ Pearl
  Ultrasound of the temporal artery may reveal a dark halo around the artery.

Reference

Liozon E et al: Risk factors for visual loss in giant cell (temporal) arteritis: a prospective study of 174 patients. Am J Med 2001;111:211. [PMID: 11530032]

Transient Ischemic Attack (TIA)

- **Essentials of Diagnosis**
  - A focal, transient, neurologic deficit associated with cerebrovascular compromise; followed by complete recovery in <24 hours
  - Limited to the neurologic dysfunction of a defined vascular supply, unless multiple embolic events occur
  - Usually not associated with headache
  - CT and MRI scans are usually normal; indicated to rule out hemorrhage and infarct
  - Evaluation for carotid artery disease is essential as is echocardiography to rule out mural thrombi, especially with atrial fibrillation
  - Vertebrobasilar events occur and can produce symptoms of vertigo, dizziness, nausea, ipsilateral facial and contralateral body numbness or weakness

- **Differential Diagnosis**
  - Migraine
  - Postictal state of epilepsy
  - Hypoglycemia
  - Tumors or mass lesions
  - Labyrinthine vertigo
  - Stroke

- **Treatment**
  - Aspirin is treatment mainstay after surgically correctable lesions of the carotid artery and cardiac mural thrombi have been ruled out
  - In the case of aspirin failure, try aspirin-dipyridamole combinations
  - Strongly consider admission for patients with hemispheric TIA symptoms such as motor deficits, speech deficits, hemianopia, and hemispatial neglect

- **Pearl**

Many TIA patients will be shown to have small lacunar infarcts on follow-up MRI.

Reference

Johnston DC, Hill MD: The patient with transient cerebral ischemia: a golden opportunity for stroke prevention. Can Med Assoc J 2004;170:1134. [PMID: 15051699]

Trigeminal Neuralgia

■ Essentials of Diagnosis

- Severe, lancinating pain in the distribution of the trigeminal nerve
- Chewing, touching the face, swallowing, or brushing the teeth may initiate paroxysms
- Careful neurologic exam to rule out compressive lesions in the posterior fossa with particular attention to the sensation of the external auditory canal supplied by the nervus intermedius; dysfunction in that distribution is an early sign of posterior fossa tumors
- Usually develops after the fourth decade
- Pain syndrome is rare in the first (ophthalmic) branch of the 5th cranial nerve

■ Differential Diagnosis

- Herpes zoster
- Maxillary sinusitis
- Acute glaucoma
- Temporomandibular joint syndrome
- Cracked tooth or dental abscess

■ Treatment

- Phenytoin, 250 mg IV, may abort some attacks
- Carbamazepine, 100 mg twice daily, increasing to 1,200 mg daily if tolerated, is effective in many cases
- For treatment failures: offer nerve block or partial nerve resection in specialty centers

■ Pearl

A cracked tooth can cause pain similar to trigeminal neuralgia; a careful dental evaluation is always warranted.

Reference

Chavin JM: Cranial neuralgias and headaches associated with cranial vascular disorders. Otolaryngol Clin North Am 2003;36:1079. [PMID: 15025008]

Wernicke-Korsakoff Syndrome

- **Essentials of Diagnosis**
  - Develops in alcoholic individuals
  - Acute neurologic dysfunction characterized by ophthalmoplegia, ataxia, and confusion
  - Sixth nerve or conjugate gaze palsies may be present
  - Truncal ataxia is a common finding; associated with a wide-based gait
  - Delirium present in 20% of cases; apathy, confusion, and Korsakoff psychosis may be manifest
  - Peripheral neuropathy is commonly associated and should be sought if the patient is able to cooperate
  - Permanent disability due to persistent confusion, ataxia, and Korsakoff psychosis is common even after immediate thiamine replacement
  - Patients with thiamine deficiency may become acutely symptomatic with ataxia, confusion, and agitation after the administration of carbohydrate load
  - May develop in patients with fasting, hyperemesis, and inability to eat from various causes

- **Differential Diagnosis**
  - Syphilis
  - HIV infection
  - Pernicious anemia
  - Drug and alcohol withdrawal
  - Psychosis

- **Treatment**
  - Thiamine, 100 mg IV, and repeated doses of 50 mg/d until adequate dietary intake is established
  - Consider adding multivitamins, including vitamin B_{12} and magnesium
  - Admit for supportive therapy and thiamine replacement

- **Pearl**

Thiamine deficiency was initially described in the 19th century as a painful polyneuropathy associated with heart disease.

Reference

Zubaran C, Fernandes JG, Rodnight R: Wernicke-Korsakoff syndrome. Postgrad Med J 1997;73:27. [PMID: 9039406]

6

Genitourinary Emergencies

Cystitis

- **Essentials of Diagnosis**
  - Common symptoms: dysuria, frequency, urgency, hesitancy, suprapubic pain
  - Most common in females of child-bearing age
  - Pregnancy, male gender, pediatric age increase risk
  - Fever, vomiting, back pain, or toxic appearance make pyelonephritis more likely
  - Catheter urine specimen preferable in pediatric patients or those not able to give good clean-catch specimen
  - Presence of leukocytes or nitrites on dip stick: 75% sensitive, 82% specific

- **Differential Diagnosis**
  - Vaginitis
  - Vulvovaginitis
  - Pyelonephritis
  - PID
  - Renal calculi

- **Treatment**
  - Nonpregnant women of child-bearing age with suspected uncomplicated cystitis: may receive 3-day course of Bactrim DS twice daily
  - Pediatric patients: trimethoprim-sulfamethoxazole (TMP-SMZ) or amoxicillin clavulanate for 7–10 days pending culture and sensitivity
  - Elderly patients: fluoroquinolone for 7–10 days to avoid possible hyperkalemic effect of TMP-SMZ in patients with baseline renal insufficiency
  - To minimize dysuric symptoms: phenazopyridine, 200 mg three times daily for 2 days

- **Pearl**

Cystitis is one of the most common presenting complaints for women of child-bearing age; be sure to exclude pregnancy.

Reference

Fihn SD: Clinical practice: acute uncomplicated urinary tract infection in women. N Engl J Med 2003;349:259. [PMID: 12867610]

Epididymitis

■ Essentials of Diagnosis

- Testicular pain
- Epididymal tenderness
- Cause in prepubertal males usually *Escherichia coli;* 50% of patients will have anatomic abnormality
- Males under age 35 years: epididymitis usually related to urethritis; *Neisseria gonorrhea* or *Chlamydia trachomatis* most common
- Males over age 35 years: usually have *E coli* from preceding urinary tract infection
- Urinalysis, urine culture, urethral swab, and culture
- Ultrasound: usually reveals increased flow and a thickened epididymis; absence of flow indicates testicular torsion

■ Differential Diagnosis

- Testicular torsion
- Torsion of testicular appendix
- Orchitis
- Urinary tract infection
- Hydrocele
- Testicular tumor

■ Treatment

- Prepubertal males: trimethoprim-sulfamethoxazole (TMP-SMZ) and urology referral
- Males under age 35 years: ceftriaxone, 250 mg IM, and doxycycline, 100 mg orally twice daily for 10–14 days
- Treatment of sexual partners and condom use should be stressed
- Males over age 35 years: TMP-SMZ or a fluoroquinolone
- Admission for intractable pain, toxic appearance

■ Pearl

Epididymitis is the most common diagnosis given when testicular torsion is missed.

Reference

Burgher SW: Acute scrotal pain. Emerg Med Clin North Am 1998;16:781. [PMID: 9889740]

Fournier Gangrene

- **Essentials of Diagnosis**
    - Rapidly progressing fascial infection of perineal, perianal, or genital areas
    - More common in men than women by 10:1
    - Usually polymicrobial; *Escherichia coli* and *Bacteroides* most common
    - Rates of fascial destruction as fast as 2 cm/h
    - Skin exam usually reveals portal of entry
    - Immunodepression from diabetes, chronic steroids, advanced age, HIV, or alcoholism can predispose to Fournier gangrene
    - Highest mortality rates with advanced age, sepsis, renal failure, or liver dysfunction
    - May see signs of sepsis, tachycardia, hypotension, or fever on physical exam
    - May observe feculent odor from anaerobes
    - Crepitus or gangrene to the scrotum/perineum may not be present early on but are diagnostic
    - CBC; electrolytes; blood, urine, and wound cultures
    - Ultrasound: may reveal air in scrotal wall
    - CT scan: typically shows soft tissue gas, thickening of soft tissues, and fat stranding; full extent of involvement seen on CT usually exceeds what is clinically evident on exam

- **Differential Diagnosis**
    - Cellulitis
    - Epididymitis
    - Testicular torsion
    - Scrotal abscess

- **Treatment**
    - Initial resuscitation with crystalloids for volume deficiency or sepsis
    - Early initiation of broad-spectrum antibiotics (ie, ampicillin-sulbactam, ticarcillin-clavulanate, piperacillin-tazobactam, or ampicillin-gentamicin-clindamycin
    - Immediate consult with general surgery and urology for definitive treatment: extensive debridement
    - Hyperbaric oxygen therapy may be beneficial

- **Pearl**

Suspect Fournier gangrene with any groin soft tissue infection in a diabetic patient.

Reference

Morpurgo E, Galandiuk S: Fournier's gangrene. Surg Clin North Am 2002;82:1213. [PMID: 12516849]

Hematuria

- **Essentials of Diagnosis**
  - Microscopic hematuria is presence of >2–5 RBCs/hpf
  - Painful hematuria suggests renal colic, but consider abdominal aortic aneurysm or renal vascular disease such as renal infarct
  - Hematuria with associated dysuria: often related to urinary tract infection
  - Painless hematuria represents numerous diseases: malignancy, hypertension, glomerulonephritis, prostate disease
  - Check blood pressure; look for flank tenderness, evidence of bladder outflow obstruction, vaginal or rectal bleeding
  - Urinalysis for RBCs/hpf and for RBC casts suggestive of glomerulonephritis; urine for myoglobin if no RBCs on microscopy
  - Electrolytes for assessment of renal function in all but uncomplicated cystitis
  - CBC and coagulation studies in patients taking Coumadin or in those with heavy bleeding and clots
  - CT scan without contrast best for stones; CT with contrast needed when looking for malignancy and vascular causes
  - Cystoscopy indicated to detect bladder cancers and localize bleeding source

- **Differential Diagnosis**
  - Renal stone
  - Genitourinary malignancy
  - Urinary tract infection
  - Hypertensive nephropathy
  - Coagulopathy
  - Menstrual bleeding or rectal bleeding
  - Myoglobinuria secondary to rhabdomyolysis
  - Factitious hematuria from patient contaminating specimen

- **Treatment**
  - Hemorrhagic cystitis: antibiotics
  - Persistent bleeding and clots may prevent bladder emptying; may require admission for three-way catheter and continuous bladder irrigation with saline
  - Transfusion: rarely needed except with large blood loss
  - Glomerulonephritis: admit with nephrology consult
  - Follow pediatric patients to exclude Wilms' tumor

- **Pearl**

Painless hematuria in elderly patients represents malignancy unless proved otherwise.

Reference

Cohen RA, Brown RS: Clinical practice: microscopic hematuria. N Engl J Med 2003;348:2330. [PMID: 12788998]

Orchitis

- **Essentials of Diagnosis**
  - Testicular swelling and pain
  - When mumps is cause, testicular swelling usually occurs 4–7 days postparotitis
  - Bacterial orchitis usually related to epididymitis; more common in sexually active males or males over age 50 years
  - Ultrasound: shows enlarged testes with normal blood flow; can exclude testicular torsion or abscess when orchitis is suspected
  - Labs not useful for viral orchitis; urine and urethral cultures as well as urinalysis indicated for suspected epididymo-orchitis

- **Differential Diagnosis**
  - Testicular torsion
  - Scrotal abscess or cellulitis
  - Epididymitis
  - Hernia
  - Hydrocele

- **Treatment**
  - Supportive therapy mainstay of viral orchitis
  - Bedrest, analgesics, cool or warm compresses as per patient preference
  - Epididymo-orchitis follows same treatment as epididymitis: under age 35 years, ceftriaxone, 250 mg IM, and doxycycline, 100 mg orally twice daily for 10–14 days; over age 35 years, cover *Escherichia coli* with trimethoprim-sulfamethoxazole or a fluoroquinolone
  - Testicular atrophy and impaired fertility may result; follow-up with a urologist indicated
  - A pyocele may develop; requires urologic drainage

- **Pearl**

Color-flow duplex ultrasound in an acutely swollen testicle will typically determine the diagnosis.

Reference

Schul MW, Keating MA: The acute pediatric scrotum. J Emerg Med 1993;11:565. [PMID: 7818620]

Paraphimosis

- **Essentials of Diagnosis**
  - Foreskin has been retracted and becomes constricted proximal to the glans
  - May occur as a result of attempts to retract a phimotic foreskin in a young male
  - Penis distal to the constriction becomes edematous, painful; ischemia and even gangrene may result if foreskin is not reduced
  - Urinary retention may develop

- **Differential Diagnosis**
  - Encircling foreign body (ie, hair, rubber band, metallic object)
  - Contact dermatitis

- **Treatment**
  - Attempt manual reduction; sedation or ring block anesthesia helpful
  - Firmly squeeze the glans for 5–10 minutes to reduce its size; then move prepuce distally while pushing glans proximally
  - If not successful, may pierce the glans up to 20 times with 26-gauge needle, express the edema, and repeat attempt (Dundee technique)
  - If reduction still unsuccessful, perform dorsal slit maneuver
  - Refer patient to a urologist for circumcision to prevent recurrence

- **Pearl**

Reduction of paraphimosis should be done promptly and requires a considerable amount of pressure, which many physicians are hesitant to apply.

Reference

Choe JM: Paraphimosis: current treatment options. Am Fam Physician 2000;62:2623. [PMID: 11142469]

Phimosis

- **Essentials of Diagnosis**
  - Inability to retract the foreskin
  - Physiologic phimosis is common in first years of life
  - In mature males, scarring or chronic balanoposthitis may lead to phimosis
  - Severe phimosis may cause urinary obstruction

- **Differential Diagnosis**
  - Balanitis
  - Balanitis xerotica obliterans
  - Physiologic phimosis
  - Contact dermatitis
  - Penile carcinoma

- **Treatment**
  - Physiologic phimosis responds to topical steroids accompanied by gentle retraction applied intermittently over the span of months
  - Be careful not to cause paraphimosis
  - Phimosis resulting from poor hygiene: cleansing, use of topical antifungals; occasionally requires antibiotics
  - Urinary retention: preputial ostia may be dilated with a hemostat, or a dorsal slit may be created in the foreskin
  - Referral to urologist for definitive treatment, an elective circumcision

- **Pearl**

Unless urinary retention is present, phimosis does not require emergent intervention.

Reference

Brown MR, Cartwright PC, Snow BW: Common office problems in pediatric urology and gynecology. Pediatr Clin North Am 1997;44:1091. [PMID 9326954]

Priapism

- **Essentials of Diagnosis**
  - Painful prolonged pathologic erection not relieved by ejaculation
  - Corpora cavernosa involved, but glans and corpus spongiosum remain flaccid
  - High-flow priapism is rare; usually results from penetrating trauma with subsequent rupture of a cavernosa artery
  - Veno-occlusive priapism more common; usually painful and may lead to fibrotic changes of the penis and subsequent impotence if not treated within 12–24 hours
  - Veno-occlusive priapism: may be caused by sickle cell anemia, use of intraurethral medications for erectile dysfunction, leukemia, multiple myeloma, or spinal cord injury
  - Common medications causing priapism: chlorpromazine, trazodone, thioridazine, hydralazine, metoclopramide, omeprazole, hydroxyzine, testosterone, calcium channel blockers, anticoagulants
  - Drugs of abuse causing priapism: marijuana, cocaine, ethanol, Ecstasy
  - CBC to exclude leukemia and type and cross for sickle cell patients who may respond to a transfusion

- **Differential Diagnosis**
  - Medications
  - Sickle cell disease
  - Leukemia

- **Treatment**
  - Subcutaneous terbutaline, 0.25–0.5 mg; repeat in 15–20 minutes if needed
  - If not successful, aspiration of 20–30 cc of blood from corpora cavernosa followed by injection of 20–30 cc of a phenylephrine–normal saline solution (10 mg phenylephrine in 500 cc normal saline)
  - Urology consult for all cases

- **Pearl**

Be sure to document a discussion with the patient about the risk of subsequent impotence associated with priapism.

Reference

Kalsi JS et al: Priapism: a medical emergency. Hosp Med 2002;63:224. [PMID: 11995273]

Prostatitis

- **Essentials of Diagnosis**
  - Several forms of prostatitis are recognized; acute bacterial prostatitis is most common form seen in the emergency department
  - Patients complain of low back, low abdominal, perineal, or rectal pain
  - Common signs and symptoms: fevers, chills, myalgias, urinary frequency, dysuria, urgency; urethral discharge may be present
  - Physical findings: fever; tender, boggy prostate on exam
  - Causes: gonococcus and *Chlamydia trachomatis* for males under age 35 years; more commonly a uropathogen in older males
  - CBC, urinalysis, urine culture

- **Differential Diagnosis**
  - Urinary tract infection
  - Benign prostatic hypertrophy
  - Prostate cancer
  - Urethritis

- **Treatment**
  - Patients under age 35 years: ofloxacin, 400 mg orally once, then 300 mg orally twice daily for 7 days; hospitalize patient if toxic appearing
  - Patients over age 35 years: consider hospitalization; treatment with a fluoroquinolone or the combination of ampicillin and an aminoglycoside
  - Urology consult
  - Analgesics and antipyretics
  - Intravenous hydration

- **Pearl**

Prostatic massage is not necessary to make the diagnosis of acute prostatitis.

Reference

Lummus WE, Thompson I: Prostatitis. Emerg Med Clin North Am 2001;19:691. [PMID: 11554282]

Pyelonephritis

- **Essentials of Diagnosis**
    - Acute pyelonephritis usually the result of cystitis that has ascended into a kidney via the ureter
    - *Escherichia coli* most common organism (>75% of cases)
    - Compared to cystitis, patients more likely to have flank pain, fever, nausea, and vomiting and often appear uncomfortable
    - Risk factors for pyelonephritis: pregnancy, diabetes, immunocompromised state, elderly, recent hospitalization, recent instrumentation, recent antibiotic use, symptoms lasting more than 7 days
    - All suspected cases of pyelonephritis: urinalysis, urine culture, and electrolytes and a pregnancy test for females
    - Urinalysis typically has >20 white blood cells per high-power field
    - Blood cultures positive in approximately 20% of patients
    - Contrast CT indicated for failure to respond to therapy or in elderly, diabetic, or severely ill patients or those with suspected renal stone to rule out perinephric abscess, renal abscess, acute bacterial nephritis, or emphysematous pyelonephritis

- **Differential Diagnosis**
    - Renal colic
    - Ectopic pregnancy
    - Acute abdomen/biliary colic
    - Cystitis
    - Pelvic inflammatory disease
    - Abdominal aortic aneurysm

- **Treatment**
    - Initial antibiotics given intravenously; emesis is common
    - Ceftriaxone or fluoroquinolone for nonpregnant patients
    - Intravenous hydration, antiemetic, and analgesics
    - Healthy, nontoxic, nonpregnant young adult females: outpatient treatment, 7–14 days of fluoroquinolone or 14 days of trimethoprim-sulfamethoxazole and follow-up guaranteed in 24–48 hours

- **Pearl**

Pregnant patients with pyelonephritis have increased risk of preterm labor and should be admitted for intravenous antibiotics.

Reference

Hooton TM: The current management strategies for community-acquired urinary tract infection. Infect Dis Clin North Am 2003;17:303. [PMID: 12848472]

Renal Colic

- **Essentials of Diagnosis**
  - Most typical presentation: acute onset of severe flank pain that radiates down to groin
  - Affects up to 10% of the population; 10-year recurrence rate approximately 50%
  - Calcium stones most common (75%)
  - Over 80% of stones pass spontaneously
  - Nearly 20% of patients are admitted for intractable pain, proximal infection, or inability to maintain hydration
  - Stone 6 mm or larger unlikely to pass spontaneously
  - Patients usually writhing in pain and appear uncomfortable
  - Fever should be absent; flank tenderness usually present
  - Patients may complain of testicular pain but should not have tenderness
  - Hematuria absent with about 10% of stones
  - Presence of white blood cells in urine should prompt search for infection
  - Non-contrast helical CT scan is imaging test of choice because of high sensitivity (95–100%), lack of exposure to intravenous contrast, and its ability to diagnose other conditions

- **Differential Diagnosis**
  - Abdominal aortic aneurysm
  - Pyelonephritis
  - Appendicitis/cholecystitis
  - Ovarian cyst/torsion
  - Ectopic pregnancy
  - Testicular torsion

- **Treatment**
  - Intravenous pain medications (narcotics, ketorolac) and antiemetics
  - Intravenous hydration for patients with signs of volume depletion or borderline creatinine and a need for intravenous pyelogram
  - Urology consult for intractable pain, solitary kidney, renal transplant, or evidence of proximal infection

- **Pearl**

Abdominal aortic aneurysms are often misdiagnosed as kidney stones in elderly patients.

Reference

Teichman JM: Clinical practice. Acute renal colic from ureteral calculus. N Engl J Med 2004;350:684. [PMID: 14960744]

Renal Failure, Acute

- **Essentials of Diagnosis**
  - Acute decline in renal function usually manifested by an increase in serum creatinine or decreased urine output
  - History: determine cause as prerenal, intrinsic, or postrenal
  - Prerenal: volume loss, diarrhea, blood loss, hypotension, poor oral intake, or congestive heart failure
  - Medications that may cause acute renal failure: intravenous contrast, angiotensin-converting enzyme inhibitors, nonsteroidal anti-inflammatory drugs, diuretics, antibiotics
  - Postrenal obstruction: usually related to prostate disease in elderly men
  - Oliguria: urine output <400 mL per 24 hours; poorer prognosis than with nonoliguric renal failure
  - Lab values associated with prerenal: BUN/Cr >20, urine osmolality >500 mOsm/kg H_2O, and fractional excretion of Na^+ <1
  - Electrocardiogram to look for hyperkalemia; chest x-ray for congestive heart failure
  - Renal ultrasound to exclude obstruction and determine kidney size; helps determine cause

- **Differential Diagnosis**
  - Urinary obstruction
  - Dehydration
  - Acute tubular necrosis
  - Renal calculi/hydronephrosis

- **Treatment**
  - Normalization of blood pressure and correction of volume status: may improve renal function in many cases
  - Foley catheter to eliminate postrenal obstruction and monitor urine output
  - Consider renal replacement therapy: hemodialysis or peritoneal dialysis for hyperkalemia not responsive to medical management, volume overload, pericarditis, encephalopathy, bleeding
  - Medications of little benefit, but removal of harmful medications may enhance recovery of function
  - Admission with nephrology consult for most cases

- **Pearl**

Acute renal failure is usually an unsuspected diagnosis; elevated creatinine is often noted on labs sent to evaluate another complaint.

Reference

Lamiere NH, De Vriese AS, Vanholder R: Prevention and nondialytic treatment of acute renal failure. Curr Opin Crit Care 2003;9:681. [PMID: 14639067]

Testicular Torsion

- **Essentials of Diagnosis**
    - Most common in teenage males but occur in all age groups
    - Early reversal of ischemia improves likelihood of salvage
    - Restoration of flow in less than 6 hours is 80–100% successful; almost 0% successful when over 12 hours
    - Pain is usually sudden in onset and severe; may follow trauma
    - Exam shows tender, swollen testicle with unilateral absent cremasteric reflex
    - Increased risk after sports, trauma, with undescended testicle, or horizontal lie
    - Ultrasound with color-flow Doppler or radionuclide scan may be helpful in equivocal cases but should not delay urologic intervention; some urologists prefer scrotal exploration as more timely and accurate

- **Differential Diagnosis**
    - Epididymitis
    - Orchitis
    - Hydrocele
    - Renal colic
    - Acute appendicitis

- **Treatment**
    - Emergent urology consult
    - Success rates of up to 70% with manual reduction of torsion
    - Initial attempts on the right testicle: examiner faces patient and rotates testicle in a counter-clockwise direction relative to the examiner
    - Left testicle should be initially rotated 180 degrees in a clockwise manner (compared to opening a book)
    - Resolution of pain signifies successful reduction
    - Up to three 180-degree rotations may be attempted
    - Definitive therapy is orchiopexy; urology consult needed even if reduction is successful

- **Pearl**

Younger males with testicular torsion may present with abdominal pain; a good scrotal exam is essential to avoid missing the diagnosis.

Reference

Shergill IS et al: Testicular torsion unravelled. Hosp Med 2002;63:456. [PMID: 12212415]

7

Vascular Emergencies

Abdominal Aortic Aneurysm

- **Essentials of Diagnosis**
  - Often asymptomatic and discovered incidentally
  - Diagnosis by pulsatile abdominal mass; present in fewer than 50% of cases
  - Acute rupture or dissection usually associated with abrupt onset of flank, abdominal, groin, or low back pain
  - Rupture results in hypotension, shock, syncope, or altered mental status
  - Abdominal CT scan with contrast: study of choice in stable patients
  - Abdominal ultrasound: can be helpful when patient is too unstable to go for CT scan or when CT scanner not available; more useful as screening test
  - Outpatient follow-up acceptable for patients with asymptomatic aneurysms smaller than 4 cm

- **Differential Diagnosis**
  - Myocardial infarction
  - Pancreatitis
  - Mesenteric ischemia
  - Gastric or peptic ulcer disease
  - Kidney stone

- **Treatment**
  - Establish good peripheral and central venous access
  - Systolic blood pressure to 100–120 mm Hg
  - Crystalloids to treat hypotension; hemodilution and further blood loss are of concern
  - Type and cross-match for 8–10 units of packed RBCs; transfuse as needed
  - Unstable patients: immediate surgical consult

- **Pearl**

Abdominal aortic aneurysm must be ruled out in elderly patients who present with signs and symptoms of kidney stone.

Reference

Prisant LM, Mondy JS: Abdominal aortic aneurysm. J Clin Hypertens 2004;6:85. [PMID: 14872146]

Acute Arterial Occlusion of Extremity Large Vessels

■ Essentials of Diagnosis

- Leads to ischemia of the limb with subsequent pain, paresthesia, pallor, and coolness of extremity
- Pulses faint or absent by palpation and Doppler
- Paralysis and paresthesia: suggest limb-threatening ischemia
- Acute occlusion leads to progressive and irreversible damage to involved tissues
- Embolic occlusion more likely with atrial fibrillation, mitral valve disease, or in patients with low ejection fraction or left ventricular aneurysm
- Thrombotic occlusion more likely in patients with atherosclerosis
- Angiography to confirm diagnosis

■ Differential Diagnosis

- Deep vein thrombosis or thrombophlebitis
- Abdominal aortic aneurysm
- Traumatic peripheral artery injury
- Compartment syndrome

■ Treatment

- Emergent restoration of flow needed for best prognosis
- Emergent surgical consult; interventional radiology may be consulted if available in conjunction with surgeon
- Intravenous heparin for full anticoagulation
- Pain medication helpful while awaiting definitive therapy

■ Pearl

A history of claudication is common in thrombotic arterial occlusion and is rare in embolic-induced arterial occlusion.

Reference

Constantini V, Lenyi M: Treatment of acute occlusion of peripheral arteries. Thromb Res 2002;106:V285. [PMID: 12359341]

Acute Arterial Occlusion of Extremity Small Vessels

- Essentials of Diagnosis
  - Abrupt onset of small painful area on affected digit
  - Tender, cool, and cyanotic
  - Usually the result of microemboli from atherosclerotic plaque or aneurysm
  - May be caused by intra-arterial procedures such as catheterization or stenting
  - Pulses typically normal in affected extremity unless prior peripheral vascular disease coexists

- Differential Diagnosis
  - Septic emboli
  - Endocarditis
  - Hematoma
  - Raynaud disease

- Treatment
  - Heparinization: may be needed to prevent further emboli
  - Consider aspirin
  - Admission for testing to identify source of emboli (ie, echocardiography, angiography)
  - Analgesics
  - Surgical consult

- Pearl

The fingers are rarely involved in acute arterial occlusion of small vessels.

Reference

Constantini V, Lenti M: Treatment of acute occlusion of peripheral arteries. Thromb Res 2002;106:V285. [PMID: 12359341]

Aortic Dissection

- **Essentials of Diagnosis**
  - Sudden, severe, tearing or ripping back pain with radiation to the back, neck, and jaw
  - Have high index of suspicion in deceleration-type traumatic injuries
  - Dissection may involve coronary arteries; electrocardiogram may show acute ST elevations
  - Dissection may involve carotid artery and result in hemiparesis
  - Unequal blood pressure in upper extremities
  - Wide mediastinum on chest x-ray
  - Contrast CT scan of chest, transesophageal echocardiogram, or aortic angiogram equally useful for diagnosis

- **Differential Diagnosis**
  - Myocardial infarction
  - Pericardial tamponade
  - Abdominal aortic aneurysm
  - Musculoskeletal chest pain
  - Pulmonary embolism

- **Treatment**
  - Control blood pressure with β-blockers (esmolol, metoprolol, propranolol) and vasodilators (nitroprusside)
  - Prompt surgical consult, especially for ascending arch or traumatic dissections
  - Dissections involving ascending portion of the arch usually treated surgically; those involving just the descending portion of the arch are more likely to be managed medically

- **Pearl**

Have a high index of suspicion in decelerating injuries, when a widened mediastinum is present, or when pressures are unequal in the extremities.

Reference

Flachskampf FA, Daniel WG: Aortic dissection. Cardiol Clin 2000;18:807. [PMID: 11236167]

Deep Vein Thrombosis

- ■ Essentials of Diagnosis
  - • Unilateral swelling, erythema, or temperature in affected extremity
  - • Physical exam unreliable
  - • Contrast venography traditional gold standard
  - • Ultrasound has largely replaced venography
  - • Risk factors: hypercoagulable state (deficiency of antithrombin, protein S, or protein C), blood flow stasis, trauma, major surgery (hip or knee)
  - • Low-risk patients: negative enzyme-linked immunoassay D-Dimer has high negative predictive value
  - • Pulmonary embolism is the most feared complication; may occur from deep vein thromboses in upper or lower extremities

- ■ Differential Diagnosis
  - • Cellulitis
  - • Lymphedema
  - • Thrombophlebitis

- ■ Treatment
  - • Proximal deep vein thromboses: anticoagulation with low-molecular-weight or unfractionated heparin; hospitalization
  - • Distal (calf) deep vein thrombosis: low-molecular-weight heparin and close outpatient follow-up
  - • Patients with contraindications to anticoagulation: inferior vena caval filters

- ■ Pearl

The superficial femoral vein is a deep vein and carries a high risk of embolization.

Reference

Heit JA: Current management of acute symptomatic deep vein thrombosis. Am J Cardiovasc Drugs 2001;1:45. [PMID: 14728051]

Mesenteric Ischemia

- ■ Essentials of Diagnosis
  - • Diffuse abdominal pain out of proportion to physical exam
  - • Gross gastrointestinal bleeding
  - • Postprandial abdominal pain
  - • Incidence increases with age
  - • Mesenteric angiography to confirm diagnosis
  - • Lactic acidosis is a late finding; associated with poorer outcomes
  - • Very high mortality; best outcomes occur with rapid diagnosis

- ■ Differential Diagnosis
  - • Acute abdomen
  - • Abdominal aortic aneurysm
  - • Kidney stone
  - • Myocardial infarction
  - • Cholecystitis
  - • Bowel obstruction
  - • Pancreatitis

- ■ Treatment
  - • Crystalloids for resuscitation from shock
  - • Broad-spectrum antibiotics to cover enteric organisms
  - • Analgesics for pain control
  - • Emergent surgical consult

- ■ Pearl

Have a high index of suspicion in elderly patients who present with severe abdominal pain and atrial fibrillation.

Reference

Burns BJ, Brandt LJ: Intestinal ischemia. Gastroenterol Clin North Am 2003;32:1127. [PMID: 14696300]

Thoracic Outlet Syndrome

- **Essentials of Diagnosis**
  - Signs and symptoms caused by compression of the neural, arterial, or venous structures at the thoracic outlet
  - Hand or arm fatigue with use, especially with abduction of the arm; cold intolerance or loss of dexterity
  - Elevated arm stress test (EAST) may elicit symptoms
  - Most common cause is compression of the C8 or T1 nerve roots against first rib
  - May have wasting of lateral muscles of hand and intrinsic hand muscles
  - Less commonly has arterial or venous cause
  - Diagnosis made clinically; rarely an emergency unless from vascular cause
  - Arterial cause suggested by decreased blood pressure in affected arm or with decreased pulses during EAST or severe pain
  - Venous cause may have associated congestion and swelling with normal pulses
  - Chest x-ray may show a cervical rib, an abnormal first rib or clavicle
  - Angiography: may be needed for evaluation of acute arterial occlusion or aneurysm
  - Ultrasound: may reveal venous cause or arterial aneurysm

- **Differential Diagnosis**
  - Acute coronary syndrome especially with left arm symptoms
  - Carpal tunnel syndrome
  - Cervical radiculopathy
  - Pancoast tumor
  - Ulnar nerve compression

- **Treatment**
  - If neurologic in origin may follow up with neurologist or thoracic surgeon
  - Patients with evidence of arterial or venous abnormality and stable symptoms: may follow up with vascular or thoracic surgeon
  - Venous thrombosis, arterial occlusion, or embolization: admission with immediate surgical consult and anticoagulation

- **Pearl**

Thoracic outlet syndrome with a neurologic cause is less likely to show improvement, whereas vascular causes usually respond well to therapy.

Reference

Mackinnon SE, Novack CB: Thoracic outlet syndrome. Curr Probl Surg 2002;39:1070. [PMID: 12407366]

Thrombophlebitis, Superficial

- ■ Essentials of Diagnosis
  - • No signs of deep vein thrombosis
  - • Tenderness, induration, and erythema along affected vein
  - • Septic thrombophlebitis: can occur after IV injection and at IV catheter sites

- ■ Differential Diagnosis
  - • Deep vein thrombosis
  - • Cellulitis
  - • Lymphangitis

- ■ Treatment
  - • Parenteral antibiotics for septic thrombophlebitis; incision and drainage possibly required
  - • Uncomplicated thrombosis: treat symptomatically with non-steroidal anti-inflammatory drugs, elevation, and elastic bandage at or above level of thrombosis

- ■ Pearl

Rule out septic thrombophlebitis and deep vein thrombosis in patients with superficial thrombophlebitis.

Reference

Decousus H et al: Superficial vein thrombosis: risk factors, diagnosis, and treatment. Curr Opin Pulm Med 2003;9:393. [PMID: 12904709]

8

Hematologic Emergencies

Autoimmune Hemolytic Anemia (AIHA)

- **Essentials of Diagnosis**
  - Presence of hemolysis, either intravascular or extravascular, with the detection of autoantibody on the patient's RBCs
  - Positive indirect Coombs test
  - Warm-type AIHA: IgG antibody directed against patient's own or transfused RBCs
  - Cold-type AIHA: IgM antibody directed; intravascular and extravascular (in the liver and spleen)
  - Often drug induced, especially from methyldopa, sulfa drugs, penicillins, and quinine
  - Routine laboratory findings consistent with anemia and hemolysis
  - Secondary causes: leukemia, systemic lupus, HIV, cancer

- **Differential Diagnosis**
  - Sickle cell anemia
  - Glucose-6-phosphate dehydrogenase (G6PD) deficiency
  - Thalassemia
  - Hereditary spherocytosis
  - Chemical-induced hemolytic anemia

- **Treatment**
  - Warm-type AIHA: prednisone, 1.0 mg/kg, and cytotoxic drugs such as azathioprine and cyclophosphamide
  - Warm- and cold-type AIHA: plasmapheresis
  - Cold avoidance
  - Treatment of underlying disease
  - Withdrawal of offending drugs

- **Pearl**

Be sure the patient does not have G6PD deficiency before starting therapy.

Reference

Gehrs BC, Friedberg RC: Autoimmune hemolytic anemia. Am J Hematol 2002;69:258. [PMID: 11921020]

Disseminated Intravascular Coagulation (DIC)

■ **Essentials of Diagnosis**

- Unexpected bleeding, either localized or profound
- Clinical evidence of thrombosis, though less severe than bleeding
- Occurring in a wide variety of settings: infection, malignancy, placental abruption, trauma, burns, snake envenomation, liver failure
- Thrombocytopenia; elevated PT, PTT, and fibrin degradation products (FDP)
- Elevated D-Dimer more specific than FDP
- Compensated minor abnormalities in patients with chronic DIC

■ **Differential Diagnosis**

- Hemolytic uremic syndrome
- Idiopathic thrombocytopenia purpura
- Thrombotic thrombocytopenia purpura

■ **Treatment**

- Treatment of underlying disease
- Supportive measures
- Consider replacement therapy for patients undergoing procedures or when bleeding is uncontrolled
- Heparin: only for those with predominating thrombotic features such as purpura fulminans

■ **Pearl**

Patient outcome depends on the underlying cause rather than the DIC; focus on stabilizing and treating the cause in the emergency department.

Reference

Levi M, Ten Cate H: Disseminated intravascular coagulation. N Engl J Med 1999;341:586. [PMID: 10451465]

Hemophilia

- **Essentials of Diagnosis**
  - Most common sites: hemarthrosis, intramuscular bleeding, gastrointestinal bleeding, genitourinary bleeding, and CNS bleeding
  - Classic hemophilia: deficiency of factor VIII (hemophilia A); Christmas disease: deficiency of factor IX (hemophilia B)
  - Types are clinically indistinguishable; diagnosis requires factor measurements
  - Sexed-linked recessive in both types; mild, moderate, and severe forms depending on amount of available clotting factor
  - Prothrombin time and partial thromboplastin time may be normal in mild forms
  - Severe: no factor activity; moderate: 2–5% of normal factor activity; mild >5% of normal

- **Differential Diagnosis**
  - Glanzmann thrombasthenia
  - Thrombocytopenia
  - Von Willebrand disease
  - Other factor deficiencies

- **Treatment**
  - Factor replacement
  - Mild factor VIII deficiency: may need only nasal desmopressin
  - Required factor VIII = kg $\times$ 0.5 $\times$ (% change factor needed)
  - Required factor IX = kg $\times$ 1.0 $\times$ (% change factor needed)
  - Aggressive workup and treatment of headache and head injury
  - Avoidance of invasive procedures and central lines
  - Patients with undiagnosed bleeding disorder: fresh frozen plasma

- **Pearl**

Most hemophilia patients have been administering their own treatment for years; listen to them.

Reference

Bolton-Maggs PH, Pasi KJ: Haemophilias A and B. Lancet 2003;361:1801. [PMID: 12781551]

Iron Deficiency Anemia

- **Essentials of Diagnosis**
    - Failure of the production of RBCs because of inadequate avail-ability of iron
    - Irritability and learning problems in children; pica, weakness, and fatigue in adults
    - Microcytic, hypochromic anemia
    - Thrombocytosis common (counts >450,000/ml)
    - Low serum iron and ferritin with an elevated total iron-binding capacity diagnostic of iron deficiency

- **Differential Diagnosis**
    - Lead poisoning
    - Thalassemia minor
    - Severe protein deficiency
    - Pyridoxine-responsive sideroblastic anemia

- **Treatment**
    - Exclusion of thalassemia minor and lead poisoning, depending on the area of the country
    - Elimination of chronic blood loss when possible
    - Ferrous sulfate dosed on reticulocyte response
    - Malabsorption or rapid blood loss: parenteral preparations and transfusions may be indicated

- **Pearl**

Always investigate the cause of the iron deficiency anemia to avoid a delayed or missed diagnosis of a cancer that is causing the anemia.

Reference

Leung AK, Chan KW: Iron deficiency anemia. Adv Pediatr 2001;48:385. [PMID: 11480764]

Immune (Idiopathic) Thrombocytopenia Purpura (ITP)

- **Essentials of Diagnosis**
  - Presence of purpura, or petechia; thrombocytopenia; and a normal bone marrow identify the disease
  - Autoantibodies are attached to platelets and thus removed by the reticuloendothelial system
  - Normal platelet function
  - May be preceded by infection
  - Anemia, hepatosplenomegaly, or evidence of hemolysis suggest another disease
  - Adults aged 20–50 years and children aged 2–4 years; 40% of all cases are in children

- **Differential Diagnosis**
  - Liver disease
  - Acute leukemia
  - Henoch-Schönlein purpura
  - Pregnancy
  - Drug-induced thrombocytopenia
  - Myelodysplastic syndrome
  - Megaloblastic anemia

- **Treatment**
  - Elimination of causes of bleeding such as procedure, drugs, and injury
  - No treatment for healthy patients with platelets >50,000/ml
  - Patients with known ITP: high-dose parenteral steroids, intravenous IgG, Rho immune globulin, and platelet transfusions may be considered if platelet count <20,000/ml, there is active bleeding, or patient has head injury
  - Patients with undiagnosed ITP: admission to rule out other causes

- **Pearl**

Inform all patients or their parents about the possible risks of severe spontaneous or traumatic bleeding, especially intracranial bleeding and its sequela.

Reference

Stasi R, Provan D: Management of immune thrombocytopenic purpura in adults. Mayo Clin Proc 2004;79:504. [PMID: 15065616]

Mononucleosis

■ Essentials of Diagnosis
- Ebstein-Barr virus infection characterized by fever, pharyngitis, adenopathy (posterior cervical), and atypical lymphocytes
- Rash develops if treated with penicillins
- Prolonged weakness may be seen in adolescents and adults
- May find splenomegaly
- Many patients do not seek treatment
- Monospot 85% sensitive
- May find elevated liver transaminases

■ Differential Diagnosis
- Streptococcal pharyngitis
- Toxoplasmosis
- Cytomegalovirus
- Rubella
- Viral hepatitis

■ Treatment
- Antibiotics not indicated
- Prednisone, 1 mg/kg/d for 5 days, indicated for associated hemolytic anemia, CNS involvement, or severe tonsillar enlargement
- Splenic rupture rare after 1 month of diagnosis; restrictions need not last longer

■ Pearl

The tonsillar enlargement associated with mononucleosis may lead to airway obstruction.

Reference

Godshall SE, Kirchner JT: Infectious mononucleosis. Complexities of a common syndrome. Postgrad Med 2000;107:175. [PMID: 10887454]

Multiple Myeloma

- **Essentials of Diagnosis**
  - Plasma cell cancer that comes in a variety of forms; all forms cause the production of monoclonal proteins
  - Presentation: bone pain (70%), pathologic fractures (90%), hypercalcemia, anemia, weakness, infection, and most acutely, spinal cord compression
  - Patients usually over age 60 years
  - Frequently diagnosed because of a large gap between total protein and albumin

- **Differential Diagnosis**
  - Other monoclonal gammopathies
  - Waldenström macroglobulinemia

- **Treatment**
  - Chemotherapy to reduce disease burden
  - Bisphosphonates for hypercalcemia
  - Spinal cord compression may require radiation
  - Fractures treated as indicated

- **Pearl**

Check albumen and protein in fracture workups in patients with a history of minimal injury.

Reference

George ED, Sadovsky R: Multiple myeloma: recognition and management. Am Fam Physician 1999;59:1885. [PMID: 10208707]

Sickle Cell Anemia: Acute Chest Syndrome

■ Essentials of Diagnosis

- Existing diagnosis of sickle cell anemia
- Presence of chest wall pain, tachypnea, and fever should raise suspicion; diagnosis by infiltrates and leukocytosis
- Bone infarction with secondary fat embolus likely pathophysiology

■ Differential Diagnosis

- Pneumonia
- Pulmonary embolism
- Asthma
- High-output heart failure
- Adult respiratory distress syndrome

■ Treatment

- Maintenance of oxygenation and ventilation
- Hydration and analgesics
- Coverage with broad-spectrum antibiotics (ceftriaxone or cefotaxime)

■ Pearl

Admit all patients with suspected acute chest syndrome; it is the leading cause of death in children with sickle cell disease.

Reference

Quinn CT, Buchanan GR: The acute chest syndrome of sickle cell disease. J Pediatr 1999;135:416. [PMID: 10518074]

Sickle Cell Anemia: Pain Crisis

- ■ Essentials of Diagnosis
  - • Painful crises, including musculoskeletal pain and hand-foot syndrome (dactylitis), reflect vaso-occlusive pathophysiology
  - • Acute pain in an extremity (bony or muscular), chest, or abdomen is common; neck and skull pain are rare
  - • Increased sickling of RBCs and evidence of hemolysis are frequent but not diagnostic
  - • Presence of swelling, other than in dactylitis, should raise suspicion of osteomyelitis
  - • Perception of pain is subjective; patients with sickle cell anemia should be given the benefit of the doubt when receiving treatment with opioids

- ■ Differential Diagnosis
  - • Cellulitis
  - • Fracture
  - • Osteomyelitis
  - • Acute abdomen
  - • Urinary tract infection

- ■ Treatment
  - • Hydration
  - • Limit use of nonsteroidal anti-inflammatory drugs due to risk of end-stage renal disease
  - • Opioid administration
  - • No proven benefit from oxygen
  - • Hydroxyurea stimulates hemoglobin F production and may be effective
  - • Transfusions as required

- ■ Pearl

Although opioid tolerance is common, true drug addiction does not occur in the sickle cell population.

Reference

Castro O: Management of sickle cell disease: recent advances and controversies. Br J Haematol 1999;107:2. [PMID: 10520020]

Sickle Cell Anemia: Aplastic Crisis

- ■ Essentials of Diagnosis
  - • Existing sickle cell anemia
  - • Profound anemia without evidence of increasing hemolysis
  - • Low or absent reticulocyte count
  - • Confirmation of parvovirus B19 infection, fifth disease
  - • No other viruses have specificity or efficacy of parvovirus B19 for sickle cell anemia patients or persons with other hemolytic anemias

- ■ Differential Diagnosis
  - • Splenic sequestration
  - • Bone marrow aplasia from other causes such as toxins or leukemia

- ■ Treatment
  - • Supportive care until bone marrow recovers
  - • Rare patients require immunoglobulin treatment
  - • Transfusion

- ■ Pearl

If you diagnose fifth disease, scour your department for potential contacts with hemolytic anemias who might be harmed.

Reference

Samuels-Reid JH: Common problems in sickle cell disease. Am Fam Physician 1994;49:1477. [PMID: 8172044]

Transfusion Reaction

■ Essentials of Diagnosis

- Occurrence within 24 hours of transfusion
- Minor symptoms: fever, chills, urticaria, and dyspnea resolving with minimal treatment
- Major symptoms: hemolysis and shock
- Distinguish between reaction and underlying disease
- Redraw blood if reaction occurs; confirm cause with blood bank
- Several types of reactions: acute hemolytic immune mediated, acute hemolytic nonimmune, febrile nonhemolytic, IgE allergic, anaphylaxis in IgA deficiency, passive antibody transfusion, volume overload, bacterial- or endotoxin-contaminated blood

■ Differential Diagnosis

- Drug reaction
- Sepsis
- Disseminated intravascular coagulation (DIC)
- Cardiogenic pulmonary edema
- Hemorrhagic shock

■ Treatment

- Acute hemolytic immune mediated: stop transfusion and prepare for impending shock, DIC, and renal failure; consider low-dose dopamine, hydration, and osmotic diuresis
- Acute hemolytic nonimmune: hydration until hemoglobinuria resolves
- Acetaminophen for fever
- Antihistamines for urticaria
- Volume overload: consider phlebotomy if diuresis not helpful
- Bacterial contamination: save blood and tubing for culture and treat with broad-spectrum antibiotics

■ Pearl

Blood transfusion is essentially organ transplantation and should never be done casually in the emergency department.

Reference

Capon SM, Goldfinger D: Acute hemolytic transfusion reaction, a paradigm of the systemic inflammatory response: new insights into pathophysiology and treatment. Transfusion 1995;35:513. [PMID: 7770905]

Thrombotic Thrombocytopenia Purpura (TTP)

- **Essentials of Diagnosis**
  - One or all of the following: thrombocytopenia, fever, renal failure, neurologic impairment, microangiopathic hemolysis
  - Physical exam: purpura, jaundice, hypertension or shock, altered mental status, splenomegaly
  - Risk factors: pregnancy, HIV infection, cancer, substance abuse, *Escherichia coli* infection

- **Differential Diagnosis**
  - Hemolytic uremic syndrome
  - Disseminated intravascular coagulation
  - Immune (idiopathic) thrombocytopenia purpura
  - Eclampsia
  - Stroke

- **Treatment**
  - Plasmapheresis
  - Fresh frozen plasma (30 ml/kg) may be helpful until plasmapheresis is done
  - Steroids have no benefit over plasmapheresis but invariably are given
  - No proven benefit from aspirin
  - Symptomatic treatment of shock, hypertension, and seizures

- **Pearl**

Platelet transfusions carry the risk of an abrupt decline in clinical condition and should be avoided.

Reference

Yarranton H, Machin SJ: An update on the pathogenesis and management of acquired thrombotic thrombocytopenic purpura. Curr Opin Neurol 2003; 16:367. [PMID: 12858075]

Von Willebrand Disease

- **Essentials of Diagnosis**
  - Bruising, gingival bleeding, prolonged bleeding, menorrhagia
  - Exacerbation with aspirin and improvement with oral contraceptives
  - Type I: 20–50% normal von Willebrand factor
  - Type II: abnormal function of von Willebrand factor
  - Type III: absent von Willebrand factor

- **Differential Diagnosis**
  - Hemophilia
  - Platelet dysfunction
  - Warfarin ingestion

- **Treatment**
  - Desmopressin (DDAVP), 0.3 µg/kg subcutaneously or IV every 12 hours for three or four doses for type I; increases circulating von Willebrand factor
  - Factor VIII concentrate has Von Willebrand factor and will treat type III
  - Type II may respond to DDAVP; factor VIII concentrate will likely be required
  - Hematologic consult needed to identify subtype of disease before specific therapy is given in newly diagnosed patient
  - Platelet transfusion and cryoprecipitate may be helpful in selected cases

- **Pearl**

Cryoprecipitate is effective in treating the bleeding in von Willebrand disease and could be used if factor VIII concentrates are not readily available.

Reference

Mannucci PM: How I treat patients with von Willebrand disease. Blood 2001;97:1915. [PMID: 11264151]

9

Infectious Disease Emergencies

Cellulitis

- **Essentials of Diagnosis**
  - Skin infection including the epidermis and dermis
  - Collective hallmarks: pain, tenderness, erythema
  - Warmth may be present, depending on size
  - Bacteremia and fever possible
  - Pruritus may occur but not a prominent feature

- **Differential Diagnosis**
  - Urticaria
  - Envenomation
  - Abscess
  - Viral exanthem
  - Fixed drug reaction

- **Treatment**
  - Treatment directed to *Streptococcus pyogenes* and *Staphylococcus aureus* (know local data for prevalence of methicillin-resistant *S aureus*)
  - Inpatient (diabetes, immunocompromised, evidence of bacteremia, significant head or neck cellulitis): nafcillin, 1–2 g IV) every 4 hours; or vancomycin, 1–1.5 g/d IV for 10–14 days
  - Outpatient: dicloxacillin, 250–500 mg orally every 6 hours; cephalexin, 500 mg orally every 6 hours; or amoxicillin-clavulanate, 875 mg–125 mg orally twice daily
  - Immunocompromised host: consider gram-negative bacteria and fungi

- **Pearl**

The more self-limited "spider bites" we treat with antibiotics, the more traps we will set for the future.

Reference

Schwartz R, Das-Young LR, Ramirez-Ronda C: Current and future management of serious skin and skin-structure infections. Am J Med 1996;100:90S. [PMID: 8678103]

Chancroid

- ■ **Essentials of Diagnosis**
  - • Ulcerative disease of the genitals
  - • Painful 1- to 2-cm ulcers with soft distortable borders
  - • Marked regional lymphadenopathy (a bubo) developing 1–2 weeks after ulcer
  - • Caused by *Haemophilus ducreyi*
  - • Mostly found in prostitutes, their clients, and intravenous drug abusers

- ■ **Differential Diagnosis**
  - • Syphilis
  - • Herpes simplex
  - • Lymphogranuloma venereum
  - • Abrasion with cellulitis

- ■ **Treatment**
  - • Azithromycin, 1 g orally once; ceftriaxone, 250 mg IM once; erythromycin, 500 mg orally four times daily for 1 week; or ciprofloxacin, 500 mg orally twice daily for 3 days
  - • Contemporaneous workup of and counseling for related sexually transmitted disease

- ■ **Pearl**

If the patient says, "This ain't my herpes," consider chancroid.

Reference

Martin DH, Mroczkowski TF: Dermatologic manifestations of sexually transmitted diseases other than HIV. Infect Dis Clin North Am 1994;8:533. [PMID: 7814834]

Chlamydia

- **Essentials of Diagnosis**
  - Genitourinary tract, respiratory tract, and ophthalmologic infections caused by *Chlamydia trachomatis* or *Chlamydia pneumonia*
  - Clinical signs of pelvic inflammatory disease or urethritis may accompany *C trachomatis* infection, the world's most common sexually transmitted disease
  - Conjunctivitis, rhinitis, and pneumonia possible in the newborn
  - Diagnosis by polymerase chain reaction (PCR) analysis of clinical specimen

- **Differential Diagnosis**
  - Gonorrhea
  - Trichomonas
  - Prostatitis
  - Influenza
  - Legionella
  - Mycoplasma
  - Tuberculosis

- **Treatment**
  - Doxycycline, 100 mg orally twice daily for 7 days
  - Azithromycin, 1 g orally once
  - Ofloxacin, 300 mg orally twice daily for 7 days

- **Pearl**

Current laboratory literature suggests that a urine specimen is sufficient in males for PCR analysis, thus banishing the transurethral swab to its rightful place, in the trash.

Reference

Hammerschlag MR: Chlamydia trachomatis and Chlamydia pneumoniae infections in children and adolescents. Pediatr Rev 2004;25:43. [PMID: 14754926]

Clostridial Myonecrosis

- ■ Essentials of Diagnosis
  - Also known as gas gangrene; occurs in three situations: post-trauma, postoperation, or spontaneous infection associated with cancer or depressed immunity
  - Anaerobic conditions in suspected area of infection capable of growing any of several *Clostridia* species
  - Rapid onset of a disproportionate amount of pain
  - Discoloration of the area from brown to dark blue
  - Frequently bulla formation with dishwater-like drainage
  - Sweet-musty odor to wound possible
  - Mental status changes possible
  - Gas formation seen by CT scan or x-ray to confirm diagnosis

- ■ Differential Diagnosis
  - Necrotizing fasciitis
  - Purpura fulminans
  - Nonclostridial myonecrosis from pyogenic organisms

- ■ Treatment
  - Mainstay of therapy: surgical debridement
  - Antibiotics: clindamycin, 900 mg IV every 8 hours, and peni-cillin G, 4 million units IV every 4 hours
  - Hyperbaric therapy presumed to be beneficial
  - Tetanus prophylaxis

- ■ Pearl

Early and aggressive surgical debridement of infected tissues is the key to management; antimicrobial therapy and hyperbaric therapy are secondary therapies.

Reference

Headley AJ: Necrotizing soft tissue infections: a primary care review. Am Fam Physician 2003;68:323. [PMID: 12892352]

Cryptococcal Meningitis

- **Essentials of Diagnosis**
  - Most often seen in patients with AIDS or other immunosuppressed states
  - Symptoms: headache, altered mental status, personality changes, confusion, lethargy, coma
  - Meningismus and fever may be absent
  - Lumbar puncture with a positive cryptococcal antigen or India ink test confirms diagnosis

- **Differential Diagnosis**
  - CNS tuberculosis
  - Bacterial meningitis
  - Cytomegalovirus
  - Neurosyphilis
  - AIDS dementia
  - CNS neoplasm
  - Stroke
  - Toxic or metabolic encephalopathy

- **Treatment**
  - Amphotericin B, 0.7–1 mg/kg/d IV, and flucytosine, 100 mg/kg/d orally
  - Involve infectious disease specialist early

- **Pearl**

The search for Cryptococcus *should be part of every diagnostic lumbar puncture.*

Reference

Apisarnthanarak A, Powderly WG: Treatment of acute cryptococcal disease. Expert Opin Pharmacother 2001;2:1259. [PMID: 11584993]

Disseminated Gonococcemia

- **Essentials of Diagnosis**

  - Subacute febrile illness followed by arthralgias, synovitis, and, in 25% of cases, frank purulent arthritis
  - Skin lesions: pustules on an erythematous base, usually on the extremities; palms, soles, and trunk usually spared
  - Gram-negative intracellular diplococci on Gram stain of mucous membranes excluding the throat may be diagnostic
  - Joint aspirate will have enough cellularity to confirm aseptic arthritis; cultures only 50% positive
  - Polymerase chain reaction identification slower but accurate
  - Meningitis and endocarditis also possible

- **Differential Diagnosis**

  - Arthritis and septic arthritis of other causes
  - Pityriasis rosea
  - Chlamydia

- **Treatment**

  - Ceftriaxone, 1–2 g IV every 12 hours; admission if patient has an arthritis or endocarditis
  - Evaluation for coexistent sexually transmitted disease
  - Debridement of joint not necessary

- **Pearl**

For any adolescent with an arthritis and no prior diagnosis, gonococcal infection should be at the top of the differential.

Reference

Ross JD: Systemic gonococcal infection. Genitourinary Medicine 1996;72:404. [PMID: 9038635]

Encephalitis

- **Essentials of Diagnosis**
  - Inflammation of the brain with neuropsychologic dysfunction that may be global or focal; may or may not include signs of meningitis
  - Two treatable acute causes: herpes simplex virus and varicella
  - Presenting complaints: fever, headache, and photophobia
  - May have cognitive deficits, seizures, movement disorder
  - CT scan findings may suggest encephalitis; MRI can be diagnostic in herpes encephalitis
  - Lumbar puncture findings: lymphocytic pleocytosis with a particularly high spinal fluid protein

- **Differential Diagnosis**
  - Meningitis
  - Subarachnoid hemorrhage
  - Leukemia
  - Rocky mountain spotted fever
  - Lyme disease
  - Brain abscess

- **Treatment**
  - Supportive measures; goal is to keep CNS pressures normal
  - Pending identification, initiate treatment with steroids for bacterial meningitis, and acyclovir, 10 mg/kg IV every 8 hours, for herpes and varicella

- **Pearl**

Initiation of acyclovir treatment is benign and should be started whenever herpetic encephalitis is suspected.

Reference

Roos KL: Encephalitis. Neurol Clin 1999;17:813. [PMID: 10517930]

Erysipelas

- **Essentials of Diagnosis**
  - Most commonly caused by *Streptococcus pyogenes* but *Staphylococcus aureus* possible
  - Febrile illness followed by onset of a rash that is well demarcated and indurated
  - Rash is tender to touch
  - Only dermis and lymphatics are involved; streaking may be present
  - Extremities and face are most commonly involved
  - Involved area most likely will have had preexisting surgery or trauma

- **Differential Diagnosis**
  - Cellulitis
  - Necrotizing fasciitis
  - Angioedema
  - Urticaria

- **Treatment**
  - Patients without diabetes or facial involvement: penicillin G, 1–2 million units IV every 6 hours
  - Patients with diabetes or facial involvement: nafcillin, 2 g IV every 4 hours, or vancomycin, 1 g IV every 12 hours
  - Symptomatic treatment for fever and volume depletion

- **Pearl**

Tenderness may be absent in the diabetic patient with neuropathy.

Reference

Bonnetblanc JM, Bedane C: Erysipelas: recognition and management. Am J Clin Dermatol 2003;4:157. [PMID: 12627991]

Genital Herpes

- **Essentials of Diagnosis**
  - Usually caused by herpes simplex type 2 virus; herpes simplex virus type 1 infection possible
  - Painful vesicular or ulcerated lesions that occur in, on, or about the genitalia or distribution of sacral nerve
  - Outbreak may occur 2 days to 2 weeks after exposure
  - Infection may be spread by asymptomatic carriers
  - Primary infection may last 3 weeks
  - Culture is positive in 85% of untreated lesions less than 48 hours old
  - Tzanck smear is positive in 50% of lesions
  - Diagnosis usually by clinical appearance

- **Differential Diagnosis**
  - Syphilis
  - Herpes zoster
  - Folliculitis

- **Treatment**
  - Oral treatment for primary infection: acyclovir, 200 mg orally 5 times a day for 10 days; valacyclovir, 1,000 mg orally twice daily for 7–10 days; or famciclovir, 250 mg orally three times daily for 7–10 days
  - Oral treatment for recurrent infection: acyclovir, 200 mg orally 5 times a day for 5 days; valacyclovir, 500 mg orally twice daily for 3 days; or famciclovir, 125 mg orally twice daily for 5 days
  - Topical antiviral agents not helpful

- **Pearl**

If it hurts, it's herpes.

Reference

Waggoner-Fountain LA, Grossman LB: Herpes simplex virus. Pediatr Rev 2004;25:86. [PMID: 14993516]

Gonorrhea

- **Essentials of Diagnosis**
  - Common sexually transmitted disease causing urethritis, vaginitis, cervicitis, proctitis, conjunctivitis, pharyngitis, endocarditis, and meningitis
  - May be asymptomatic
  - Exposure may produce disease in 2–7 days
  - Diagnosis by gram-negative intracellular diplococci on smear, positive culture, or polymerase chain reaction (PCR)
  - PCR on urine is promising as replacement for urethral swabs

- **Differential Diagnosis**
  - Chlamydia
  - Meningococcemia
  - Disseminated gonococcemia
  - Other bacterial conjunctivitis

- **Treatment**
  - Ceftriaxone, 125 mg IM once; ciprofloxacin, 500 mg orally once; or cefixime, 400 mg orally once
  - Consider treatment for chlamydia, syphilis, and HIV

- **Pearl**

The exudates of gonococcal conjunctivitis will reaccumulate in the time it takes to take off exam gloves.

Reference

Tapsall J: Current concepts in the management of gonorrhoeae. Expert Opin Pharmacother 2002;3:147. [PMID: 11829728]

Infective Endocarditis

- **Essentials of Diagnosis**
  - Multifaceted infection of the endocardium and valves, including prosthetic valves
  - Fever is most common symptom but is intermittent
  - Neurologic symptoms present in 40% of cases
  - Heart murmurs or changed murmurs in 90% of cases
  - Petechiae, splinter hemorrhages, Janeway lesions, Osler nodes, and Roth spots possible
  - Suspect in the presence of prior rheumatic fever, congenital heart disease, valvular implantation, or intravenous drug abuse
  - Diagnosis by positive blood cultures or echocardiography; made in the emergency department only rarely

- **Differential Diagnosis**
  - Fever of unknown origin
  - Rheumatologic disease
  - Lung abscess from other causes
  - Stroke
  - Brain abscess

- **Treatment**
  - Prompt admission based on suspected diagnosis
  - Stabilization of systemic abnormalities
  - Cardiology and infectious disease consults
  - Antibiotic therapy, after blood cultures, depending on type of predisposing risks for endocarditis, such as intravenous drug abuse or rheumatic heart disease

- **Pearl**

Consider antibiotic prophylaxis against endocarditis before draining the "shooter's abscess."

Reference

Bayer AS et al: Diagnosis and management of infective endocarditis and its complications. Circulation 1998;98:2936. [PMID: 9860802]

Lyme Disease

- ■ Essentials of Diagnosis
  - Tick-borne spirochetal (*Borrelia burgdorferi*) disease found throughout the United States but most prevalent in the northeast and midwest
  - Stage I: begins 3 days to a month after a tick bite; rash characterized by a nontender migrating erythematous border with central clearing (erythema migrans)
  - Stage II: dissemination of the spirochete, causing multisystemic symptoms such as fever, splenomegaly, lymphadenopathy, myalgias, arthralgias
  - About 15% of stage II patients will progress to more severe manifestations: meningitis, cardiac involvement, peripheral neuropathies (most commonly facial nerve palsy)
  - Stage III: chronic persistent infection that occurs years after primary infection; manifested by chronic arthritis, myocarditis, central and peripheral neurologic abnormalities
  - Serologic diagnosis unreliable

- ■ Differential Diagnosis
  - Arthritis of all types
  - Bacterial meningitis
  - Pericarditis
  - Infectious mononucleosis
  - Rocky mountain spotted fever
  - Atherosclerotic cardiovascular disease

- ■ Treatment
  - Stage I or II: doxycycline, 100 mg orally for 10–21 days or as long as symptoms persist; amoxicillin for children under age 12 years
  - CNS involvement, serious cardiac involvement: ceftriaxone, 1 g IV every 12 hours for 21 days; or penicillin G, 20 million units/d IV for 21 days
  - Stage III: often unresponsive to aggressive antibiotic therapy

- ■ Pearl

It is easier to treat Lyme disease or the fear of Lyme disease than it is to confirm the diagnosis.

Reference

Edlow JA: Lyme disease and related tick-borne illnesses. Ann Emerg Med 1999;33:680. [PMID: 10339684]

Meningitis

- ■ Essentials of Diagnosis
  - • Inflammation of the meninges from one or multiple infectious organisms
  - • Characterized by fever, headache, altered mental status, nuchal rigidity, and a spinal fluid pleocytosis
  - • Lumbar puncture: confirms clinical diagnosis
  - • Empiric treatment needed immediately if lumbar puncture is contraindicated or delayed
  - • Contraindications to lumbar puncture: shock, focal neurologic findings, evidence of very high intracranial pressure

- ■ Differential Diagnosis
  - • Stroke
  - • Subarachnoid hemorrhage
  - • Brain abscess
  - • Toxic encephalopathy
  - • CNS vasculitis

- ■ Treatment
  - • Antimicrobial treatment based on age and likely organism
  - • Empiric therapy of bacterial meningitis: <1 month of age, ampicillin and cefotaxime, 50 mg/kg each, given in emergency department; >1 month of age, vancomycin (15 mg/kg) and either cefotaxime (75mg/kg) or ceftriaxone (50 mg/kg), given in emergency department; age 18–50 years, ceftriaxone, 2 g IV every 12 hours, and vancomycin, 1–1.5 g IV q 12 hours; over age 50, ceftriaxone, 2 g IV every 12 hours and vancomycin, 1–1.5 g IV every 12 hours; add ampicillin, 2 g IV every 4 hours, to cover *Listeria monocytogenes*
  - • Suspected cases of pneumococcal meningitis: dexamethasone prior to antibiotics provided that antibiotics are not being delayed for results of tests; children, 0.15 mg/kg; adults, 10 mg IV

- ■ Pearl

Never delay the administration of antibiotics if the completion of a lumbar puncture will be delayed.

Reference

Saez-Llorens X, McCracken GH Jr: Antimicrobial and anti-inflammatory treatment of bacterial meningitis. Infect Dis Clin North Am 1999;13:619. [PMID: 10470558]

Meningococcemia

- **Essentials of Diagnosis**
  - Acute febrile illness characterized by fever, shock, and a petechial rash (85%)
  - Severe headache, fever, nausea, vomiting, mental status changes possible
  - Meningitis may be present
  - Confirmed by blood, nasopharyngeal culture, or polymerase chain reaction in spinal fluid or urine
  - Patients with meningitis present sooner

- **Differential Diagnosis**
  - Other forms of sepsis with purpura fulminans
  - Thrombotic thrombocytopenia purpura
  - Rocky mountain spotted fever
  - Immune thrombocytopenia purpura
  - Leukemia
  - Henoch-Schönlein purpura

- **Treatment**
  - Ceftriaxone, 2 g IV, and vancomycin, 1 g IV, in emergency department
  - Remainder of treatment directed to supportive care
  - Prophylaxis of close contacts with ciprofloxacin or rifampin recommended

- **Pearl**

Meningococcemia patients without meningitis have a higher mortality rate than those with meningitis.

Reference

Kirsch EA, Barton RP, Kitchen L: Pathophysiology, treatment and outcome of meningococcemia: a review and recent experience. Pediatr Infect Dis J 1996;15:967. [PMID: 8933544]

Necrotizing Fasciitis

- ■ Essentials of Diagnosis
  - Infection of the deep fascia with rapid necrosis of subcutaneous tissue
  - Mostly occurs in mildly immunocompromised individuals such as diabetics
  - Mixed infection of gram-negative and gram-positive organisms that frequently results in gas production
  - *Streptococcus pyogenes* has notoriety but alone causes few cases
  - Occurs at a portal of entry such as trauma or surgery but may have no source such as seen in Fournier gangrene, a type of necrotizing fasciitis
  - Rapidly spreading area of poorly demarcated erythema that develops a necrotic area at the origin
  - Patient may be toxic appearing but not necessarily septic

- ■ Differential Diagnosis
  - Cellulitis
  - Toxic shock syndrome
  - Other causes of gas gangrene

- ■ Treatment
  - Supportive care with aggressive fluid resuscitation
  - Prompt surgical consult
  - Consider hyperbaric therapy
  - Antibiotic therapy should not forestall surgical debridement
  - Penicillin G, 4 million units every 4 hours, plus clindamycin, 900 mg IV every 8 hours

- ■ Pearl

Necrotizing fasciitis caused by group A streptococci does not cause gas formation and does not respond well to hyperbaric therapy.

Reference

Jallali N: Necrotising fasciitis: its aetiology, diagnosis and management. J Wound Care 2003;12:297. [PMID: 14533236]

Osteomyelitis

- ■ Essentials of Diagnosis
  - Acute or chronic infection of bone from direct invasion of microorganisms or by hematogenous seeding
  - Fever, malaise, and pain over the site of infection in acute or chronic osteomyelitis
  - Diabetic neuropathy may blunt pain
  - X-rays may be normal for 2 weeks
  - Elevation of erythrocyte sedimentation rate or C-reactive protein is common but not diagnostic
  - Bone scan or MRI may aid in diagnosis
  - Diagnosis by biopsy and culture of infected bone

- ■ Differential Diagnosis
  - Cellulitis
  - Gout
  - Toxic synovitis
  - Congenital bone cyst
  - Discitis
  - Metastatic disease of the spine

- ■ Treatment
  - Accurate culture is critical: treatment initiation is urgent, and antibiotics usually sustained for 6–8 weeks
  - Consultation to obtain biopsy if diagnosis is suspected
  - Empiric treatment against *Staphylococcus aureus,* with additional coverage depending on clinical situation (eg, age, comorbidity, culture result)
  - Surgical debridement frequently necessary

- ■ Pearl

Osteomyelitis from direct inoculation may be prevented by proper techniques of wound management and consideration of the use of prophylactic antibiotic when the acute injury is treated.

Reference

Bamberger DM: Diagnosis and treatment of osteomyelitis. Compr Ther 2000;26:89. [PMID: 10822787]

Pneumocystis Pneumonia

- **Essentials of Diagnosis**
  - Cough, fever, dyspnea, and tachypnea in the presence of an immunocompromised state of T-cell deficiency
  - May have no or only minor ausculatory findings
  - Patients with HIV tend to be less toxic appearing
  - Diagnosis suggested by elevated LDH, chest x-ray with perihilar interstitial infiltrates, and hypoxemia
  - Sputum for direct fluorescent antibody may be positive

- **Differential Diagnosis**
  - Cytomegalovirus
  - *Legionella*
  - Tuberculosis
  - Other pneumonia
  - Pulmonary embolism

- **Treatment**
  - Trimethoprim-sulfamethoxazole (TMP-SMZ), 5 mg/kg TMP IV every 8 hours; or clindamycin, 600 mg IV every 8 hours, plus primaquine 15 mg/d orally
  - Prednisone, 40 mg twice daily, added to above regimens

- **Pearl**

HIV patients with cough and more hypoxemia than clinically suspected have pneumocystis until proved otherwise.

Reference

Levine S: Pneumocystis carinii. Clin Chest Med 1996;17:665. [PMID: 9016371]

Rocky Mountain Spotted Fever

- ■ Essentials of Diagnosis
  - • Caused by *Rickettsia rickettsii*
  - • Fever, arthralgias, headache followed by a rash that appears first on the wrist and ankles and then spreads to the extremities and trunk; face is generally spared
  - • Rash may involve palms and soles
  - • History of tick exposure or risk for tick exposure
  - • Serologic testing or direct biopsy of skin lesions confirms diagnosis

- ■ Differential Diagnosis
  - • Enterovirus
  - • Meningococcemia
  - • Infectious mononucleosis
  - • Lyme disease
  - • Syphilis
  - • Thrombotic thrombocytopenia purpura
  - • Henoch-Schönlein purpura
  - • Measles
  - • Toxic shock syndrome

- ■ Treatment
  - • Doxycycline, 100 mg orally or IV twice daily; or chloramphenicol, 100 mg/kg/d divided every 6 hours
  - • Initiation of treatment as soon as diagnosis is suspected
  - • Hospitalization of patients with significant systemic symptoms; intravenous antibiotics with supportive care

- ■ Pearl

The occurrence of an acute febrile illness with tick exposure may be sufficient to start treatment.

Reference

Thorner AR, Walker DH, Petri WA Jr: Rocky mountain spotted fever. Clin Infect Dis 1998;27:1353. [PMID: 9868640]

Syphilis

- ■ Essentials of Diagnosis
  - • Caused by *Treponema pallidum*
  - • Disease occurs in three stages
  - • Primary stage: typified by a painless chancre at the site of inoculation that heals in 3–6 weeks
  - • Secondary stage: begins weeks after resolution of the chancre; characterized by a nonpruritic rash that starts on the torso and then spreads to extremities and involves the palms and soles, lymphadenopathy, fever, and malaise
  - • Tertiary syphilis: develops 3–10 years after the primary infection with typical gumma lesions and neurologic involvement
  - • Positive serologic test for syphilis: VDRL, RPR, or FTA-ABS

- ■ Differential Diagnosis
  - • Chancroid
  - • Drug reaction
  - • Rubella
  - • Tinea

- ■ Treatment
  - • Benzathine penicillin G, 2.4 million units IM once
  - • Skin test documentation of penicillin allergy recommended before selecting alternative antibiotic such as doxycycline, 100 mg orally twice daily for 14 days, or erythromycin, 500 mg orally four times daily for 14 days

- ■ Pearl

Consider congenital syphilis in immigrant infants younger than 2 months old with profuse rhinorrhea.

Reference

Garnett GP et al: The natural history of syphilis. Implications for the transmission dynamics and control of infection. Sex Transm Dis 1997;24:185. [PMID: 9101629]

Toxic Shock Syndrome

- **Essentials of Diagnosis**
  - Syndrome of high fever, diffuse rash, hypotension, and multi-organ involvement
  - May be seen most commonly with *Staphylococcus aureus* but similar syndrome occurs with *Streptococcus pyogenes*
  - If these symptoms occur with three organs involved, diagnosis can be made after considering alternatives

- **Differential Diagnosis**
  - Rocky mountain spotted fever
  - Leptospirosis
  - Measles
  - Hepatitis B
  - Syphilis
  - Ebstein-Barr virus
  - Kawasaki disease
  - Toxic epidermal necrolysis
  - Staphylococcal scalded skin syndrome

- **Treatment**
  - Fluid resuscitation
  - Removal of tampon or offending packing or dressing
  - Dopamine may be necessary for hypotension not responsive to aggressive fluid resuscitation
  - Initiation of antibiotic therapy directed against *S aureus:* nafcillin, 2 g IV every 4 hours; cefazolin, 2 g IV every 6 hours; vancomycin, 1.5 g IV every 12 hours; or clindamycin, 600 mg IV every 8 hours
  - ICU admission

- **Pearl**

Consider toxic shock syndrome in young adult patients who have a cast and a wound underneath.

Reference

Stevens DL: The toxic shock syndromes. Infect Dis Clin North Am 1996;10:727. [PMID: 8958166]

Trichomoniasis

- **Essentials of Diagnosis**
  - Caused by the protozoan parasite *Trichomonas vaginalis*
  - Yellow-green vaginal discharge, odor, vaginal pain or itching
  - Associated abdominal pain possible
  - Infection likely asymptomatic in men
  - Nonvenereal transmission is rare but occurs
  - Diagnosis by trichomonads seen in urine or wet prep specimens

- **Differential Diagnosis**
  - Gonorrhea
  - Chlamydia
  - Pelvic inflammatory disease
  - Prostatitis

- **Treatment**
  - Most effective therapy: metronidazole, 2 g orally once
  - Treat patient's sexual partner(s)

- **Pearl**

Metronidazole gel is not nearly as effective as the oral formulation in achieving a cure; the gel has up to a 50% failure rate.

Reference

Schwebke JR: Update of trichomoniasis. Sex Transm Infect 2002;78:378. [PMID: 12407245]

10

Metabolic & Endocrine Emergencies

Adrenal Insufficiency, Acute

- **Essentials of Diagnosis**
  - History of abrupt discontinuation of chronic glucocorticoid administration (moon facies, buffalo hump)
  - Hypotension (particularly refractory to fluids), hypoglycemia, orthostasis, severe weakness, weight loss, anorexia, lethargy, abdominal cramps, nausea, vomiting, diarrhea, mental depression, and, if chronic, skin hyperpigmentation changes
  - Patients with sepsis who have rapid or unexplained deterioration
  - Altered mental status ranging from lethargy to obtundation and coma
  - Manifestations of a hypothalamic or pituitary tumor (including headache, bitemporal visual field defects, or enlargement of the sella turcica) in patients with hypothalamic or pituitary disorders
  - CBC, electrolytes (classically hyponatremia and hyperkalemia occur together with mineralocorticoid deficiency), glucose level, renal and hepatic function test; consider cultures of blood, urine, and cerebrospinal fluid; serum cortisol; perform an ACTH (Cortrosyn) stimulation test

- **Differential Diagnosis**
  - Sepsis and other causes of shock

- **Treatment**
  - Careful attention to ABCs; ICU admission indicated in all cases
  - Intravenous fluid (0.9% normal saline) administration to correct hypovolemia and hypotension
  - Rapid administration of dexamethasone, 4 mg IV (do not delay treatment while awaiting diagnostic studies)
  - Consider antibiotics if fever present

- **Pearl**

Initially treat acute adrenal insufficiency with dexamethasone instead of hydrocortisone because dexamethasone will not affect cortisol levels and therefore can be used while a Cortrosyn stimulation test is being conducted.

Reference

Zolga GP, Marik P: Hypothalamic-pituitary-adrenal insufficiency. Crit Care Clin 2001;17:25. [PMID: 11219233]

Central Diabetes Insipidus

■ Essentials of Diagnosis

- Multiple causes: head trauma, neurosurgery, tumors, infections, and CNS catastrophes
- Lethargy, altered mental status, irritability, hyperreflexia, and spasticity related to antidiuretic hormone deficiency
- Profound polydipsia and polyuria (sometimes 45 mL/kg/d), which may lead to nocturia, incontinence, or enuresis
- Urine osmolarity <150 mOsm/kg in the setting of serum hypertonicity and polyuria is generally diagnostic of diabetes insipidus
- Hypernatremia with serum sodium >160 mEq/L can occur in severe cases
- Trial of desmopressin will differentiate central versus nephrogenic diabetes insipidus (DI)
- CT and MRI of the brain are indicated
- Renal and thyroid function tests, serum calcium, glucose, cortisol, antidiuretic hormone, and osmolality studies; measure urine osmolality and specific gravity

■ Differential Diagnosis

- Severe dehydration with associated hypernatremia although urine will be concentrated
- Nephrogenic DI

■ Treatment

- Administer fluids by oral, nasogastric, or intravenous (0.45% normal saline or 5% dextrose in water) routes for rehydration
- Calculate the free water deficit (FWD): FWD = 0.6 × premorbid body weight in kg × (1 − [140/plasma sodium in mmol/L])
- Replace half the deficit in the first 12–24 hours; when serum sodium <150 mEq/L, use 0.45% or 0.9% saline
- Desmopressin is the drug of choice for central DI
- Hospitalization for definitive diagnosis and initiation of therapy
- Patients with severe hypernatremia or symptoms: admission to ICU advised

■ Pearl

Be careful not to reduce the serum sodium more than 1 mEq/L/h to avoid inducing cerebral edema.

Reference

Singer I, James OR, Fishman LM: The management of diabetes insipidus in adults. Arch Intern Med 1997;157:1293. [PMID: 9201003]

Hyperglycemia without Ketosis

- **Essentials of Diagnosis**
  - Common symptoms: polydipsia, polyuria, weakness, fatigue, blurred vision, headache, lightheadedness, frequent recurrent infections, varying degrees of dehydration
  - Risk factors: age > 45 years, obesity, family history of first-degree relative, sedentary lifestyle, most non-Caucasian ethnic groups, gestational diabetes, polycystic ovarian syndrome, hypertension, dyslipidemia, or vascular disease
  - Random plasma glucose >200 mg/dL in the setting of symptoms of hyperglycemia or fasting plasma glucose >126 mg/dL on repeat occasions is suggestive of diabetes
  - Patients with plasma glucose ≥400 mg/dL: carefully consider impending metabolic decompensation and look for precipitating stressors such as infections or cardiac ischemia
  - Electrolytes, BUN, and creatinine to assess metabolic status

- **Differential Diagnosis**
  - Early DKA or hyperglycemic hyperosmolar nonketotic syndrome

- **Treatment**
  - If hyperglycemia is mild (<300 mg/dL), patient is well hydrated, no specific cause is identified, and medical follow-up is readily available, no specific treatment is required other than referral to primary care for diabetes testing
  - If blood glucose >300 mg/dL, consider intravenous fluids; insulin (lispro, Humalog, or insulin aspart, NovoLog), 0.1 unit/kg subcutaneously, can be administered to mildly dehydrated patients; for moderately to severely dehydrated patients, use intravenous regular insulin
  - Treatment of underlying infections
  - Hyperglycemia with serious underlying causes or resistant to treatment: hospitalization for further work-up and treatment

- **Pearl**

The "1500 rule" can be used for adults to estimate the dosage of regular insulin required to lower the blood glucose to a desirable level. For example, if a patient takes a total of 100 units of insulin per day, the blood sugar will be lowered by 1,500/100 or 15 mg/dL for every unit of insulin administered.

Reference

Report of the Expert Committee on the Diagnosis and Classification of Diabetes Mellitus. Diabetes Care 2003;26(Suppl. 1):S5. [PMID: 12502614]

Hyperglycemic Hyperosmolar Nonketotic Syndrome (HHNS)

- ■ Essentials of Diagnosis
  - • Most symptoms relate to severe dehydration
  - • Polyuria, polydipsia, polyphagia, weakness, altered mental status (confusion to lethargy or coma)
  - • Unlike in diabetic ketoacidosis (DKA), Kussmaul respirations and abdominal pain are unusual findings in HHNS
  - • Usually no acidosis (pH ≥7.3 and serum bicarbonate >15), small or absent serum ketones, hyperglycemia usually ≥600 mg/dL, and serum osmolarity ≥320 mOsm/kg
  - • Hyponatremia may be related to osmotic shifts; correct for these shifts by adding 1.8 mg/dL sodium for every 100 mg/dL of glucose above normal
  - • Risk factors: age >65, resident of long-term care facility, dementia, recent change in medication or addition such as steroids, recent or current infection; another precipitating factor to consider is myocardial ischemia

- ■ Differential Diagnosis
  - • Uncontrolled hyperglycemia without severe dehydration or metabolic decompensation
  - • DKA

- ■ Treatment
  - • Careful attention to ABCs
  - • Continuous cardiac monitoring and frequent reassessment of vital signs
  - • Intravenous fluid resuscitation (initial bolus of 0.9% normal saline) and insulin drip (0.1 units/kg/h)
  - • Frequent monitoring of electrolytes and serum osmolarity, being careful not to drop the serum osmolarity >3 mOsm/kg/h
  - • Admission to an ICU or intermediate care area (with continuous cardiac monitoring) for at least 24 hours for patients with all but the mildest cases of HHNS

- ■ Pearl

In contrast to DKA, HHNS is more likely to occur in elderly, obese type II diabetics and can develop more slowly, over days to weeks.

Reference

Kitabchi AE et al: Management of hyperglycemic crises in patients with diabetes mellitus. Diabetes Care 2001;24:131. [PMID: 11194218]

Hypoglycemia

- **Essentials of Diagnosis**
  - Irritability, diaphoresis, and tachycardia related to increased circulating catecholamines and hypothermia
  - Severe hypoglycemia: neuroglycopenic effects include focal neurologic deficits such as diplopia, paresthesias, seizures, lethargy, or coma
  - Children are particularly susceptible to hypoglycemia
  - Consider precipitating factors: infection, myocardial infarction, stroke, alcohol use, pregnancy, drug use, occult trauma, depression (poor caloric intake or insulin or oral agent overdose), other endocrinopathies (Addison disease, myxedema, thyrotoxicosis, pituitary insufficiency)

- **Differential Diagnosis**
  - Other causes of mental status changes or adrenergic response in diabetics (stroke, myocardial infarction)

- **Treatment**
  - Severe hypoglycemia: administer intravenous 50% dextrose in water (50 cc = approximately 25 g of glucose, which is enough to resolve most hypoglycemic episodes); give thiamine, 100 mg IV or IM, to alcoholic patients prior to administration of glucose to prevent Wernicke encephalopathy
  - Recheck fingerstick glucose every 30 minutes, bolus with intravenous 50% dextrose as needed
  - If intravenous access not readily available, 1 mg IM glucagon
  - Admission for patients with persistent or recurrent hypoglycemia despite appropriate therapy, hypoglycemia in patients taking oral agent or long-acting insulin, related serious ancillary cause (eg, severe infection, persistent nausea and vomiting)
  - Discharge is appropriate if a responsible adult is with patient for 8–12 hours, patient is able to take oral fluids and food, medical follow-up is available within 24–48 hours, and patient has ability and understanding to perform blood glucose checks, especially if changes are made in therapeutic regimen

- **Pearl**

Check the fingerstick blood glucose measurement on every patient presenting with altered mental status or who appears acutely ill.

Reference

McAulay V, Deary IJ, Frier BM: Symptoms of hypoglycaemia in people with diabetes. Diabet Med 2001;18:690. [PMID: 11606166]

Inappropriate Secretion of Antidiuretic Hormone (SIADH)

- **Essentials of Diagnosis**
  - Syndrome with multiple causes including CNS disorders, medication side effects, neoplasms, and pulmonary disorders in which excess antidiuretic hormone acts on the kidney to resorb free water
  - Anorexia, nausea, vomiting, personality changes, depressed tendon reflexes, and muscle weakness; severe cases: coma, seizures, delirium, cranial nerve palsies, hypothermia, and altered patterns of respiration (Cheyne Stokes) may be evident
  - Classic feature: hyponatremia; other findings: reduced plasma osmolality, persistent urinary secretion of sodium (>20 mEq/L), and inappropriately high urine osmolality
  - Lab studies for serum sodium and other electrolytes, creatinine, BUN, osmolality, cortisol levels, and thyroid function studies (TSH and free T_4), send urine for urinalysis and measurement of urinary osmolality, electrolytes, and specific gravity

- **Differential Diagnosis**
  - Water intoxication from psychogenic polydipsia or children given inappropriately large amounts of free water

- **Treatment**
  - Degree of hyponatremia and patient symptomatology determine the treatment
  - Severe (serum sodium <105 mEq/L or at any level if the patient develops neurologic complications such as coma or seizures): administer hypertonic saline 3% solution at 1–2 mL/kg/h for the first 3–4 hours; furosemide, 1 mg/kg IV, may be used to counteract volume overload; monitor sodium and potassium every 1–2 hours and adjust fluids or replace as needed; correction should average 0.5–2.0 mEq/L/h and no more than 12 mEq/L in the first 24 hours to a serum sodium level of 125 mEq/L or resolution of CNS involvement; treatment in ICU
  - Moderate hyponatremia: admission
  - Asymptomatic, mild hyponatremia: outpatient treatment with fluid restriction and close follow-up

- **Pearl**

Correction of the serum sodium at too rapid a rate can increase the risk for central pontine myelinolysis. Symptoms of tetraparesis and bulbar palsy are seen.

Reference

Miller M: Syndromes of excess antidiuretic hormone release. Crit Care Clin 2001;17:11. [PMID: 11219224]

Ketoacidosis, Alcoholic (AKA)

- ■ Essentials of Diagnosis
  - Usually associated with recent or ongoing alcohol binge with poor food intake; nausea, vomiting, and abdominal pain
  - Clinical findings: tachypnea (Kussmaul respirations are common), tachycardia, abdominal tenderness, poor skin turgor, delayed capillary refill
  - Metabolic acidosis: low pH (often <7.2) and low serum bicarbonate are common
  - Check serum for ketones
  - Electrolyte disorders: hyponatremia, hyperkalemia, hypokalemia, hypophosphatemia, hypomagnesemia, and hypocalcemia frequently occur with AKA
  - Glucose: ranges from hypoglycemia to moderately elevated (up to 250 mg/dL) in the absence of diabetes
  - Alcohol levels: may not be elevated by time of presentation as patient may not have been able to maintain oral intake of even alcohol for some time; be alert for signs and symptoms of alcohol withdrawal or delirium tremens

- ■ Differential Diagnosis
  - Diabetic ketoacidosis
  - Lactic acidosis
  - Toxic alcohol ingestion

- ■ Treatment
  - Glucose: After giving thiamine, 100 mg IV or IM, give 5% dextrose solution in 0.9% normal saline at rate of 1 L/h for the first 1–2 hours; 5% dextrose in 0.45% normal saline is then appropriate at 250 cc/h
  - Correct significant electrolyte imbalances
  - Metabolic problems tend to correct reasonably rapidly with intravenous fluids and glucose administration, but most AKA patients are extremely unreliable and would have difficulty complying with outpatient treatment and follow-up
  - Alcohol withdrawal may complicate course as patient improves; hospitalization for observation is prudent for patients with AKA

- ■ Pearl

Most of the ketone bodies produced in AKA are β-hydroxybutyrate, which does not show up on standard tests for ketones in serum or urine. A negative initial ketone test does not rule out AKA.

Reference

Adrogue HJ, Madias NE: Management of life-threatening acid-base disorders. N Engl J Med 1998;338:26. [PMID: 9414329]

Ketoacidosis, Diabetic (DKA)

- ■ Essentials of Diagnosis
  - Fatigue, weakness, tachypnea (Kussmaul respiration), tachycardia, altered mental status, abdominal pain (related to degree of acidosis), vomiting, polyuria and polydipsia, fruity or acetone-like breath
  - High anion gap metabolic acidosis with arterial pH <7.3
  - Serum glucose ≥250 mg/dL and serum bicarbonate ≤15 mEq/L
  - Look for precipitating stressors such as occult infection or myocardial infarction, noncompliance with insulin therapy
  - Electrocardiogram for all adults with DKA, to look for myocardial ischemia or severe hyperkalemia
  - Ketonemia is unreliable unless β-hydroxybutyrate is measured

- ■ Differential Diagnosis
  - Other causes of metabolic acidosis
  - An acute abdominal catastrophe in a diabetic (cholangitis, perforated peptic ulcer, severe pancreatitis, ischemic bowel, or appendicitis)

- ■ Treatment
  - Careful attention to ABCs
  - Continuous cardiac monitoring and frequent reassessment of vital signs
  - Intravenous fluid resuscitation and insulin drip (1 unit/kg/h)
  - Careful monitoring of serum potassium; replacement as soon as urine output is documented, unless serum potassium ≥5.0
  - Sodium bicarbonate for severe acidosis (pH <6.9)
  - Careful monitoring of serum glucose, changing to 5% dextrose in normal saline or 5% dextrose in half-normal saline (depending on corrected serum sodium) when the serum glucose ≤250 mg/dL
  - Admission to an ICU or intermediate care area (with continuous cardiac monitoring) for at least 24 hours for patients with all but the mildest cases of DKA

- ■ Pearl

Check a bedside fingerstick blood glucose level on severely dehydrated children with tachypnea, altered mental status, or vomiting because this can be a presentation of undiagnosed diabetes.

Reference

Kitabchi AE et al: Management of hyperglycemic crises in patients with diabetes mellitus. Diabetes Care 2001;24:131. [PMID: 11194218]

Lactic Acidosis

- **Essentials of Diagnosis**
  - Complication of critical illness; often associated with respiratory, hepatic, renal, or heart failure; sepsis; shock; cancer (ie, leukemia); acute infarction of lung, bowel, or extremities; severe abdominal or multisystem trauma; alcohol, methanol, or ethylene glycol poisoning; or drugs (cocaine, metformin, isoniazid)
  - Hyperventilation, generalized weakness, abdominal pain, tachycardia, and hypotension
  - Diagnostic studies: serum lactic acid >5 (specimen must be on ice) and pH <7.35 (often <7.2), elevated anion gap >15, often associated hyperphosphatemia

- **Differential Diagnosis**
  - Acidosis related to diabetic ketoacidosis or alcoholic ketoacidosis

- **Treatment**
  - Careful attention to ABCs
  - Supplemental oxygen and ventilator support to improve tissue oxygenation
  - Fluid resuscitation to reverse hypovolemia and improve tissue perfusion
  - Sodium bicarbonate is controversial but advocated by some if pH <6.9
  - Support of perfusion may require inotropic agents such as dopamine or dobutamine; drugs with more vasoconstrictive properties, such as norepinephrine, can worsen tissue hypoxia and lactic acidosis; afterload reduction may improve tissue perfusion
  - Treatment of underlying cause: antibiotics and fluids for septic shock; hemorrhage control and blood replacement for hemorrhagic shock

- **Pearl**

Discontinue medications such as metformin, which may be causing or exacerbating lactic acidosis.

Reference

Adrogue HJ, Madias NE: Management of life-threatening acid-base disorders. N Engl J Med 1998;338:26. [PMID: 9414329]

Myxedema Coma

- **Essentials of Diagnosis**
  - Clinical diagnosis in which manifestations of severe hypothyroidism are accompanied by disturbances of consciousness, hypothermia, hypoventilation, and hypotension
  - Cardinal features: hypothermia (in 80% of patients), CNS depression, generalized weakness, delayed deep tendon reflexes, disorientation, apathy, ataxia, inappropriate humor (myxedema wit), psychosis, grand mal seizures, lethargy, and coma; bradycardia and pericardial effusion; respiratory depression (decreased respiratory drive and muscle weakness) may lead to hypoxemia
  - Cutaneous findings: periorbital edema, ptosis, cutaneous myxedema, coarse, dry skin, macroglossia, thyroidectomy scar or a goiter, coarse or sparse hair
  - Often insidious onset, especially in the elderly
  - Free T_4, free T_3, TSH, cortisol, CBC, renal and hepatic function tests, arterial blood gas, electrolyte and glucose levels; chest x-ray and electrocardiogram in search for precipitating cause

- **Differential Diagnosis**
  - Other causes of altered mental status such as sepsis, meningitis, or CNS catastrophe
  - Primary respiratory failure with hypercarbia and hypoxemia

- **Treatment**
  - Intravenous fluid resuscitation for severe dehydration or hypotension; if hypotension persists despite volume replacement, vasopressors may be required
  - Identify and rapidly treat any precipitating causes such as associated hypoglycemia (ie, intravenous bolus of 50% dextrose initially)
  - Administer intravenous corticosteroids as associated adrenal insufficiency can occur
  - Intravenous thyroid hormone replacement (exact regimen is controversial); some favor administering both T_3 and T_4
  - Hospitalization in an ICU is indicated for all cases

- **Pearl**

Consider the diagnosis in any patient with a thyroidectomy scar and hypotension or abnormal mental status.

Reference

Wall CR: Myxedema coma: diagnosis and treatment. Am Fam Physician 2000;11:2485. [PMID: 11130234]

Pheochromocytoma

■ Essentials of Diagnosis

- Headache, palpitations, diaphoresis, flushing, apprehension, nausea, vomiting, or abdominal pain associated with hypertension (often severe; ≥120 mm Hg diastolic)
- Symptoms often intermittent (asymptomatic periods between episodes)
- Complications associated with severe hypertension: aortic dissection, myocardial infarction, encephalopathy, cardiomyopathy, pulmonary edema
- Associated neurocutaneous syndromes: neurofibromatosis, von Hippel-Lindau disease, ataxia-telangiectasia, tuberous sclerosis, Sturge-Weber syndrome
- Cutaneous findings: café-au-lait spots, telangiectasias
- CBC, electrolytes, glucose, 24-hour urine collection for catecholamines and catecholamine metabolites
- Localization of catecholamine-secreting tumor by CT, MRI, or nuclear scan only after lab confirmation of excess catecholamine state

■ Differential Diagnosis

- Monoamine oxidase inhibitor crisis
- Sympathomimetic overdose such as from cocaine or methamphetamine

■ Treatment

- Careful attention to ABCs, including continuous cardiac monitoring
- Supplemental oxygen administration and intravenous access
- Intravenous phentolamine (for α-adrenergic blockade), nitroprusside, fenoldopam, β-blockers (although controversial), benzodiazepines
- Hospitalization in an ICU for all cases, whether suspected or confirmed
- Surgical resection is only treatment that can offer cure

■ Pearl

In the treatment of pheochromocytoma, initiate β-blockade only after the patient has been adequately treated with α-blockade drugs so as not to precipitate severe hypertensive crisis from unopposed α stimulation.

Reference

Liao WB et al: Cardiovascular manifestations of pheochromocytoma. Am J Emerg Med 2000;18:622. [PMID: 10999582]

Pituitary Apoplexy

- ■ Essentials of Diagnosis
  - • Diagnosis is challenging; rare disease with varied presentations
  - • Headache (retroorbital, subacute and worsening, or a sudden thunderclap), other neurologic symptoms of paresthesias, ataxia or unilateral weakness (mimicking stroke), mild lethargy to coma; ophthalmologic disturbances such as particularly bitemporal hemianopsia or ophthalmoplegia; nausea, vomiting, and central fever
  - • Associated life-threatening adrenal insufficiency or respiratory depression possible
  - • CT and MRI are imaging studies of choice; acute hemorrhage appears hyperdense on CT; blood appears hypodense on T2-weighted MRI; MRI is helpful in detecting hemorrhage in the subacute setting
  - • Thyroid function tests, cortisol levels, growth hormone levels, and prolactin levels to assess global pituitary function; renal and hepatic function studies, serum glucose, and routine cultures

- ■ Differential Diagnosis
  - • Other CNS catastrophes such as subarachnoid hemorrhage or large cerebrovascular accident
  - • Sepsis, meningitis

- ■ Treatment
  - • Patients with respiratory depression related to elevated intracranial pressure: emergent intubation
  - • Associated adrenal insufficiency: intravenous hydrocortisone or dexamethasone
  - • Definitive treatment for pituitary apoplexy is neurosurgical decompression, generally accomplished by transsphenoidal approach; indications for surgery: decreasing consciousness, progressive vision loss, or increasing extraocular motor palsy indicating cavernous sinus compression
  - • Hospitalization in an ICU for all cases, whether suspected or confirmed

- ■ Pearl

Sheehan syndrome is pituitary apoplexy that occurs as a complication of hemorrhage and hypotension in postpartum women.

Reference

Lee CC et al: Emergency department presentation of pituitary apoplexy. Am J Emerg Med 2000;18:328. [PMID: 10830692]

Thyroid Storm

- **Essentials of Diagnosis**
  - Clinical diagnosis: fever (>38.5°C); tachycardia out of proportion to fever; nausea, vomiting, diarrhea, abdominal pain, and in rare cases jaundice; sinus tachycardia, atrial arrhythmias, and congestive heart failure; confusion/agitation/delirium (rather than lethargy/obtundation/coma), agitation, tremor, generalized weakness (especially in the proximal muscles), and periodic paralysis
  - Common triggers: infection, recent surgery, trauma, pregnancy, stroke, metabolic disorders such as diabetic ketoacidosis, radioiodine therapy, drug or alcohol abuse, iodinated contrast material, discontinuation of antithyroid medications
  - Often patients have history of partially treated hyperthyroidism or signs and symptoms of antecedent thyroid disease such as thyromegaly, proptosis, stare, myopathy, or myxedema
  - Lab studies are typically unavailable acutely; most helpful are TSH, which will be markedly low in most patients with thyroid storm, and free T_4, which will be elevated; blood cultures, urine cultures, chest x-ray, CBC with differential, chemistry panel, and electrocardiogram and cardiac enzymes generally indicated to look for precipitating causes
  - Head CT indicated in evaluating delirious or comatose patients

- **Differential Diagnosis**
  - Sepsis or meningitis
  - Often misdiagnosed initially as primary psychosis

- **Treatment**
  - Monitor ABCs carefully; hospitalization in ICU
  - Thioamides (propylthiouracil) administered orally or by nasogastric tube
  - Oral iodine therapy is a therapeutic adjunct to propylthiouracil
  - Intravenous β-adrenergic antagonists (propanolol or esmolol)
  - Intravenous corticosteroids (hydrocortisone, dexamethasone)

- **Pearl**

Thyroid storm is a clinical diagnosis. Never delay treatment for a patient with suspected thyroid storm while awaiting confirmatory lab studies; untreated mortality is nearly 100%.

Reference

Dabon-Almirante CL, Surks MI: Clinical and laboratory diagnosis of thyrotoxicosis. Endocrinol Metab Clin North Am 1998;27:25. [PMID: 9534025]

11

Electrolyte & Acid-Base Emergencies

Hypercalcemia

- **Essentials of Diagnosis**
  - Serum calcium concentration >11 mg/dL
  - Patients usually aren't symptomatic until serum concentration >12 mg/dL
  - Symptoms may become severe at serum concentration >15 mg/dL
  - Symptoms usually nonspecific and may easily be missed
  - Anorexia, vomiting, constipation, abdominal pain
  - Altered mentation, stupor, coma
  - Impaired renal function eventually leads to azotemia
  - Electrocardiographic changes: prolonged PR interval, shortened QT interval, widened T waves

- **Differential Diagnosis**
  - Endocrine: primary or secondary hyperparathyroidism, adrenal insufficiency, acromegaly
  - Malignancy: parathyroid hormone–producing tumors, metastases to bone, lymphoproliferative disease, secretion of prostaglandin and osteolytic factors
  - Increased intake: milk-alkali syndrome, vitamin A or D excess
  - Miscellaneous: thiazide diuretics, sarcoidosis, Paget disease, hypophosphatemia, immobilization, familial, iatrogenic

- **Treatment**
  - Prompt treatment if serum calcium concentration >12 mg/dL
  - Intravenous fluids for volume expansion
  - Loop diuretics such as furosemide, 40 mg IV, to increase excretion of calcium after fluids
  - Bisphosphonates, mithramycin, calcitonin, phosphate, glucocorticoids, dialysis
  - Treatment of underlying disorder

- **Pearl**

Hypercalcemia is most commonly caused by hyperparathyroidism or malignancy.

Reference

Carroll MF, Schade DS: A practical approach to hypercalcemia. Am Fam Physician 2003;67:1959. [PMID: 12751658]

Hyperkalemia

- ■ Essentials of Diagnosis
  - Serum potassium >5.5 mEq/L
  - More common in patients with renal disease
  - Symptoms usually neuromuscular and cardiac
  - Generalized weakness and paresthesias
  - Cardiac dysrhythmias correlate loosely with level of hyperkalemia
  - Hyperacute T waves in mild hyperkalemia
  - PR interval and QRS duration prolongation in moderate disease
  - Severe hyperkalemia leads to ST depression, continued prolongation of the QRS and T waves, and eventual sine wave electrocardiogram and cardiac arrest

- ■ Differential Diagnosis
  - Spurious hyperkalemia (hemolysis, thrombocytosis, fist-clenching during blood draw)
  - Renal disease
  - Adrenal insufficiency
  - Drug induced (potassium supplements, aldosterone antagonists)
  - Crush injuries or burns (usually not acute)

- ■ Treatment
  - Intravenous calcium preparation to stabilize the myocardial cell: calcium chloride, 5–10 cc of a 10% solution, or calcium gluconate, 10–20 cc
  - Insulin, 10–20 units with one amp of 50% dextrose in water IV
  - Sodium bicarbonate, 1–2 amps IV
  - Nebulized β-agonists to force a temporary shift of potassium to the intracellular space
  - Sodium polystyrene sulfate (Kayexalate), 15–30 g orally or rectally as a binding resin for the potassium
  - Hemodialysis
  - Correction of underlying disorder

- ■ Pearl

Always obtain an electrocardiogram in a patient at risk for hyperkalemia, while waiting for the potassium level from the lab.

Reference

Gennari FJ: Disorders of potassium homeostasis. Hypokalemia and hyperkalemia. Crit Care Clin 2002;18:273. [PMID: 12053834]

Hypermagnesemia

- **Essentials of Diagnosis**
  - Usually associated with renal failure
  - Signs and symptoms correlate with degree of hypermagnesemia
  - Peripheral vasodilation, nausea, hypotension develop with serum magnesium concentration of 3–4 mEq/L
  - Drowsiness, confusion, and depressed or absent deep tendon reflexes develop with serum concentration of 5–7 mEq/L
  - Coma and death occur with serum concentration >10 mEq/L
  - Electrocardiographic findings: prolonged PR interval, wide QRS, elevated T waves

- **Differential Diagnosis**
  - Renal failure
  - Excessive magnesium intake (antacids, magnesium sulfate, green vegetables, nuts, peas, beans)
  - Iatrogenic

- **Treatment**
  - Hospitalization
  - Treatment depends on renal function
  - Patients with renal insufficiency or failure: dialysis
  - Patients with normal renal function: intravenous fluids for volume expansion; loop diuretics such as furosemide, 20–40 mg IV, and calcium chloride, 5 cc of a 10% solution IV
  - Treatment of underlying cause

- **Pearl**

Remember to check for magnesium disorders when faced with a calcium or phosphate disorder.

Reference

Whang R: Clinical disorders of magnesium metabolism. Compr Ther 1997;23:168. [PMID: 9113454]

Hypernatremia

- ■ Essentials of Diagnosis
  - • Serum sodium concentration >150 mEq/L
  - • Usually associated with loss of free water; rarely due to excess salt gain
  - • Common in extremes of age
  - • Signs and symptoms are associated with severity and rate of rise of the serum sodium: thirst, lethargy, tachycardia, hypotension, fever, confusion, seizures, coma
  - • Intracerebral hemorrhage occurs occasionally when shrinking brain tissue tears bridging veins
  - • Measurement of urine osmolarity

- ■ Differential Diagnosis
  - • Inadequate water intake
  - • Renal causes (tube feeding syndrome; diabetes insipidus; hypercalcemia; renal failure; and toxicity, usually drugs)
  - • Excessive water loss (prolonged fever, burns, thyrotoxicosis)
  - • Massive salt ingestion

- ■ Treatment
  - • Initial treatment of hypovolemic patient with isotonic saline
  - • Switch to 5% dextrose in water to replace the free water deficit
  - • Calculate the water deficit: water deficit (L) = total body water (1 − measured sodium/desired sodium)
  - • Do not correct hypernatremia faster than 1–2 mEq/L/h
  - • Correction of underlying disorder

- ■ Pearl

A general rule is that each liter of water deficit causes the sodium level to increase 3–5 mEq/L.

Reference

Halperin ML, Bohn D: Clinical approach to disorders of salt and water balance. Emphasis on integrative physiology. Crit Care Clin 2002;18:249. [PMID: 12053833]

Hyperphosphatemia

- **Essentials of Diagnosis**
  - Serum phosphate concentration >7 mg/dL
  - No symptoms directly referable to the hyperphosphatemia
  - Hypocalcemia and hypomagnesemia may develop because of tissue deposition of calcium phosphate

- **Differential Diagnosis**
  - Ingestion of large amounts of phosphate, vitamin D, or laxatives
  - Chronic or acute renal disease
  - Hypoparathyroidism
  - Growth hormone excess
  - Rhabdomyolysis
  - Cytolysis of chemotherapy
  - Excessive enemas with phosphate-containing solutions

- **Treatment**
  - Administer 50% dextrose in water and regular insulin as in hyperkalemia to induce an intracellular shift in phosphate
  - Volume expansion with intravenous crystalloid
  - Acetazolamide, 500 mg every 6 hours
  - Oral phosphate-binding antacids (aluminum hydroxide)
  - Hemodialysis in patients with renal failure

- **Pearl**

If patients with hyperphosphatemia need hospitalization, it is usually because of the precipitating event such as renal failure.

Reference

Shiber JR, Mattu A: Serum phosphate abnormalities in the emergency department. J Emerg Med 2002;23:395. [PMID: 12480022]

Hypocalcemia

- ■ Essentials of Diagnosis
  - • Ionized calcium concentration <2.0 mEq/L
  - • Mild hypocalcemia: may be asymptomatic
  - • More severe signs and symptoms: tetany, weakness, fatigue, cramps, carpopedal spasm, muscle fasciculations, convulsions, diplopia, laryngospasm
  - • Positive Chvostek sign (tapping over cranial nerve VII causing twitching of the corner of the mouth) and Trousseau sign (carpal spasm induced by a blood pressure cuff inflated above the systolic pressure for 3 minutes)
  - • Electrocardiographic findings: may show prolonged QT without U waves
  - • Coexisting abnormalities of potassium and magnesium common
  - • Check renal function
  - • Hypercapnia: may be associated with severe hypocalcemia

- ■ Differential Diagnosis
  - • Decreased intake or absorption of calcium
  - • Increased loss of calcium
  - • Endocrine disease (hypoparathyroidism, pseudohypoparathyroidism, calcitonin secretion from carcinoma)
  - • Low serum albumin
  - • Hyperphosphatemia
  - • Decreased tissue response to vitamin D
  - • Iatrogenic (aminoglycosides, loop diuretics, mithramycin)

- ■ Treatment
  - • Calcium chloride, 10 cc of a 10% solution, or calcium gluconate, 10–20 cc IV, then 1 ampule in 500 cc normal saline every 8 hours, to keep calcium concentration at 7–8 mg/dL
  - • Treatment of other electrolyte disorders, if present
  - • Calcium chloride, 10 cc for every 4–6 units of packed RBCs in massive transfusions
  - • Oral supplements with calcium and vitamin D may be needed
  - • Admission unless very mild disease

- ■ Pearl

Correct the hyperphosphatemia before correcting the hypocalcemia to prevent metastatic calcifications.

Reference

Fukugawa M, Kurokawa K: Calcium homeostasis and imbalance. Nephron 2002;92(Suppl 1):41. [PMID: 12425329]

Hypokalemia

- **Essentials of Diagnosis**
  - Serum potassium concentration <3.5 mEq/L
  - Signs and symptoms: weakness, paralysis, ileus, rhabdomyolysis, cardiac dysrhythmias
  - Electrocardiographic findings: ST depression, T wave flattening, U waves
  - Common dysrhythmias: atrioventricular dissociation and ventricular tachycardia or fibrillation
  - Most commonly seen with diuretic therapy
  - Potassium cation is predominantly intracellular; serum potassium accounts for only 2% of total body stores

- **Differential Diagnosis**
  - Increased potassium loss (diuretics, renal tubular acidosis, diarrhea)
  - Reduced absorption (malabsorption, short bowel syndrome)
  - Poor intake of potassium-containing foods and fluids
  - Hypokalemia without deficit (anything such as alkalosis, insulin, or β-agonists), which causes potassium shift into the cell
  - Familial periodic paralysis (hypokalemia)

- **Treatment**
  - Correction of underlying condition, such as alkalosis or hypomagnesemia, causing the hypokalemia
  - Administration of oral (preferred) or intravenous potassium salts to replenish total body potassium stores
  - If intravenous potassium is administered, infuse slowly; no more than 0.2 mEq/kg/h, never IV push
  - Use dextrose-free solution to prevent stimulating insulin release
  - Administration of 20 mEq of potassium will cause 0.25 mEq/L rise in serum potassium

- **Pearl**

Because hypokalemia may occur with academia or alkalosis, identification of the metabolic abnormality is important in determining the proper initial treatment.

Reference

Gennari FJ: Disorders of potassium homeostasis. Hypokalemia and hyperkalemia. Crit Care Clin 2002;18:273. [PMID: 12053834]

Hypomagnesemia

- **Essentials of Diagnosis**
  - Serum magnesium concentration <1.2 mg/dL
  - Frequently associated with abnormalities of calcium, potassium, and phosphate
  - Signs and symptoms similar to those of hypocalcemia: carpopedal spasm, tetany, athetoid movements, tremors, weakness, hyperexcitable reflexes, hypertension, positive Babinski sign
  - Mental status changes: confusion, disorientation, psychotic behavior
  - Electrocardiographic findings: QT prolongation leading to ventricular tachycardia and fibrillation

- **Differential Diagnosis**
  - Decreased absorption (malabsorption, laxatives, small bowel bypass, prolonged gastrointestinal suction)
  - Decreased intake (malnutrition, alcoholism)
  - Increased loss (diarrhea, diuretics, renal wasting, diabetic ketoacidosis)
  - Idiopathic (usually associated with calcium or potassium abnormalities)

- **Treatment**
  - Oral (preferred) or intravenous replacement; intramuscular magnesium replacement is painful and should be avoided unless absolutely necessary
  - Magnesium oxide, 400 mg, orally four times daily; or magnesium sulfate, 1 g IV, every 6 hours except in the face of ventricular dysrhythmias, when 200 mg may be given over 1–2 minutes
  - Correction of other electrolyte abnormalities
  - Symptomatic patients: admission

- **Pearl**

Hypocalcemia and hypokalemia associated with hypomagnesemia will respond well when magnesium is replaced.

Reference

Whang R: Clinical disorders of magnesium metabolism. Compr Ther 1997; 23:168. [PMID: 9113454]

Hyponatremia

- **Essentials of Diagnosis**
  - Serum sodium concentration <130 mEq/L
  - Disorder of free water balance
  - Initial evaluation for volume status (hyper-, hypo-, or euvolemic)
  - Patients with hypovolemia: may need initial volume resuscitation
  - Severity of symptoms related to duration and rate of fall of serum sodium
  - Nonspecific signs and symptoms: weakness, confusion, cramps, seizures, coma, increased deep tendon reflexes
  - Measurement of urine and serum osmolality
  - Hyperglycemia can cause a pseudohyponatremia; sodium may be corrected by adding 1.54 mEq/L for every 100 mg/dL over 200 mg/dL of serum glucose
  - Hyperlipidemia and hyperproteinemia may also cause pseudo-hyponatremia

- **Differential Diagnosis**
  - Hypervolemic (nephrotic syndrome, heart, liver, or renal failure)
  - Euvolemic (adrenal insufficiency, syndrome of inappropriate antidiuretic hormone, hypothyroidism, drugs and toxins, psychogenic polydipsia)
  - Hypovolemic (diuretics, adrenal insufficiency, vomiting, diarrhea, burns, muscle trauma, excessive sweating, peritonitis)

- **Treatment**
  - Treatment of underlying disorder
  - Restoration of volume status with isotonic saline
  - Water restriction
  - Diuretics only in patients with volume overload
  - Hypertonic saline only in the ICU in severe cases (serum sodium <110 mEq/L with coma or seizures)
  - Hyponatremic patients with renal failure: dialysis may be needed
  - Significantly symptomatic patients or patients in whom the hyponatremia developed abruptly: admission

- **Pearl**

Symptoms are related to the rate of change of serum sodium, not the absolute level.

Reference

Yeates KE, Singer M, Morton AR: Salt and water: a simple approach to hyponatremia. Can Med Assoc J 2004;170:365. [PMID: 14757675]

Hypophosphatemia

- ■ Essentials of Diagnosis
  - Serum phosphorous concentration <2 mg/dL
  - Signs and symptoms vague and nonspecific
  - Fatigue, weakness, irritability, paresthesias, dysarthria, confusion, seizures, coma possible
  - Hemolysis, decreased delivery of oxygen to tissues, rhabdomyolysis, and impaired neutrophil phagocytosis may occur below 1 mg/dL

- ■ Differential Diagnosis
  - Alcoholism
  - Primary hyperparathyroidism
  - Ingestion of phosphate-binding antacids
  - Metabolic or respiratory alkalosis
  - Severe burns
  - Recovery from diabetic ketoacidosis
  - Starvation and phosphorous-deficient parenteral nutrition

- ■ Treatment
  - Oral (preferred) or intravenous replacement of phosphorous
  - Oral replacement: milk, aluminum phosphate gel, neutral phosphate salts
  - Intravenous replacement: patient should be in ICU with careful monitoring of other electrolytes
  - Potassium phosphate, 8 mmol IV every 6 hours
  - Patients with severe hypophosphatemia (<1 mg/dL): admission; all others: close follow up

- ■ Pearl

An isolated serum phosphate level doesn't necessarily reflect total body stores, because phosphorous is prone to shifting.

Reference

Shiber JR, Mattu A: Serum phosphate abnormalities in the emergency department. J Emerg Med 2002;23:395. [PMID: 12480022]

Metabolic Acidosis

- **Essentials of Diagnosis**
  - Plasma concentration of HCO_3^- <22 mmol/L; pH <7.35
  - Separated into increased anion gap and nonanion gap metabolic acidosis
  - Anion gap = sodium − [chloride + HCO_3^-]; normal = 8–14 mEq/L
  - Created with an imbalance between hydrogen ions and HCO_3^-
  - Increased anion gap caused by overproduction of acids or reduced clearance by kidneys
  - Nonanion gap acidosis caused by loss of HCO_3^- with reciprocal increase in chloride ions
  - Symptoms are nonspecific and associated with underlying cause of metabolic acidosis
  - Calculate the pCO_2 using the Winter formula:

  $$pCO_2 = (1.5([HCO_3^-]) + 8) \pm 2$$

  - If measured pCO_2 is below the calculated level, a respiratory alkalosis is present; if it is higher, a respiratory acidosis is present

- **Differential Diagnosis**
  - Increased anion gap (diabetic or alcoholic ketoacidosis; uremia; lactic acidosis; toxins such as ethylene glycol, methanol, salicylates, paraldehyde, iron, ibuprofen, isoniazid)
  - Normal anion gap with hypokalemia (diarrhea, small bowel or pancreatic fistula, ureteral diversion, ileal loop, type 1 renal tubular acidosis, carbonic anhydrase inhibitors)
  - Normal anion gap with hyperkalemia (type 4 renal tubular acidosis, early renal failure, hydronephrosis, hypoaldosteronism)

- **Treatment**
  - Treatment of underlying cause
  - Restoration of tissue perfusion by optimizing respiratory and cardiovascular support, frequently with volume resuscitation

- **Pearl**

Treatment of the underlying cause is the key to treating metabolic acidosis.

Reference

Kraut JA, Madias NE: Approach to patients with acid-base disorders. Respir Care 2001;46:392. [PMID: 11262558]

Metabolic Alkalosis

- ■ Essentials of Diagnosis
  - Plasma concentration of HCO_3^- >28 mmol/L; pH >7.45
  - Majority of cases come from volume depletion
  - Signs and symptoms nonspecific and generally caused by underlying disorder or electrolyte derangement
  - Hypokalemia, hypocalcemia, and hypomagnesemia commonly seen with metabolic alkalosis
  - Respiratory system will compensate for a metabolic alkalosis by hypoventilation; each 1 mmol/L increase in the HCO_3^- will increase the pCO_2 by 0.7 mm Hg up to about 55 mm Hg
  - Metabolic alkalosis may be divided into saline-responsive and saline-resistant causes
  - Check urine electrolytes

- ■ Differential Diagnosis
  - Saline responsive: vomiting, diarrhea, nasogastric suction, villous adenoma, diuretics, cystic fibrosis, alkali syndrome, posthypercapnia
  - Saline resistant: mineralocorticoid excess, Cushing syndrome, severe hypokalemia, congenital adrenal hypoplasia
  - Other causes: massive blood transfusion, hypercalcemia, refeeding alkalosis

- ■ Treatment
  - Urine chloride <10 mEq/L: volume expansion should correct alkalosis
  - Correction of other electrolyte disorders (potassium, calcium, magnesium)
  - Urine chloride >20 mEq/L: treatment of underlying disorder because patients will be resistant to volume expansion

- ■ Pearl

Metabolic alkalosis usually results from vomiting or excess diuresis.

Reference

Khanna A, Kurtzman NA: Metabolic alkalosis. Respir Care 2001;46:354. [PMID: 11262555]

Respiratory Acidosis

- **Essentials of Diagnosis**
  - pCO_2 >45 mm Hg; pH <7.35
  - May be caused by any disorder that causes alveolar hypoventilation
  - Primary clinical finding: alteration in level of consciousness; level depends on severity of hypercapnia present and its chronicity
  - Other symptoms: fatigue, irritability, confusion, coma
  - Acute respiratory acidosis: HCO_3^- will increase 1.0 mEq/L for every 10 mm Hg increase in pCO_2
  - Chronic respiratory acidosis: HCO_3^- will increase 3.5 mEq/L for every 10 mm Hg increase in pCO_2

- **Differential Diagnosis**
  - Respiratory center depression (narcotics, cardiac arrest)
  - Paralysis of respiratory muscles (toxins, neuromuscular disease)
  - Airway obstruction (spasm, edema, aspiration, neoplasm)
  - Primary pulmonary disorders inhibiting exchange of gases
  - Extreme disorders of the chest wall preventing adequate ventilation (kyphosis, obesity)

- **Treatment**
  - Reversal or stabilization of underlying disorder
  - Aggressive airway management
  - Positive airway pressure to improve exchange of gases (PEEP, BiPAP)
  - Rapid correction of the pCO_2 can cause hypocalcemia
  - Admission decisions depend on patient's clinical condition

- **Pearl**

If the pH is compensated back to normal, consider a mixed acid-base disturbance to be present.

Reference

Epstein SK, Singh N: Respiratory acidosis. Respir Care 2001;46:366. [PMID: 11262556]

Respiratory Alkalosis

- **Essentials of Diagnosis**
  - pCO_2 <35; pH >7.45
  - Circumoral and digital paresthesias common
  - Associated hypocalcemia may cause tetany or carpopedal spasm
  - May progress to lightheadedness, confusion, and loss of consciousness (cerebral vasoconstriction)
  - Respiratory alkalosis causes a metabolic compensation: acutely, a 10 mm Hg decrease will decrease HCO_3^- by 2.5 mEq/L; chronically, a 10 mm Hg decrease will decrease HCO_3^- by 5 mEq/L
  - Mild hypokalemia may result from chronic respiratory acidosis by shifting potassium into the cells

- **Differential Diagnosis**
  - Early shock states (sepsis, trauma)
  - Pulmonary disease (especially pulmonary embolism)
  - Cerebrovascular accident
  - CNS infection
  - Acute salicylate ingestion
  - Pregnancy, liver disease, or hyperthyroidism

- **Treatment**
  - Treatment of underlying cause
  - Rebreathing devices may be helpful for psychogenic causes of respiratory alkalosis

- **Pearl**

Remember to search for the serious underlying causes of respiratory alkalosis such as pulmonary embolism and early shock states.

Reference

Kraut JA, Madias NE: Approach to patients with acid-base disorders. Respir Care 2001;46:392. [PMID: 11262558]

12

Rheumatologic Emergencies

Ankylosing Spondylitis

- **Essentials of Diagnosis**
  - Patient under 40 years of age
  - Back pain of gradual onset
  - Stiffness worse in morning; improves with exercise or stooping forward
  - X-rays show sacroiliitis, "bamboo spine"
  - May present with cauda equina syndrome
  - Enthesitis common, especially Achilles tendonitis or plantar fasciitis
  - May have systemic inflammatory manifestations such as uveitis
  - Joint fluid: low viscosity; 2,000–50,000 WBCs; culture negative

- **Differential Diagnosis**
  - Septic arthritis
  - Psoriatic arthritis
  - Viral illness with fever and malaise
  - Osteoarthritis
  - Traumatic arthritis
  - Gout
  - Rheumatoid arthritis
  - Reiter syndrome
  - Systemic lupus erythematosus
  - Neoplastic back pain

- **Treatment**
  - Nonsteroidal anti-inflammatory drugs
  - Analgesia
  - Steroids for severe refractory cases
  - Strengthening exercises
  - Rheumatology follow-up

- **Pearl**

Patients with ankylosing spondylitis are at increased risk of traumatic spinal injury, even from minor injury.

Reference

van der Linden S, van der Heijde D: Ankylosing spondylitis. Clinical features. Rheum Dis Clin North Am 1998;24:663. [PMID: 9891705]

Arthritis, Psoriatic

- ■ Essentials of Diagnosis
  - Arthritis associated with psoriasis
  - Joint swelling, tenderness, warmth, restricted movement
  - "Sausage digits" due to interphalangeal involvement
  - Predominant age at onset: 30–35 years
  - Rheumatoid factor negative
  - X-ray findings: gross destructive changes of isolated small joints
  - Joint fluid: low viscosity; 2,000–50,000 WBCs; culture negative

- ■ Differential Diagnosis
  - Septic arthritis
  - Rheumatoid arthritis
  - Viral illness with fever and malaise
  - Osteoarthritis
  - Traumatic arthritis
  - Gout
  - Reiter syndrome
  - Ankylosing spondylitis
  - Systemic lupus erythematosus

- ■ Treatment
  - Nonsteroidal anti-inflammatory drugs
  - Immobilizing splints
  - Isometric exercises and swimming
  - Heat therapy
  - Psoriatic skin care (treatment of skin lesions sometimes improves arthritic symptoms)
  - Dermatology referral

- ■ Pearl

Arthritis occurs before psoriasis in 15% of patients. Nail changes, which include pitting, dystrophy, and onycholysis, are a clue to diagnosis.

Reference

Salvarani C et al: Psoriatic arthritis. Curr Opin Rheumatol 1998;10:299. [PMID: 9725090]

Arthritis, Rheumatoid

- ■ Essentials of Diagnosis
    - • Often subacute joint pain; in acute presentation, joints warm, tender, and swollen
    - • Usually symmetric polyarthritis
    - • Most commonly proximal interphalangeal and metacarpophalangeal joints
    - • X-rays show juxta-articular osteoporosis and later cartilage erosions
    - • Joint fluid: low viscosity; 2,000–50,000 WBCs; culture negative

- ■ Differential Diagnosis
    - • Septic arthritis
    - • Psoriatic arthritis
    - • Viral illness with fever and malaise
    - • Osteoarthritis
    - • Traumatic arthritis
    - • Gout
    - • Reiter syndrome
    - • Ankylosing spondylitis
    - • Systemic lupus erythematosus

- ■ Treatment
    - • Aspirin and nonsteroidal anti-inflammatory drugs
    - • Urgent rheumatology follow-up

- ■ Pearl

Only 85% of patients with rheumatoid arthritis are rheumatoid factor positive.

Reference

Newsome G; American College of Rheumatology: Guidelines for the management of rheumatoid arthritis: 2002 update. J Am Acad Nurse Pract 2002;14:432. [PMID: 12426799]

Arthritis, Septic

- **■ Essentials of Diagnosis**
  - Painful, erythematous, and tender joint
  - Fever and chills common
  - Definitive diagnosis by joint aspiration, Gram stain, and culture
  - Large joints most often affected
  - Joint fluid: low viscosity; >50,000 WBCs; culture usually positive

- **■ Differential Diagnosis**
  - Traumatic arthritis
  - Gout
  - Pseudogout
  - Osteoarthritis
  - Psoriatic arthritis
  - Rheumatoid arthritis
  - Reiter syndrome
  - Ankylosing spondylitis
  - Systemic lupus erythematosus

- **■ Treatment**
  - Empiric intravenous antibiotics for suspected organism: ceftriaxone for gonorrhea; penicillinase-resistant agent plus aminoglycoside for intravenous drug use; antipseudomonal β-lactam plus aminoglycoside for gram-negative organisms
  - Analgesia
  - Hospitalization with orthopedic consult
  - Once diagnosis is established, joint washout in the operating room is usually indicated (exception is gonococcal septic arthritis)

- **■ Pearl**

  Joint fluid in gonococcal septic arthritis often does not demonstrate organisms. Typical pustular skin lesions; tenosynovitis; or positive cervical, throat, or rectal cultures suggest the diagnosis.

Reference

Pioro MH, Mandell BF: Septic arthritis. Rheum Dis Clin North Am 1997;23:239. [PMID: 9156391]

Arthritis, Traumatic

- **Essentials of Diagnosis**
  - Effusions often develop immediately after trauma
  - Fever or other systemic signs or symptoms not present
  - Presence of noninflammatory or hemorrhagic synovial fluid
  - Joint fluid: variable viscosity; variable WBCs; culture negative

- **Differential Diagnosis**
  - Septic arthritis
  - Gout
  - Pseudogout
  - Osteoarthritis
  - Early inflammatory arthritis

- **Treatment**
  - Splinting
  - Ice
  - Elevation
  - Aspiration of large effusions may provide pain relief
  - Protection from weight bearing
  - Nonsteroidal anti-inflammatory drugs
  - Analgesia
  - Follow-up care

- **Pearl**

Traumatic hemarthrosis has a high association with ligamentous injury or intra-articular fracture.

Reference

Fredberg U, Bolvig L: Traumatic arthritis in sport. Scand J Med Sci Sports 2001;11:251. [PMID: 11476432]

Bursitis

- **Essentials of Diagnosis**
  - Inflammation localized to the bursa, not the entire joint
  - Pain worsens with movement of adjacent structures
  - Common sites: olecranon of the elbow and prepatellar area of the knee

- **Differential Diagnosis**
  - Infectious causes of inflammation
  - Osteoarthritis
  - Tendonitis
  - Fracture
  - Gout
  - Avascular necrosis

- **Treatment**
  - Nonsteroidal anti-inflammatory drugs
  - Analgesia
  - Rest
  - Ice versus heat
  - Aspiration and antibiotics if infectious cause suspected
  - Local injection of steroids if skilled in procedure
  - Treatment of associated diseases (eg, gout)
  - Septic bursitis may require repeated aspiration
  - Orthopedic or rheumatology referral for recurrent bursitis

- **Pearl**

Consider infection as cause of inflammation if fever and chills are present.

Reference

Stell IM: Management of acute bursitis: outcome study of a structured approach. J R Soc Med 1999;92:516. [PMID: 10692903]

Gout

- **Essentials of Diagnosis**
  - Sudden onset of warmth and pain, most commonly metatar-sophalangeal joint of the great toe (podagra) and knee; often recurrent
  - Arthrocentesis needed for initial diagnosis
  - Increased incidence with alcoholism, loop diuretics, renal failure, obesity
  - Joint fluid: low viscosity; 2,000–50,000 WBCs; culture negative
  - Presence of negative birefringent urate crystals; negative Gram stain and culture

- **Differential Diagnosis**
  - Pseudogout
  - Septic arthritis
  - Rheumatoid arthritis
  - Bursitis
  - Cellulitis
  - Dislocations
  - Osteomyelitis
  - Reiter syndrome
  - Tenosynovitis

- **Treatment**
  - Nonsteroidal anti-inflammatory drugs (NSAIDs)
  - Colchicine
  - Steroids for patients who cannot take NSAIDs or colchicine
  - Allopurinol and probenecid not for acute therapy

- **Pearl**

Uric acid level is not helpful for diagnosis in an acute attack.

Reference

Monu JU, Pope TL Jr: Gout: a clinical and radiologic review. Radiol Clin North Am 2004;42:169. [PMID: 15049530]

Osteoarthritis

■ Essentials of Diagnosis

- Usually polyarticular
- Most common joints: hips, knees, spine, distal interphalangeal, proximal interphalangeal
- Fever and chills should be absent
- X-rays show cartilage changes with osteophytes
- Prolonged morning stiffness
- Pain relieved by rest
- More common in obese individuals
- Joint fluid: high viscosity; <4,000 WBCs; culture negative

■ Differential Diagnosis

- Septic arthritis
- Traumatic arthritis
- Gout
- Pseudogout
- Rheumatoid arthritis

■ Treatment

- Acetaminophen or nonsteroidal anti-inflammatory drugs
- Range of motion exercise
- Weight-bearing exercise

■ Pearl

Clinical diagnosis of osteoarthritis is based on pain; decreased movement; muscle wasting; and x-ray findings of joint space narrowing, osteophytes, and bony sclerosis.

Reference

Schnitzer TJ: Update of ACR guidelines for osteoarthritis: role of the coxibs. J Pain Symptom Manage 2002;23(4 Suppl):S24. [PMID: 11992747]

Pseudogout

- ■ Essentials of Diagnosis
  - • Calcium pyrophosphate crystals in the joint
  - • Most common site is knee; wrist is also common location
  - • Increased incidence in the elderly (rarely occurs in those under age 50), trauma, surgery, hyperparathyroidism
  - • Joint fluid: low viscosity; 2,000–50,000 WBCs; culture negative
  - • X-rays may demonstrate chondrocalcinosis (calcification of fibro-cartilage within the joint)

- ■ Differential Diagnosis
  - • Gout
  - • Septic arthritis
  - • Rheumatoid arthritis
  - • Bursitis
  - • Cellulitis
  - • Dislocations
  - • Osteomyelitis
  - • Reiter syndrome
  - • Tenosynovitis

- ■ Treatment
  - • Aspiration often adequate for relief of symptoms
  - • Nonsteroidal anti-inflammatory drugs

- ■ Pearl

Unlike in the treatment of gout, colchicine is not usually helpful.

Reference

Hammoudeh M, Siam AR: Pseudogout in a young patient. Clin Rheumatol 1998;17:242. [PMID: 9694062]

Reiter Syndrome

- ■ Essentials of Diagnosis
  - Usually affects young males
  - Classic triad (although rare): arthritis, conjunctivitis, urethritis
  - Oligoarticular and asymmetric arthritis, developing 2–6 weeks after chlamydial infection or other bacterial gastroenteritis (*Shigella, Salmonella, Yersinia, Campylobacter*)
  - Synovial fluid: inflammatory and culture negative

- ■ Differential Diagnosis
  - Septic arthritis
  - Psoriatic arthritis
  - Viral illness with fever and malaise
  - Osteoarthritis
  - Traumatic arthritis
  - Gout
  - Rheumatoid arthritis
  - Ankylosing spondylitis
  - Systemic lupus erythematosus

- ■ Treatment
  - Nonsteroidal anti-inflammatory drugs
  - Analgesia
  - Tetracycline: decreases recovery time for arthritis due to chlamydia but not enteral causes

- ■ Pearl

Typically the arthritis lasts 4–5 months, but patients may develop chronic or recurrent arthritis.

Reference

Kataria RK, Brent LH: Spondyloarthropathies. Am Fam Physician 2004;69:2853. [PMID: 15222650]

Systemic Lupus Erythematosus

- **Essentials of Diagnosis**
  - Arthritis associated with malar or discoid rash and fever
  - Two or more peripheral joints with warmth, tenderness, or effusion
  - Multisystem involvement
  - Female to male ratio of 9:1
  - More common in African Americans
  - Peak onset: ages 15–25 years
  - Positive anti-double-stranded DNA or antinuclear antibody test
  - Joint fluid: low viscosity; 2,000–50,000 WBCs; culture negative

- **Differential Diagnosis**
  - Septic arthritis
  - Psoriatic arthritis
  - Viral illness with fever and malaise
  - Osteoarthritis
  - Traumatic arthritis
  - Gout
  - Rheumatoid arthritis
  - Reiter syndrome
  - Ankylosing spondylitis
  - Neoplastic back pain

- **Treatment**
  - Nonsteroidal anti-inflammatory drugs
  - Steroids
  - Rheumatology follow-up
  - Treatment of complications in other organ systems
  - Patients should receive treatment as for immunocompromised

- **Pearl**

Multisystem involvement: ask about signs and symptoms of life-threatening complications in other systems (such as pulmonary involvement with pleurisy, coughing, or dyspnea as common symptoms).

Reference

American College of Rheumatology: Guidelines for referral and management of systemic lupus erythematosus in adults. Arthritis Rheum 1999;42:1785. [PMID: 10513791]

Tendonitis

■ **Essentials of Diagnosis**

- Pain and tenderness localized to the tendon
- Pain reproduced by stretching the affected tendon
- Caused by overuse and repetitive motion
- Achilles tendonitis associated with fluoroquinolones (but also associated with other tendonitis sites)

■ **Differential Diagnosis**

- Infectious causes of inflammation (suppurative tenosynovitis)
- Osteoarthritis
- Bursitis
- Osteomyelitis
- Phlebitis or deep venous thrombosis
- Myositis
- Avascular necrosis

■ **Treatment**

- Rest
- Ice
- Nonsteroidal anti-inflammatory drugs
- Analgesia
- Exercise program
- Identification and avoidance of inciting activity
- Local injection of steroids if skilled in procedure

■ **Pearl**

Always consider infectious causes of inflammation, although such causes are rare.

Reference

Almekinders LC, Temple JD: Etiology, diagnosis, and treatment of tendonitis: an analysis of the literature. Med Sci Sports Exerc 1998;30:1183. [PMID: 9710855]

13

Obstetric & Gynecologic Emergencies

Adnexal Torsion

- **Essentials of Diagnosis**
  - Occurs in females of any age; most patients are young
  - Single or recurrent episodes of moderate to severe unilateral pelvic pain often of sudden onset
  - Nausea; vomiting; back, groin, or thigh pain may accompany episodes of pelvic pain
  - With infarction of the ovary, fever and leukocytosis often develop
  - Patient may be predisposed to adnexal torsion because of large cyst or mass on the ovary; in 20% of cases, no ovarian pathology exists
  - 20% of cases occur in pregnant patients
  - Pelvic ultrasound is diagnostic if Doppler flow studies demonstrate reduced or absent flow to the ovary; other findings: enlarged ovary and enlarged follicles at the periphery of the ovary

- **Differential Diagnosis**
  - Ruptured ovarian cyst
  - Ectopic pregnancy
  - Pelvic inflammatory disease or tuboovarian abscess
  - Appendicitis
  - Diverticulitis
  - Cystitis or pyelonephritis

- **Treatment**
  - Emergent gynecologic consultation for exploration and correction of the torsion
  - Pain control with narcotic medications usually indicated
  - Delayed diagnosis can lead to ovarian necrosis and peritonitis

- **Pearl**

The most common cause of adnexal torsion is a benign cystic ovarian tumor; malignant tumors twist less often because of associated inflammatory reaction and scarring in the pelvis.

Reference

Challoner K, Incerpi M: Nontraumatic abdominal surgical emergencies in the pregnant patient. Emerg Med Clin North Am 2003;21:971. [PMID: 14708815]

Bartholin Abscess

- **Essentials of Diagnosis**
  - Severe labial pain, swelling and tenderness at one of the Bartholin glands (usually located at the 4 and 8 o'clock positions on the posterolateral aspect of the vestibule)
  - Endocervical and abscess cultures or other tests for *Neisseria gonorrhea* and *Chlamydia trachomatis* cultures

- **Differential Diagnosis**
  - Infected sebaceous cyst or Skene gland abscess
  - Vulvar and vaginal noninfectious lesions

- **Treatment**
  - Nonfluctuant lesions: intramuscular ceftriaxone and broad-spectrum oral antibiotics with sitz baths and warm compresses; follow up in 1 or 2 days with a gynecologist for reevaluation and possible incision and drainage
  - Fluctuant lesions: sterile prep, administer local anesthesia and make incision along the inside of the labium, drainage and packing with a Word catheter; antimicrobials and follow-up as above

- **Pearl**

Bartholin gland abscesses are polymicrobial infections occurring in patients with many of the same risk factors as those with sexually transmitted diseases (10–15% of Bartholin abscesses are caused by N gonorrhea).

Reference

Zeger W, Holt K: Gynecologic infections. Emerg Med Clin North Am 2003;21:631. [PMID: 12962350]

Cervicitis, Mucopurulent

- **Essentials of Diagnosis**
  - Classically greenish-yellow endocervical or vaginal discharge, pruritus, or nonspecific abdominal or back pain
  - Associated symptoms: dysuria, urinary frequency and urgency, pelvic pain, vaginal bleeding
  - Mucopurulent endocervical exudates, cervical friability
  - *Neisseria gonorrhoeae* and *Chlamydia trachomatis* enzyme immune assay antigen identification or genetic DNA probe amplification techniques
  - Urine pregnancy test

- **Differential Diagnosis**
  - Vaginitis

- **Treatment**
  - For chlamydia: azithromycin single dose; or erythromycin, doxycycline, ofloxacin, or levofloxacin for 7 days
  - For gonorrhea: one intramuscular ceftriaxone dose or single-dose oral therapy with cefixime
  - Patient should be instructed to encourage her partner to be tested and treated
  - Referral for RPR and HIV testing

- **Pearl**

Patients with mucopurulent cervicitis should be treated for gonorrhea and chlamydia because it is difficult to definitively differentiate the cause until cultures or other methods of identification are available.

Reference

Zeger W, Holt K: Gynecologic infections. Emerg Med Clin North Am 2003;21:631. [PMID: 12962350]

Dysmenorrhea (Painful Menstruation)

- **Essentials of Diagnosis**
  - Recurrent, crampy lower abdominal or back pain that occurs at the onset of menstruation and usually last a few days
  - Associated symptoms: headache, nausea, vomiting, diarrhea
  - Associated findings: no pelvic pathology or associated conditions such as chronic pelvic inflammatory disease or endometriosis
  - Uterine tenderness on pelvic exam but specific cervical motion tenderness usually absent
  - Normal vital signs
  - Symptoms usually begin in adolescence and can be moderately severe or debilitating
  - Absence of systemic signs of infection
  - Ultrasound: useful to exclude other causes of abdominal pain

- **Differential Diagnosis**
  - Ruptured ovarian cyst
  - Pelvic inflammatory disease
  - Tuboovarian abscess
  - Appendicitis
  - Diverticulitis
  - Pyelonephritis or cystitis

- **Treatment**
  - Symptomatic relief with nonsteroidal anti-inflammatory medications or narcotics; gynecologic referral for follow-up
  - Chronic oral contraceptives may control symptoms

- **Pearl**

Dysmenorrhea should be diagnosed only after more serious causes of pelvic pain have been excluded.

Reference

Harel Z: A contemporary approach to dysmenorrhea in adolescents. Paediatr Drugs 2002;4:797. [PMID: 12431132]

Eclampsia

- **Essentials of Diagnosis**
  - First step in evaluating a woman (not known to be pregnant) after a seizure is to obtain a urine pregnancy test
  - Headache or visual changes frequently precede the seizure and may be the only symptoms of preeclampsia
  - Complication of severe preeclampsia (pregnancy-induced hypertension), in which seizures occur usually in the third trimester and in the postpartum period (although it can occur before 20 weeks especially with molar pregnancy)
  - Risk factors: non-white race, multiparity, preeclampsia or eclampsia with previous pregnancy, mean arterial pressure >161 mm Hg
  - Clinical diagnosis based on seizures or coma occurring without other identifiable causes in the setting of preeclampsia
  - CT scan of the head to evaluate other causes of seizures or altered consciousness

- **Differential Diagnosis**
  - Intracranial pathology such as hemorrhage, cerebrovascular ischemia, intracranial tumor, meningitis, or encephalitis
  - Metabolic derangements such as hypoglycemia, hyperglycemia, or electrolyte imbalances
  - Hematologic disorders such as thrombotic thrombocytopenia purpura

- **Treatment**
  - Start with ABCs and control the airway if needed
  - Intravenous magnesium sulfate (2–3 g IV push every 15 minutes up to 6 g) or diazepam (5–10 mg IV push every 5 minutes) to control seizure or for prophylaxis of recurrence
  - Emergent obstetric consultation; delivery of fetus is only definitive treatment available
  - For hypertension: hydralazine, labetalol, or nitroprusside

- **Pearl**

The absence of proteinuria or peripheral edema cannot be used to rule out preeclampsia or eclampsia because a significant percentage of women have no proteinuria or edema associated with an eclamptic seizure.

Reference

Abbrescia K, Sheridan B: Complications of second and third trimester pregnancies. Emerg Med Clin North Am 2003;21:695. [PMID: 12962354]

Ectopic Pregnancy

- ■ Essentials of Diagnosis
  - • Life-threatening complication of pregnancy with varied presentations from minimal symptoms to hemorrhagic shock
  - • Most patients present 6–8 weeks after a missed menstrual period; almost all have a positive urine pregnancy test
  - • Common presenting complaints: pelvic pain (often unilateral) or vaginal bleeding early in pregnancy
  - • Risk factors: previous ectopic pregnancy, pelvic inflammatory disease, use of an intrauterine device, smoking, infertility treatments, tubal surgery
  - • Unilateral adnexal tenderness or mass may be present; absence of those findings cannot exclude ectopic pregnancy
  - • Pelvic ultrasound findings: obvious ectopic, or suggestion of ectopic based on secondary signs such as abnormal pelvic fluid, adnexal mass, or empty uterus
  - • Urinalysis, urine pregnancy test, hemogram, Rh blood type, quantitative hCG; consider cross-matching blood

- ■ Differential Diagnosis
  - • Threatened, incomplete, or complete spontaneous abortion
  - • Early normal intrauterine pregnancy or heterotopic pregnancy (especially in women undergoing infertility treatment)
  - • Ruptured corpus luteum cyst or adnexal torsion
  - • Appendicitis, diverticulitis, cystitis, pyelonephritis, or renal colic

- ■ Treatment
  - • Emergency consultation with gynecologist
  - • Unstable patients: resuscitate with isotonic fluids or blood and arrange for immediate laparoscopy or laparotomy
  - • Stable, reliable patients with low quantitative hCG level (<5,000) and small ectopics: some gynecologists will treat with single-dose intramuscular methotrexate if close follow-up is available (90% success rate)
  - • Patients with Rh-negative blood type: administer RhoGAM

- ■ Pearl

Syncope in a female of child-bearing age can be the initial presenting symptom of ectopic pregnancy.

Reference

Bouyer J et al: Risk factors for ectopic pregnancy: a comprehensive analysis based on a large case-control, population-based study in France. Am J Epidemiol 2003;157:185. [PMID: 12543617]

Endometriosis

- **Essentials of Diagnosis**
    - Usually cyclical or recurrent pelvic, flank, or abdominal pain and cramps with menses (dysmenorrhea), dyspareunia
    - Tenderness on pelvic exam (worse at menses); uterus may be less mobile due to inflammatory adhesions
    - Often associated with painful defecation or dyspareunia
    - Major cause of chronic pelvic pain; acute exacerbations usually prompt emergency department visit
    - Negative urine pregnancy test
    - Absence of systemic signs of infection
    - Urinalysis and cervical cultures
    - Ultrasound or CT scan may be suggestive but results usually not definitive
    - Laparoscopy: gold standard for diagnosis

- **Differential Diagnosis**
    - Ruptured ovarian cyst
    - Pelvic inflammatory disease
    - Tuboovarian abscess
    - Appendicitis
    - Diverticulitis
    - Pyelonephritis or cystitis
    - Pelvic tumor

- **Treatment**
    - Symptomatic relief with nonsteroidal anti-inflammatory medications or narcotics and gynecologic referral for follow-up
    - Gynecologists use hormonal agents to induce at least temporary remission of symptoms

- **Pearl**

Endometriosis is a major risk factor for infertility: 20–50% of infertile women have endometriosis.

Reference

Winkel CA: Evaluation and management of women with endometriosis. Obstet Gynecol 2003;102:397. [PMID: 12907119]

Endometritis, Postpartum

■ Essentials of Diagnosis

- Recent delivery (more common with cesarean than vaginal delivery)
- Abdominal pain, vaginal discharge, systemic signs of infection (fever)
- Peritoneal signs
- Boggy, exquisitely tender uterus and purulent foul-smelling lochia
- Risk factors: cesarean section, prolonged labor, prolonged rupture of membranes, multiple vaginal exams, presence of meconium, diabetes, bacterial vaginosis, colonization with group B streptococci
- Blood culture, hemogram, and endocervical cultures for aerobic and anaerobic organisms

■ Differential Diagnosis

- Appendicitis
- Diverticulitis
- Pyelonephritis or cystitis

■ Treatment

- Emergent gynecologic consultation
- Emergent broad-spectrum antibiotics (usually gentamicin and clindamycin); infections usually polymicrobial
- Watch for signs of complications such as septic pelvic thromboembolism or sepsis

■ Pearl

With the trend toward shorter postpartum hospital stays, patients with endometritis are more likely now to present to the emergency department with fever or abdominal pain than in the past.

Reference

Ledjer WJ: Post-partum endomyometritis diagnosis and treatment: a review. J Obstet Gynaecol Res 2003;29:364. [PMID: 14641683]

Hyperemesis Gravidarum

■ Essentials of Diagnosis

- Unlike minor cases of pregnancy-associated vomiting, hyperemesis gravidarum is a severe form of persistent vomiting often associated with postural dizziness, presyncope, or other signs of dehydration
- Usually occurs in first or early second trimester and resolves by week 16
- Risk factors: multiple gestation, gestational trophoblastic disease, triploidy, trisomy 21, hydrops fetalis
- Ultrasound: to confirm normal pregnancy and rule out molar pregnancy; look for gallbladder or kidney disorders
- Search for other causes; hyperemesis gravidarum is a diagnosis of exclusion
- Physical exam usually shows evidence of dehydration: tachycardia and dry mucous membranes; record weight
- Serum electrolytes and urinalysis; consider liver function tests and lipase if indicated by history

■ Differential Diagnosis

- Pyelonephritis, gastritis, or peptic ulcer disease
- Diabetic ketoacidosis
- Preeclampsia and fatty liver

■ Treatment

- Rehydration with isotonic intravenous fluids and correction of electrolyte abnormalities
- Antiemetics for severe vomiting after discussion of risk-benefit ratio with patient; common choices include prochlorperazine, 5–10 mg, or promethazine, 25 mg intravenously (both category C; safety in pregnancy has not been established); or ondansetron 2–4 mg IV or IM (category B, animal studies do not suggest toxicity or human studies have not shown any problems)
- Trial of pyridoxine (vitamin B_6) may be beneficial (category A, presumed safe in pregnancy)
- Patients with uncontrolled emesis or severe dehydration: hospitalization

■ Pearl

Just as in conditions such as peptic ulcer disease, which are associated with vomiting, Helicobacter pylori *may play a role in the cause of hyperemesis gravidarum.*

Reference

Quinlan JD, Hill DA: Nausea and vomiting of pregnancy. Am Fam Physician 2003;68:121. [PMID: 12887118]

Mastitis, Postpartum

- ■ Essentials of Diagnosis
  - Postpartum localized, usually unilateral breast pain
  - Variable systemic signs of infection (eg, fever, chills)
  - Localized tenderness, redness, induration, or warmth
  - Rare after third postpartum month
  - Risk factors: skin or nipple damage, poor hygiene, fatigue, primiparity, milk stasis
  - Abscess formation may occur

- ■ Differential Diagnosis
  - Breast abscess
  - Normal, noninfectious breast pain related to engorgement or nipple irritation
  - Plugged duct or galactocele

- ■ Treatment
  - Continue breast feeding or pumping on affected side to decompress ductal system
  - If severe, hospitalization with intravenous antibiotics such as nafcillin is recommended
  - Outpatient management: warm compresses to breast, oral antiinflammatory agents, and 7–10 days of antibiotics (cloxacillin or dicloxacillin) or, if penicillin allergic, clindamycin
  - If abscess develops, aspiration is indicated

- ■ Pearl

The source of the infection in postpartum mastitis is frequently the infant's mouth, and the most common organism is Staphylococcus aureus; *continuation of breast feeding is not harmful to the infant.*

Reference

Michie C, Lockie F, Lynn W: The challenge of mastitis. Arch Dis Child 2003;88:818. [PMID: 12937109]

Miscarriage (Spontaneous Abortion)

- **Essentials of Diagnosis**
  - Vaginal bleeding early in pregnancy often with associated pelvic and back pain (uterine cramps) in a patient with a positive urine pregnancy test may represent a miscarriage
  - Variable pelvic exam findings: often suprapubic tenderness on palpation, vaginal bleeding ranging from spotting to severe hemorrhage; status of the cervical os (open versus closed) can be important for management
  - Pelvic ultrasound often used to evaluate presence of retained products of conception or the possibility of ectopic pregnancy and to determine if fetal cardiac activity is present; findings consistent with impending miscarriage are abnormal gestational sac size, small embryo for gestation, and slow fetal heart rate
  - Baseline hemogram; quantitative hCG; Rh blood type
  - Types of spontaneous miscarriage: *threatened,* pregnancy in jeopardy; *inevitable,* open cervix or passage of some or all of products of conception; *complete/incomplete,* depends on the presence of retained products of conception; *missed abortion,* retained conceptus
  - Submit to pathology any tissue passed or removed during exam

- **Differential Diagnosis**
  - Ectopic pregnancy (presentation can be similar)
  - Normal menses or early intrauterine pregnancy with bleeding associated with implantation

- **Treatment**
  - If vaginal bleeding or abdominal or back pain is severe and diagnosis of spontaneous abortion is confirmed clinically, dilation and curettage of the uterus can be performed to decrease symptoms and slow bleeding
  - Usually patient is discharged from the emergency department with close gynecologic follow-up and instructions to return for fever, worsening abdominal or back pain, heavy vaginal bleeding, or syncope
  - Treatment of pain symptoms with narcotic medications if necessary
  - Patients with Rh-negative blood type: administer RhoGAM

- **Pearl**

Only 5% of women with an intrauterine pregnancy and fetal heart tones noted by ultrasound will miscarry.

Reference

Coppola PT, Coppola M: Vaginal bleeding in the first 20 weeks of pregnancy. Emerg Med Clin North Am 2003;21:667. [PMID: 12962352]

Ovarian Cyst, Ruptured

- **Essentials of Diagnosis**
  - Sudden, moderate to severe unilateral pelvic pain
  - Possible history of initial nausea, diaphoresis, near syncope
  - Lack of systemic signs of infection
  - Usually negative urine pregnancy test
  - Unilateral adnexal tenderness with or without mass
  - Baseline hemogram, urinalysis, pelvic exam with cervical cultures
  - Transvaginal pelvic ultrasound can be diagnostic; Doppler flow analysis used to exclude adnexal torsion

- **Differential Diagnosis**
  - Ectopic pregnancy
  - Pelvic inflammatory disease or tuboovarian abscess
  - Adnexal torsion
  - Appendicitis
  - Diverticulitis
  - Cystitis or pyelonephritis

- **Treatment**
  - Pay close attention to vital signs to identify significant ongoing hemorrhage
  - Rarely, ruptured ovarian cysts can be associated with significant hemoperitoneum requiring surgical exploration for control of hemorrhage
  - Most patients can be treated as outpatients with close gynecologic follow-up arranged
  - Pain control with narcotic medications may be indicated
  - Instructions to return for syncope or worsening abdominal or pelvic pain

- **Pearl**

The most common types of ruptured ovarian cysts include dermoid, cystadenoma, and endometrioma cysts; unlike corpus luteum cysts, these cysts do not have the potential to cause significant hemoperitoneum with rupture, although the contents that spill into the peritoneal cavity can cause local irritation and pelvic pain.

Reference

Hertzberg BS, Kliewer MA, Paulson EK: Ovarian cyst rupture causing hemoperitoneum: imaging features and the potential for misdiagnosis. Abdom Imaging 1999;24:304. [PMID: 10227900]

Pelvic Inflammatory Disease (PID; Salpingitis)

- ■ Essentials of Diagnosis
  - Lower abdominal pain of gradual or sudden onset, either continuous or crampy
  - Vaginal discharge or bleeding
  - Symptoms usually occur during or shortly after menstruation
  - Fever often present; other common symptoms: anorexia, nausea, vomiting
  - Lower abdominal tenderness; cervical motion and bilateral lower adnexal tenderness often with peritoneal signs
  - Risk factors: young age, multiple sexual partners, intrauterine device insertion, vaginal douching, tobacco smoking, chlamydial or gonococcal infection, bacterial vaginosis
  - Pelvic ultrasound: may demonstrate thickened fluid-filled tubes with or without free fluid or a tuboovarian abscess
  - Laparoscopy is gold standard for diagnosis; diagnosis usually made on clinical criteria

- ■ Differential Diagnosis
  - Tuboovarian abscess (usually a complication)
  - Ruptured ovarian cyst or adnexal torsion
  - Appendicitis or diverticulitis
  - Cystitis or pyelonephritis

- ■ Treatment
  - Indications for admission: uncertain diagnosis, pelvic abscess, pregnancy, adolescence, severe illness, inability to tolerate outpatient oral regimen, failure of outpatient management, inability to arrange follow-up, HIV-positive status
  - Intravenous antibiotics: (1) cefoxitin or cefotetan with doxycycline, (2) clindamycin and gentamicin, (3) a fluoroquinolone (ofloxacin) plus metronidazole, or (4) ampicillin-sulbactam plus doxycycline
  - For patients who meet outpatient treatment criteria: (1) administer an intramuscular injection of a third-generation cephalosporin and prescribe a 14-day regimen of doxycycline or (2) prescribe a 14-day regimen of a fluoroquinolone with metronidazole
  - Referral for RPR and HIV testing

- ■ Pearl

Pelvic inflammatory disease should be treated aggressively in an effort to reduce the complications related to scarring, including infertility.

Reference

Zeger W, Holt K: Gynecologic infections. Emerg Med Clin North Am 2003;21:631. [PMID: 12962350]

Placenta Previa

- ■ Essentials of Diagnosis
  - Painless bright red vaginal bleeding in the third trimester related to placental location in the lower uterine segment at or near the cervical os
  - Uterine contractions may occur in association with the bleeding
  - Sudden massive hemorrhage can occur, posing a threat to the lives of the fetus and the mother
  - Risk factors: previous cesarean section, increased age, smoking, minority race, multiparity, multiple gestations, previous placenta previa, previous abortion
  - To avoid precipitating a severe hemorrhage, never perform a speculum or bimanual exam in patients with third-trimester bleeding
  - Ultrasound: useful for identifying position of placenta in relation to the cervical os; previa, by definition, is implantation of the placenta in the lower uterine segment either partially or completely covering the cervical os
  - Baseline hemogram; send clot of blood for typing and cross-matching

- ■ Differential Diagnosis
  - Placental abruption
  - Vasa previa
  - Lower genital tract bleeding
  - Systemic coagulopathy

- ■ Treatment
  - Emergent obstetric consultation and admission
  - Close monitoring of mother and fetus
  - Resuscitation with intravenous fluids or blood if indicated
  - Maternal complications: hysterectomy, antepartum hemorrhage, blood transfusions, septicemia, thrombophlebitis
  - Emergent delivery by cesarean section required if fetal distress occurs

- ■ Pearl

Unlike placental abruption, the uterus usually remains soft with bleeding associated with placenta previa, although associated contractions occur in 20% of patients.

Reference

Abbrescia K, Sheridan B: Complications of second and third trimester pregnancies. Emerg Med Clin North Am 2003;21:695. [PMID: 12962354]

Placental Abruption

■ Essentials of Diagnosis
  - Clinical triad of external (or occult) vaginal bleeding, uterine tenderness (and hyperactivity), and fetal distress (or death)
  - Risk factors: hypertension, advanced maternal age, multiparity, multifetal gestation, smoking, blunt abdominal trauma, cocaine use, poor nutrition, preterm premature rupture of membranes, polyhydramnios, chorioamnionitis, previous abruption
  - Grade I: minimal placental separation, usually asymptomatic (40%)
  - Grade II: moderate vaginal bleeding or hematoma formation, uterine tenderness, and prolonged contractions; may have signs of maternal shock or fetal distress (45%)
  - Grade III: severe vaginal bleeding, extreme uterine tenderness, fetal demise, maternal shock, risk for disseminated intravascular coagulation (DIC)
  - CBC, coagulation studies (fibrinogen, fibrin degradation products, PT, PTT, blood typing and cross-matching
  - Ultrasound: used in evaluation but results can be nondiagnostic in 50% of cases; negative ultrasound cannot be used to rule out abruption

■ Differential Diagnosis
  - Placenta previa
  - Vasa previa
  - Lower genital tract bleeding
  - Systemic coagulopathy

■ Treatment
  - Emergent obstetric consultation and admission
  - Emergent cesarean section if fetal distress
  - Close monitoring of mother and fetus (even after minor trauma in the second and third trimesters)
  - Resuscitation with intravenous fluids or blood if indicated
  - Watch for maternal complications including DIC, acute renal failure from hypovolemia, and death

■ Pearl

With a fetal mortality rate of 35%, abruption is the most common cause of intrapartum fetal death.

Reference

Abbrescia K, Sheridan B: Complications of second and third trimester pregnancies. Emerg Med Clin North Am 2003;21:695. [PMID: 12962354]

Preeclampsia

- **Essentials of Diagnosis**
  - Development during pregnancy (or early postpartum) of hypertension (blood pressure ≥140/90) and proteinuria or pathologic edema
  - As blood pressure, proteinuria, and edema worsen, creatinine becomes elevated (>1.2) and the hemolysis, elevated liver enzymes, low platelets (HELLP) syndrome may develop
  - Eclampsia (seizure) is most dangerous complication of preeclampsia
  - Risk factors: nulliparity, age over 35 years, diabetes, personal or family history of pregnancy-induced hypertension, multiple gestations, obesity, African-American ethnicity, chronic hypertension, renal disease
  - Headache, visual changes or vertigo, or upper abdominal pain
  - Physical findings: elevated blood pressure or frank hypertension, abdominal tenderness, hyperreflexivity, peripheral edema, decreased urine output or anuria
  - Laboratory findings: elevated BUN, serum creatinine, and urate; proteinuria; disseminated intravascular coagulation; thrombocytopenia

- **Differential Diagnosis**
  - Gestational hypertension: isolated hypertension that develops during pregnancy without any of the findings or complications of preeclampsia
  - Chronic hypertension: hypertension existing before and continuing after pregnancy

- **Treatment**
  - Emergent obstetric consultation
  - For hypertension: hydralazine, labetalol, or nitroprusside
  - For hyperreflexia: magnesium sulfate
  - Definitive treatment: delivery of fetus

- **Pearl**

Symptoms of preeclampsia are so variable that whenever a woman in the third trimester of pregnancy or up to 1 month following delivery presents to the emergency department with any complaint, her blood pressure should be taken and her urine checked for proteinuria.

Reference

Abbrescia K, Sheridan B: Complications of second and third trimester pregnancies. Emerg Med Clin North Am 2003;21:695. [PMID: 12962354]

Septic Abortion

- Essentials of Diagnosis
  - History of recent pregnancy may be withheld, check urine pregnancy test, which should still be positive
  - Recent surgical (especially nonsterile, nontherapeutic abortion) or spontaneous abortion
  - Diffuse pelvic tenderness with foul-smelling vaginal discharge
  - Systemic signs of infection including fever and leukocytosis; clinical spectrum may include shock
  - Baseline hemogram, serum chemistries; coagulation studies including PT/PTT, fibrin split products, and fibrinogen level; blood, urine, and cervical cultures and gram stains
  - Pelvic ultrasound may demonstrate intrauterine material, CT scan may demonstrate uterine emphysema or intraperitoneal free air from uterine perforation
  - Rapid diagnosis is essential because complications such as bacteremia, pelvic abscess, septic pelvic thrombophlebitis, disseminated intravascular coagulopathy, septic shock, renal failure, and death occur more commonly if diagnosis is delayed

- Differential Diagnosis
  - Incomplete abortion with pain and tenderness
  - Other causes of intra-abdominal infections such as appendicitis, diverticulitis, cystitis, or pyelonephritis
  - Missed ectopic pregnancy

- Treatment
  - Emergent gynecologic consultation for evacuation of uterine contents or hysterectomy
  - Rapid administration of broad-spectrum intravenous antibiotics (after appropriate cultures), such as ampicillin, 2–3 g IV every 6 hours, plus clindamycin, 900 mg IV every 8 hours, and gentamicin, loading dose of 2 mg/kg
  - Treat septic shock with fluid resuscitation and watch for complications mentioned above

- Pearl

The morbidity and mortality of septic abortion are rare in countries where induced abortion is legal but is significant in the many developing countries where it is either illegal or inaccessible.

Reference

Tamussino K: Postoperative infection. Clin Obstet Gynecol 2002;45:562. [PMID: 12048413]

Sexual Assault

- **Essentials of Diagnosis**
  - As with any form of trauma, always start with the ABCs and then perform a secondary survey
  - Law enforcement officials should be notified of any sexual assault complaint, if required by law
  - The evaluation should occur in a quiet location and in a non-threatening manner; obtain an appropriate history
  - If the assault occurred within 72 hours of the evaluation, and only if the patient consents, perform the rape exam (a systematic, thorough physical exam in which evidence is collected carefully and passed off to police to ensure proper chain of custody)
  - Obtain culture swabs from various sites as indicated based on history; urine pregnancy test; obtain or refer for testing for RPR, HIV, and hepatitis B titer
  - Pelvic exam may not reveal any physical signs of injury

- **Differential Diagnosis**
  - In the case of a child with vaginal irritation, vulvovaginitis may be a cause unrelated to sexual abuse

- **Treatment**
  - Ideally a counselor will accompany the patient in the emergency department to provide additional emotional support
  - Treatment of associated injuries as appropriate
  - Prophylaxis for sexually transmitted diseases, including bacterial vaginosis (oral metronidazole), gonorrhea (intramuscular ceftriaxone or oral ciprofloxacin), chlamydia (oral azithromycin or doxycycline), and hepatitis B (vaccine)
  - Pregnancy prophylaxis (if urine pregnancy test is negative): norgestrel with an antiemetic to control nausea associated with high-dose norgestrel
  - Medically stable patients with a safe place to go: arrange outpatient follow-up prior to discharge
  - Follow up with primary care physician or health department for further testing

- **Pearl**

Sexual assault is an unfortunately common occurrence; almost 18% of women admit to being raped, but only 16% of cases are ever reported to police.

Reference

Cantu M, Coppola M, Lindner AJ: Evaluation and management of the sexually assaulted woman. Emerg Med Clin North Am 2003;21:737. [PMID: 12962356]

Tuboovarian Abscess (TOA)

- ■ Essentials of Diagnosis
  - • A complication of pelvic inflammatory disease (PID), although other conditions such as ruptured appendicitis and diverticulitis can cause TOA
  - • Pelvic pain with severe lower abdominal tenderness and fever often present
  - • Pelvic ultrasound: test of choice (sensitivity 93%, specificity 98%) to evaluate a patient with PID; recommended for those patients ill enough to require admission, those not responding to appropriate therapy, or those with a palpable mass on pelvic exam
  - • Abdominal CT scan can be used for initial evaluation or to better define the abscess

- ■ Differential Diagnosis
  - • Uncomplicated PID
  - • Ruptured ovarian cyst
  - • Adnexal torsion
  - • Pelvic neoplasm
  - • Endometriosis
  - • Appendicitis
  - • Diverticulitis
  - • Pyelonephritis or cystitis

- ■ Treatment
  - • Aggressive inpatient therapy, including intravenous fluids and broad-spectrum intravenous antibiotics; antibiotic regimens include (1) ofloxacin, 400 mg IV every 12 hours, and metronidazole, 500 mg every 8 hours, or (2) ampicillin-sulbactam, 3 g IV every 8 hours, and doxycycline, 100 mg IV or orally every 12 hours
  - • Close monitoring for the development of sepsis; rupture and subsequent sepsis are associated with a mortality rate of 25%
  - • Surgical drainage options include laparoscopy or laparotomy
  - • Ultrasound-guided drainage has become another option for some patients
  - • Referral for RPR and HIV testing

- ■ Pearl

The treatment of TOA has changed significantly with the development of percutaneous drainage techniques utilizing ultrasound.

Reference

Zeger W, Holt K: Gynecologic infections. Emerg Med Clin North Am 2003;21:631. [PMID: 12962350]

Uterine Prolapse

- ■ Essentials of Diagnosis
  - • Prior vaginal deliveries
  - • History of pelvic heaviness, vaginal mass (sensation of sitting on lump), low back pain, dyspareunia
  - • Diagnosis made by speculum exam
  - • Patient may present with urinary retention or other urinary symptoms
  - • Firm muscular mass protruding from vagina especially with bearing down in the lithotomy position
  - • Vaginal pain, bleeding, or discharge
  - • Cystocele, rectocele, and enterocoele are commonly associated with procidentia

- ■ Differential Diagnosis
  - • Vaginal tumor
  - • Cystocele
  - • Rectocele
  - • Enterocoele

- ■ Treatment
  - • Acute postpartum prolapse is an emergency requiring immediate obstetric consultation
  - • Urgent gynecologic consultation for patients with uterine prolapse and ureteral obstruction, urinary retention, or procidentia (complete rectal prolapse)
  - • Nonsurgical treatment: use of pessary inserted into the vagina in addition to vaginal estrogen cream
  - • Patients with mild prolapse: refer for gynecologic evaluation within 5–7 days for possible surgery

- ■ Pearl

Uterine prolapse is not associated with ischemia to the tissues that have been displaced from their normal anatomic position by weaknesses in the supporting ligaments (sacrouterine and cardinal).

Reference

Harrison BP, Cespedes RD: Pelvic organ prolapse. Emerg Med Clin North Am 2001;19:781. [PMID: 11554287]

Vaginitis

- ■ Essentials of Diagnosis
  - • Abnormal vaginal discharge
  - • Vulvovaginal pruritus, irritation, odor
  - • Inflamed cervix
  - • Causes can be infectious, estrogen deficiency (atrophic vaginitis), or chemical irritation
  - • Consider vaginal foreign bodies, especially in young girls
  - • Ask about recent antibiotics
  - • Potassium hydroxide and normal saline wet preps may yield diagnosis (candida, trichomoniasis, bacterial vaginosis): candida: buds and hyphae on KOH; trichomoniasis: motile, flagellated trichomonads; bacterial vaginosis: "clue cells" = epithelial cells with a finely granulated cytoplasm and indistinct borders as if the cell were covered with a light coating of sand
  - • Urinalysis (urethral catheterization preferred), urine pregnancy test, cervical cultures for gonorrhea and chlamydia, consider fingerstick blood glucose
  - • Consider sexual abuse in all pediatric patients with vaginitis

- ■ Differential Diagnosis
  - • Associated pelvic inflammatory disease
  - • Mucopurulent cervicitis
  - • Vaginal neoplasm

- ■ Treatment
  - • Based on underlying cause: candida (antifungal), bacterial vaginosis (metronidazole topical or oral), atrophic (topical estrogen)
  - • Wear loose-fitting cotton underpants with skirts
  - • Sitz baths for possible relief
  - • Avoidance of sexual intercourse for a few days after treatment; ensure partners are also treated
  - • Follow up with gynecologist or primary care physician for further evaluation and to discuss results of cultures

- ■ Pearl

In patients with recurrent candidal vaginitis, consider undiagnosed diabetes.

Reference

Anderson MR, Klink K, Cohrssen A: Evaluation of vaginal complaints. JAMA 2004;291:1368. [PMID: 15026404]

14

Eye Emergencies

Acute Angle Closure Glaucoma

- **Essentials of Diagnosis**
  - Acute onset of moderate to severe, unilateral eye pain
  - Eye redness that is more pronounced in perilimbal area
  - May be provoked by a dark or low-light environment
  - Haloes around lights
  - Blurred vision
  - Nausea and vomiting
  - Mid-dilated unreactive pupil, often with irregular margins
  - Hazy (steamy) cornea due to corneal edema
  - Shallow anterior chamber
  - Increased intraocular pressure

- **Differential Diagnosis**
  - Uveitis (iritis and iridocyclitis)
  - Conjunctivitis
  - Corneal ulcer

- **Treatment**
  - Immediate ophthalmologic consult
  - Sedation and analgesia to control pain and agitation
  - Reduce intraocular pressure by using one or more of the following: timolol 0.5%, 1 drop; pilocarpine 2%, 2 drops every 15 minutes; mannitol 20%, 1–2 g/kg IV over 2–3 hours; acetazolamide, 500 mg orally or IV; glycerin, 1g/kg orally in cold 50% solution mixed with chilled lemon juice

- **Pearl**

Acute pain and a unilateral red eye is acute angle closure glaucoma until proved otherwise.

Reference

Leibowitz HM: The red eye. N Engl J Med 2000;343:345. [PMID: 10922425]

Cavernous Sinus Thrombosis

- **Essentials of Diagnosis**
  - Decreased vision associated with headache, nausea, fever, chills, and other signs of systemic infection
  - Unilateral or bilateral exophthalmos, absent pupillary reflexes and papilledema
  - Cranial nerve (CN) palsies, especially of CN III, CN IV, CN VI, or the ophthalmic branch of CN V
  - High-resolution thin-slice CT or MRI is invaluable in making the diagnosis

- **Differential Diagnosis**
  - Orbital cellulitis
  - Preseptal cellulitis
  - Cranial nerve palsy
  - Meningitis
  - Ophthalmoplegic migraine

- **Treatment**
  - Hospitalization
  - Ophthalmologic and neurologic consult
  - Intravenous antibiotics to cover *Staphylococcus aureus,* pneumococci, streptococci, gram-negative bacteria and anaerobes: nafcillin or oxacillin, 2.0 g IV every 4 hours, plus third-generation cephalosporin or imipenem, 0.5 g IV every 6 hours; consider vancomycin if methicillin-resistant *S aureus* is a possibility
  - Use of anticoagulants and steroids is controversial, but heparin is generally recommended

- **Pearl**

Do not be fooled by the name; cavernous sinus thrombosis is a life-threatening infection with a 30% mortality rate, not a primary coagulation problem.

Reference

Ebright JR, Pace MT, Niazi AF: Septic thrombosis of the cavernous sinuses. Arch Intern Med 2001;161:2671. [PMID: 11732931]

Central Retinal Artery Occlusion

- **Essentials of Diagnosis**
  - Sudden, painless, complete loss of vision in one eye
  - Ophthalmoscopy reveals pallor of the optic disk, retinal edema, cherry-red fovea, and "boxcar" segmentation of the blood in the retinal veins
  - Bloodless constricted arterioles may be difficult to visualize
  - Occurs primarily in patients at increased risk for other thromboembolic diseases (eg, those with hypertension, diabetes, vascular disease, sickle cell anemia, or other hypercoagulable states; IV drug abusers)
  - Normal-appearing retinal vessels do not rule out central retinal artery occlusion

- **Differential Diagnosis**
  - Acute angle closure glaucoma
  - Retinal detachment
  - Retinal hemorrhage
  - Retinal vein occlusion
  - Optic neuritis or papillitis
  - Methanol poisoning
  - Vitreous hemorrhage
  - Cerebrovascular accident
  - Complicated migraine
  - Temporal (giant cell) arteritis
  - Hysterical blindness

- **Treatment**
  - Ophthalmologic consult
  - Ocular massage: intermittent pressure for 10 seconds with 5-second pauses
  - Acetazolamide, 500 mg IV
  - Timolol 0.5%, 1 drop

- **Pearl**

Central retinal artery occlusion should be thought of as an "eye stroke" or "eye attack" and should be treated with the same urgency as an ischemic cerebrovascular accident or acute coronary syndrome.

Reference

Beatty S, Au Eong KG: Acute occlusion of the retinal arteries: current concepts and recent advances in diagnosis and management. J Accid Emerg Med 2000;17:324. [PMID: 11005400]

Central Retinal Vein Occlusion

■ Essentials of Diagnosis

- Sudden, painless, unilateral loss of vision
- Most common risk factors: advanced age, hypertension, diabetes, glaucoma
- Ophthalmoscopy reveals dilated, tortuous veins; retinal and macular edema; retinal hemorrhages; and attenuated arterioles
- Episodes of amaurosis fugax may precede retinal vein occlusion
- Patient may describe floaters

■ Differential Diagnosis

- Retinal hemorrhage
- Retinal vasculitis
- Optic neuritis or papillitis
- Retinal detachment
- Retinal artery occlusion
- Vitreous hemorrhage
- Acute angle closure glaucoma
- Cerebrovascular accident
- Complicated migraine
- Methanol poisoning
- Temporal (giant cell) arteritis
- Hysterical blindness

■ Treatment

- Urgent ophthalmologic consult or referral
- No currently accepted specific or effective therapy

■ Pearl

Central retinal vein occlusion is second only to diabetic retinopathy as the most common cause of vision loss.

Reference

Sharma A, D'Amico DJ: Medical and surgical management of central retinal vein occlusion. Int Ophthalmol Clin 2004;44:1. [PMID: 14704516]

Conjunctivitis

- **Essentials of Diagnosis**
  - Most frequent cause of a red eye
  - Multiple causes including bacteria, viruses, chlamydia, allergens, and irritants
  - Scratchy, "sand in the eye" discomfort
  - Purulent or mucopurulent discharge that causes matted eyelids after sleeping
  - Preauricular adenopathy may be present
  - Vision is preserved

- **Differential Diagnosis**
  - Acute angle closure glaucoma
  - Viral keratoconjunctivitis
  - Subconjunctival hemorrhage
  - Blepharitis
  - Episcleritis or scleritis
  - Acute anterior uveitis

- **Treatment**
  - Eye drops four times a day for daytime use: trimethoprim/polymyxin B, 1 mg/mL; sulfacetamide 10%; or ciprofloxacin, 0.3%
  - Eye ointment for use at bedtime: erythromycin 0.5% or gentamicin 0.3%
  - For suspected chlamydial conjunctivitis, also give an appropriate oral medication for 1–3 weeks: erythromycin, 250 mg four times a day; or doxycycline, 100 mg twice a day
  - For gonococcal conjunctivitis, add ceftriaxone, 125 mg IM
  - Warm compresses may provide symptomatic relief and assist with the matted lids

- **Pearl**

A review of 6,872 references on conjunctivitis published in the British Medical Journal *in 2004 concluded there was no evidence in the world's literature to support any signs or symptoms that would distinguish bacterial from viral conjunctivitis.*

Reference

Leibowitz HM: The red eye. N Engl J Med 2000;343:345. [PMID: 10922425]

Corneal Abrasions

- **Essentials of Diagnosis**
  - Pain, photophobia, and blurred vision almost universally present
  - History of minor eye trauma generally offered
  - Proparacaine or tetracaine 0.5% gives patient prompt, significant relief and facilitates examination
  - Fluorescein stain reveals corneal epithelial defect
  - Eversion of upper lid to inspect for foreign body is essential

- **Differential Diagnosis**
  - Corneal ulcer
  - Corneal foreign body
  - Viral keratoconjunctivitis
  - Keratitis

- **Treatment**
  - Achieve cycloplegia and mydriasis for pain relief: cyclopentolate 0.5% or tropicamide 0.5%; avoid using atropine due to prolonged duration of action
  - Oral analgesics as needed
  - Nonsteroidal ophthalmic drops may provide pain relief: ketorolac 0.5% solution
  - Eye drops four times a day for daytime use: trimethoprim/ polymyxin B, 1 mg/ml; sulfacetamide sodium 10%; or ciprofloxacin 0.3%
  - Eye ointment for use at bedtime: erythromycin 0.5% or gentamicin 0.3%; avoid corticosteroid-containing ointments
  - Ophthalmologic referral for abrasions that do not heal within 48–72 hours

- **Pearl**

Never use anesthetic drops for ongoing symptomatic relief of pain due to toxicity that may delay healing or contribute to the formation of a corneal ulcer.

Reference

Weaver CS, Terrell KM: Update: Do ophthalmic nonsteroidal anti-inflammatory drugs reduce the pain associated with simple corneal abrasion without delaying healing? Ann Emerg Med 2003;41:134. [PMID: 12514694]

Corneal Foreign Bodies

■ Essentials of Diagnosis
  - Pain and foreign body sensation
  - Slit-lamp examination to identify foreign body
  - Upper eyelid eversion to rule out additional foreign bodies
  - Fluorescein exam to rule out other injury
  - May need to consider X-ray or CT to rule out intraocular foreign bodies in the case of high-speed (drill) injuries

■ Differential Diagnosis
  - Corneal abrasion
  - Intraocular foreign body

■ Treatment
  - Removal of foreign body by a moist cotton swab, eye spud, or small-bore (25- or 27-gauge) needle after instillation of anesthetic drops
  - After foreign body removal, treat like a corneal abrasion
  - Achieve cycloplegia and mydriasis for pain relief: cyclopentolate 0.5% or tropicamide 0.5%; avoid using atropine due to prolonged duration of action
  - Oral analgesics as needed
  - Nonsteroidal eye drops may provide pain relief: ketorolac 0.5% solution
  - Eye drops four times a day for daytime use: trimethoprim/polymyxin B, 1 mg/ml; sulfacetamide sodium 10%; OR ciprofloxacin 0.3%
  - Eye ointment for use at bedtime: erythromycin 0.5% or gentamicin 0.3%; avoid corticosteroid-containing ointments
  - Ophthalmologic referral for abrasions that do not heal within 48–72 hours

■ Pearl

Rust rings that form from iron-containing metallic foreign bodies should be removed completely to avoid permanent staining of the corneal stroma.

Reference

Reich J: Investigating a foreign body. Part 2—removal. Aust Fam Physician 2000;29:1086. [PMID: 11127070]

Corneal Ulcer

- **Essentials of Diagnosis**
  - Eye pain, photophobia, blurry vision, eye irritation
  - Conjunctival hyperemia, chemosis
  - Ulceration or infiltrate seen on slit-lamp examination with fluorescein

- **Differential Diagnosis**
  - Corneal abrasion
  - Recurrent corneal abrasion (corneal erosion)
  - Conjunctivitis
  - Iritis
  - Acute glaucoma
  - Corneal foreign body

- **Treatment**
  - Ophthalmologic consult for urgent and ongoing care
  - Cultures of the ulcer, eyelid margins, and conjunctivae
  - Gram stain of corneal scrapings
  - Broad-spectrum antibiotic drops as directed by ophthalmologist
  - Oral analgesics

- **Pearl**

Contact lens wearers with what appears to be an atraumatic corneal abrasion should receive treatment as though they have a corneal ulcer.

Reference

Benson WH, Lainer JD: Current diagnosis and treatment of corneal ulcer. Curr Opin Ophthalmol 1998;9:45. [PMID: 10387468]

Dacryocystitis, Dacryoadenitis

- **Essentials of Diagnosis**
  - Dacryocystitis: swelling, pain, redness, and tenderness over the lacrimal sac, inferior and medial to the eye on the proximal lateral portion of the nose
  - Dacryoadenitis: swelling, pain, redness, and tenderness over the lacrimal gland, at the temporal aspect of the upper eyelid

- **Differential Diagnosis**
  - Cutaneous abscess
  - Preseptal cellulitis
  - Mumps
  - Sjögren syndrome
  - Malignancy
  - Sarcoidosis

- **Treatment**
  - Warm compresses
  - Antibiotics: cephalexin, 250 mg orally four times daily; amoxicillin/clavulanate, 875/125 mg orally every 12 hours
  - Antibiotic eye drops and ointment
  - Dacryocystitis: drain and collect pus for culture and sensitivity by massage and expression from the punctum
  - Dacryoadenitis: drain and collect pus for culture and sensitivity by incision and drainage
  - Discharge with referral to an ophthalmologist in 1–3 days

- **Pearl**

Beware of that "superficial abscess on the side of the nose"; it may be acute dacryocystitis.

Reference

Greenberg MF, Pollard ZF: The red eye in childhood. Pediatr Clin N Am 2003;50:105. [PMID: 12713107]

Hordeolum

- **Essentials of Diagnosis**
  - Pain, redness, and swelling over the eyelid
  - A localized, pointing abscess may be seen at either the skin or the conjunctiva
  - Usually caused by *Staphylococcus aureus*
  - Internal hordeolum: caused by infection of meibomian gland
  - External hordeolum: caused by infection of gland of Zeis or Moll

- **Differential Diagnosis**
  - Preseptal cellulitis
  - Blepharitis
  - Dacryocystitis
  - Chalazion

- **Treatment**
  - Warm compresses
  - Antibiotic ointment: erythromycin 0.5% or gentamicin 0.3%
  - Oral antibiotics may be necessary for lesions not improving with conservative care
  - If pus is localized and pointing to the skin: may be drained through a horizontal incision
  - If pus is localized and pointing to the conjunctiva: a vertical incision may be made

- **Pearl**

A hordeolum is painful and can be differentiated from a chalazion based on tenderness.

Reference

Lederman C, Miller M: Hordeola and chalazia. Pediatr Rev 1999;20:283. [PMID: 10429150]

Hyphema

- **Essentials of Diagnosis**
  - Generally results from direct blunt trauma to the globe
  - Blood can be seen in the anterior chamber and settles out when the patient remains upright
  - Sudden decrease in visual acuity
  - Symptoms of acute glaucoma may occur with increased intraocular pressure
  - Conjunctiva is hyperemic with perilimbal injection

- **Differential Diagnosis**
  - Glaucoma
  - Ruptured globe
  - Hypopyon
  - Iritis
  - Corneal abrasion

- **Treatment**
  - Emergent ophthalmologic evaluation
  - Elevation of patient's head to 30 degrees
  - Shielding of the affected eye
  - Measurement of intraocular pressure

- **Pearl**

A completely filled anterior chamber with black clots has been referred to as an "eight-ball hemorrhage."

Reference

Sankar PS et al: Traumatic hyphema. Int Ophthalmol Clin 2002;42:57. [PMID: 12131583]

Ocular Chemical Burns

■ Essentials of Diagnosis
  - History of toxic exposure
  - Alkali burns are the most serious due to rapid penetration into the corneal stroma and saponification
  - Corneal haze and edema with or without concomitant eyelid injury
  - Varied degrees of fluorescein uptake depending on severity of exposure

■ Differential Diagnosis
  - Corneal abrasion
  - Corneal ulcer
  - Keratitis
  - Corneal foreign body

■ Treatment
  - Topical anesthetic drops to facilitate examination: proparacaine 0.5% or tetracaine 0.5%
  - Copious irrigation with water or isotonic solution after instillation of topical anesthetic until pH is 6.8–7.4
  - Particular attention directed at removing any solid particles
  - Narcotic or non-narcotic analgesics
  - Topical mydriatic
  - Antibiotic ointment
  - Emergent ophthalmologic consult

■ Pearl

Never attempt to neutralize an alkali or acid chemical exposure due to the resultant exothermic reaction and subsequent further injury.

Reference

Kuckelkorn R et al: Emergency treatment of chemical and thermal eye burns. Acta Ophthalmol Scand 2002;80:4. [PMID: 11906296]

Ocular Thermal Burns

■ **Essentials of Diagnosis**
- History of thermal exposure
- Injury may be obvious and include any and all structures of the eye, or may be more subtle and demonstrated only by slit-lamp examination with fluorescein

■ **Differential Diagnosis**
- Chemical burns
- Corneal abrasion
- Corneal foreign body
- Corneal ulcer
- Conjunctivitis
- Keratitis

■ **Treatment**
- Topical anesthetic drops to facilitate examination: proparacaine 0.5% or tetracaine 0.5%
- Narcotic or non-narcotic analgesics as needed
- Ophthalmologic consult

■ **Pearl**

Superficial corneal burns from curling irons were fairly common injuries until manufacturers began to place protective caps on the ends of the irons.

Reference

Kuckelkorn R et al: Emergency treatment of chemical and thermal eye burns. Acta Ophthalmol Scand 2002;80:4. [PMID: 11906296]

Ocular Ultraviolet Burns

- **Essentials of Diagnosis**
  - Onset 6–12 hours after exposure to an ultraviolet light source, usually a welder's arc, tanning light, or intense sunlight
  - Intense pain, photophobia, conjunctival hyperemia, copious tearing
  - Corneal edema with diffuse superficial punctate uptake of fluorescein on slit-lamp examination

- **Differential Diagnosis**
  - Dry eye syndrome
  - Corneal ulcer
  - Acute angle closure glaucoma
  - Viral keratoconjunctivitis
  - Conjunctivitis
  - Corneal foreign body
  - Corneal abrasion

- **Treatment**
  - Topical anesthetic drops to facilitate examination: proparacaine 0.5% or tetracaine 0.5%
  - Short-acting cycloplegic drop to relieve ciliary spasm: cyclopentolate 0.5% or tropicamide 0.5%
  - Oral narcotic and non-narcotic analgesics
  - Eye ointments (drops burn too much to be helpful): erythromycin 0.5% or gentamicin 0.3%
  - Ophthalmologic referral for burns that do not heal within 24–48 hours

- **Pearl**

Ultraviolet keratitis is also known as snowblindness, welder's flash, arc eye, actinic keratitis, and flash burn.

Reference

Schein OD: Phototoxicity and the cornea. J Natl Med Assoc 1992;84:579. [PMID: 1620021]

Orbital Cellulitis

- **Essentials of Diagnosis**
  - Periorbital swelling and redness
  - Proptosis
  - Painful, limited extra-ocular muscle movement
  - Systemic signs of infection
  - Most commonly the result of direct extension of paranasal sinusitis
  - CT of the head and orbit to rule out abscess
  - Primary organisms: *Streptococcus pneumoniae, Staphylococcus aureus,* non-typeable *Haemophilus influenzae,* anaerobes, and polymicrobial infections
  - Can be caused by phycomycosis (*Mucor, Rhizopus*) in diabetics and immunocompromised patients
  - Can spread to the cavernous sinus or meninges

- **Differential Diagnosis**
  - Preseptal cellulitis
  - Cavernous sinus thrombosis
  - Orbital abscess
  - Sinusitis
  - Odontogenic infection
  - Malignancy, especially retinoblastoma

- **Treatment**
  - Hospitalization
  - Intravenous broad-spectrum antibiotics: ceftriaxone, 1–2 g IV, plus vancomycin, 1 g IV; piperacillin/tazobactam, 3.375 g IV.
  - Antifungals if appropriate and surgical consult for suspected orbital phycomycosis

- **Pearl**

The incidence of Haemophilus influenzae *as the cause of orbital cellulitis in children has all but disappeared since the introduction of an effective immunization.*

Reference

Jain A, Rubin PAD: Orbital cellulitis in children. Int Ophthalmol Clin 2001;41:71. [PMID: 11698739]

Penetrating Eye Trauma

- ■ Essentials of Diagnosis
  - • History of trauma
  - • Examination may be complicated by concurrent injury to periorbital structures
  - • Visual acuity and pupillary response should be tested and followed
  - • CT or x-rays may be needed to rule out intraocular foreign body
  - • High-speed projectiles can leave deceptively trivial-appearing entrance wounds

- ■ Differential Diagnosis
  - • Corneal abrasion
  - • Corneal laceration
  - • Subconjunctival hemorrhage

- ■ Treatment
  - • Emergent ophthalmologic consult
  - • Prepare patient for surgery
  - • Avoid needless examination or manipulation of the globe
  - • Cover injured eye with solid eye shield
  - • Patch uninjured eye to minimize ocular movement
  - • Do not apply any eye drops or ointments
  - • Prophylactic intravenous antibiotics
  - • Intravenous analgesia and sedation as needed
  - • Consider tetanus prophylaxis

- ■ Pearl

It has been quoted that up to one-fifth of patients with intraocular foreign bodies can have intact vision and no pain.

Reference

Mester V, Kuhn F: Intraocular foreign bodies. Ophthalmol Clin North Am 2002;15:235. [PMID: 12229240]

Preseptal Cellulitis

- ### Essentials of Diagnosis
  - Pain, tenderness, edema, and erythema surrounding the eye
  - No pain with ocular movement
  - Normal visual acuity
  - Commonly caused by *Staphylococcus aureus* and *Streptococcus* spp.
  - No systemic signs of infection

- ### Differential Diagnosis
  - Orbital cellulitis
  - Herpes zoster
  - Trauma
  - Insect bite or sting
  - Dacryocystitis
  - Dacryoadenitis
  - Allergic reaction

- ### Treatment
  - Oral antibiotics: amoxicillin/clavulanate, 500/125 to 875/125 mg orally every 12 hours; cephalexin, 250–500 mg orally every 6 hours
  - Cleansing of the area to remove debris
  - Oral analgesics as needed

- ### Pearl

It can sometimes be difficult to differentiate between a significant insect bite and preseptal cellulitis: when in doubt, prescribe antibiotics.

Reference

Mawn LA, Jordan DR, Donahue SP: Preseptal and orbital cellulitis. Ophthalmol Clin North Am 2000;13:633.

Retinal Detachment

- **Essentials of Diagnosis**
  - Painless decrease in vision
  - Flash of light followed by a curtain in the visual field
  - Central vision is spared if the macula is not involved
  - Normal intra-ocular pressure
  - The detachment may sometimes be visualized with an indirect ophthalmoscope
  - Elderly and highly myopic people are at increased risk
  - May be caused by mild trauma in persons with predisposing factors
  - Concomitant vitreous hemorrhage may occur

- **Differential Diagnosis**
  - Central retinal artery occlusion
  - Central retinal vein occlusion
  - Retinal hemorrhage
  - Retrobulbar optic neuritis
  - Cerebrovascular accident
  - Vitreous hemorrhage
  - Temporal arteritis
  - Endophthalmitis
  - Complicated migraine
  - Hysterical blindness

- **Treatment**
  - Immediate ophthalmologic consult for surgical repair

- **Pearl**

Retinal detachment can be a complication of cataract surgery, although newer surgical techniques have decreased the incidence.

Reference

Banker AS, Freeman WR: Retinal detachment. Ophthalmol Clin North Am 2001;14:695. [PMID: 11787748]

Retinal Hemorrhage

- **Essentials of Diagnosis**
  - Can be asymptomatic and found on routine ophthalmoscopy
  - May cause painless loss of vision if macula is involved
  - Usually due to one of multiple underlying systemic conditions that cause inflammation, neovascularization, vascular sludging, or hyperviscosity: hypertension, diabetes, hemoglobinopathy, malignancy, infection
  - Superficial retinal hemorrhages: bright red and flame shaped
  - Deep retinal hemorrhages: dark red and round
  - Subhyaloid hemorrhage: boat shaped

- **Differential Diagnosis**
  - Central retinal artery occlusion
  - Central retinal vein occlusion
  - Retinal detachment
  - Retrobulbar optic neuritis
  - Cerebrovascular accident
  - Giant cell arteritis
  - Endophthalmitis
  - Complicated migraine
  - Hysterical blindness

- **Treatment**
  - No specific treatment
  - Investigation of underlying disease processes if none are identified previously
  - Ophthalmologic consult

- **Pearl**

Retinal hemorrhages can occur in normal healthy individuals who are not acclimated and ascend above 6,500 feet.

Reference

Tolls DB: Peripheral retinal hemorrhages: a literature review and report on thirty-three patients. J Am Optom Assoc 1998;69:563. [PMID: 9785731]

Subconjunctival Hemorrhage

- **Essentials of Diagnosis**
  - Generally unilateral, well-circumscribed redness with normal surrounding conjunctiva
  - May be atraumatic or caused by trauma as trivial as a cough or sneeze
  - Due to rupture of conjunctival or episcleral blood vessels
  - Painless
  - Vision is unaffected
  - May be accompanied by significant chemosis if blood volume is large

- **Differential Diagnosis**
  - Globe perforation
  - Conjunctivitis
  - Episcleritis
  - Scleritis

- **Treatment**
  - Cold compresses initially, then may change to warm compresses
  - May use lubricating ointment at bedtime if chemosis causes conjunctiva to protrude beyond closed lids
  - Follow-up with primary care physician
  - Workup for underlying coagulopathies or hypertension for recurrent hemorrhages or if other systemic symptoms warrant

- **Pearl**

Patients tend to be quite distressed and require a great deal of reassurance regarding the benign nature of this condition and should be advised that the conjunctiva will go through the usual color changes of a bruise over a period of 2–3 weeks.

Reference

Leibowitz HM: The red eye. N Engl J Med 2000;343:345. [PMID: 10922425]

Uveitis

- **Essentials of Diagnosis**
  - Photophobia, pain, blurred vision, and constricted pupil due to ciliary spasm
  - Pain described as a deep ache
  - Absence of discharge, although tearing may be present due to photophobia
  - Tender globe
  - No uptake with fluorescein staining
  - "Cell and flare" is seen on slit-lamp examination due to cellular and protein components in the anterior chamber
  - If enough cells are present, a hypopyon may form
  - Chronic or recurrent uveitis warrants workup for systemic inflammatory disease

- **Differential Diagnosis**
  - Acute angle closure glaucoma
  - Corneal abrasion
  - Corneal foreign body
  - Conjunctivitis
  - Scleritis
  - Episcleritis
  - Keratitis

- **Treatment**
  - Cycloplegic mydriatic agents: tropicamide 0.5% or cyclopentolate 0.5%
  - Ophthalmologic referral for further evaluation and consideration of steroid eye drops
  - Oral analgesics

- **Pearl**

That guy wearing sunglasses and asking for a work excuse on Monday morning may be there for his acute traumatic iritis left over from the weekend fight.

Reference

Haupert CL, Jaffe GJ: New and emerging treatments for patients with uveitis. Int Ophthalmol Clin 2000;40:205. [PMID: 10791266]

Vitreous Hemorrhage

- **Essentials of Diagnosis**
  - Sudden painless loss or decrease of vision accompanied by floaters
  - Occurs secondary to trauma, retinal detachment, retinal vein occlusion, or diabetic retinopathy
  - Loss or haziness of the red reflex of the fundus
  - Retina obscured on ophthalmoscopic exam
  - Eye is not red; no discharge, tearing, or photophobia is present

- **Differential Diagnosis**
  - Acute angle closure glaucoma
  - Retinal detachment
  - Retinal hemorrhage
  - Retinal vein occlusion
  - Optic neuritis or papillitis
  - Methanol poisoning
  - Central retinal artery occlusion
  - Cerebrovascular accident
  - Complicated migraine
  - Temporal (giant cell) arteritis
  - Hysterical blindness

- **Treatment**
  - Emergent ophthalmologic consult
  - No emergency department treatment

- **Pearl**

If the patient cannot see out of his or her eye and you cannot see in and see only red or black, the patient has a vitreous hemorrhage.

Reference

Spraul CW, Grossniklaus HE: Vitreous hemorrhage. Surv Ophthalmol 1997;42:3. [PMID: 9265701]

15

ENT Emergencies

Benign Positional Vertigo

- **Essentials of Diagnosis**
  - Associated with true vertigo symptoms of room-spinning sensation with exaggerated sense of motion
  - Symptoms and nystagmus associated with head movement
  - Symptoms occur acutely and are severe with associated nausea and vomiting
  - Normal neurologic exam (particularly cerebellar exam)
  - Examiner should be able to reproduce symptoms with the Dix-Hallpike test, which is specific for the diagnosis: While the patient is sitting, his or her head is turned to either side by about 45 degrees; next, a rapid move from a sitting to a supine position is made with the head hanging off of the back of the examining table, keeping the head in the same 45-degree position; a positive test results in vertigo, after a latency of 5–10 seconds and lasting 30 seconds to a minute, and rotary nystagmus along with complaints of dizziness

- **Differential Diagnosis**
  - Ménière disease, labyrinthitis
  - Foreign body in the external auditory canal
  - Acoustic neuroma
  - Central causes (cerebrovascular accident, toxic, tumor, CNS infection, multiple sclerosis, temporal lobe epilepsy)

- **Treatment**
  - Meclizine, 25–50 mg every 8–12 hours
  - Diazepam, 2–10 mg (lower doses for the elderly)
  - Scopolamine, 0.5-mg patch
  - Other drugs with anticholinergic effects may be helpful in controlling the vertigo and vomiting
  - Patients may need admission if unable to tolerate oral medications

- **Pearl**

Benign positional vertigo must be differentiated from central vertigo on the basis of history and physical exam.

Reference

Parnes LS, Agrawal SK, Atlas J: Diagnosis and management of benign paroxysmal positional vertigo (BPPV). CMAJ 2003;169:681. [PMID: 14517129]

Croup

- ■ Essentials of Diagnosis
  - Also referred to as laryngotracheobronchitis
  - Seen most commonly in children aged 6 months to 3 years, but may occur in older children
  - Pathognomonic "seal" or "barking" cough
  - Often associated with viral upper respiratory symptoms such as rhinorrhea and low-grade fever
  - Stridor is common, usually seen with exertion or crying
  - Resting stridor is a more ominous sign; indicates severe narrowing of the subglottic trachea
  - Caused by parainfluenza virus, which also causes laryngitis in adults
  - Leads to subglottic swelling of the trachea, which is seen as a "steeple" sign on anteroposterior neck x-rays
  - Mild WBC elevations may be seen
  - Pharyngeal exam should be benign without exudates or unilateral swelling
  - Course is usually 5–7 days with symptoms peaking on day 2 or 3

- ■ Differential Diagnosis
  - Epiglottitis
  - Aspirated foreign body
  - Peritonsillar or retropharyngeal abscess
  - Bacterial tracheitis
  - Tracheal atresia
  - Tracheal ring

- ■ Treatment
  - Cool, nebulized saline (humidifier at home)
  - Steroids orally or parenterally; dexamethasone, 0.6 mg/kg
  - Racemic epinephrine for resting stridor or if patient does not improve quickly
  - Observe the child after giving racemic epinephrine for at least 2 hours prior to discharge to avoid rebound symptoms
  - Most children can be discharged after resolution of symptoms
  - Children with persistent or severe symptoms after adequate treatment should be admitted for observation

- ■ Pearl

Heliox may prevent the need for intubation in patients with severe croup.

Reference

Fitzgerald DA, Kilham HA: Croup: assessment and evidence-based management. Med J Aust 2003;179:372. [PMID: 14503904]

Dental Pain

- ■ Essentials of Diagnosis
  - • Simple dental pain must be differentiated from serious infectious sources as well as other serious causes
  - • Most common cause: dental caries
  - • Pain usually limited to one tooth or a specific area of the mouth and worse while chewing
  - • Recent instrumentation would suggest noninfectious cause
  - • Insidious onset with localized swelling suggests infectious cause
  - • Examine oral and gingival mucosa carefully

- ■ Differential Diagnosis
  - • Acute myocardial infarction
  - • Acute necrotizing ulcerative gingivitis
  - • Ludwig's angina
  - • Temporomandibular joint (TMJ) syndrome
  - • Periapical infection or abscess
  - • Pulpitis
  - • Drug-seeking behavior

- ■ Treatment
  - • Pain medications (nonsteroidal anti-inflammatory drugs, opioids)
  - • Dental block for severe pain
  - • Antibiotics to cover mouth flora; oral penicillin adequate for most, but sicker patients may require a cephalosporin and clindamycin
  - • Dental referral

- ■ Pearl

The absence of pain relief with a well-placed dental block implies a diagnosis other than tooth pain (eg, acute myocardial infarction, drug seeking).

Reference

Douglass AB, Douglass JM: Common dental emergencies. Am Fam Physician 2003;67:511. [PMID: 12588073]

Epiglottitis

- **Essentials of Diagnosis**
  - Fever, throat pain, odynophagia
  - Decreased incidence in children with *Haemophilus influenzae* type B vaccine
  - Children will appear very toxic, with stridor, drooling, and tripod position
  - Young adults are now the most commonly affected; generally do not appear toxic
  - Instead of stridor, adults usually have "hot potato" voice
  - Lateral soft tissue x-ray of the neck shows a thickened epiglottis "thumb" sign; normal x-ray does not rule out diagnosis
  - Definitive diagnosis made by visualizing the epiglottis, usually through endoscopy

- **Differential Diagnosis**
  - Croup
  - Bacterial tracheitis
  - Foreign body
  - Peritonsillar and retropharyngeal abscess
  - Streptococcal pharyngitis

- **Treatment**
  - Leave a child with a patent airway in the parent's lap with blow-by nebulized saline while rapid preparations are made for airway control in the operating room
  - Immediate consult for ENT and anesthesiology
  - Adults: intravenous pain medication; endoscopy in emergency department; admit for intravenous antibiotics, usually broad-spectrum such as ceftriaxone, 1 g IV

- **Pearl**

Be very suspicious of epiglottitis in the patient with fever, throat pain, and trouble swallowing in whom you see no pathology on physical exam.

Reference

Bansal A, Miskoff J, Lis RJ: Otolaryngologic critical care. Crit Care Clin 2003;19:55. [PMID: 12688577]

Epistaxis

- ■ Essentials of Diagnosis
  - • Usually caused by trauma or environmental factors
  - • Most common area of bleeding is anterior in Kiesselbach plexus
  - • History may include nasal trauma, nose picking, dry environmental conditions, warfarin or platelet-inhibiting drug use, renal failure, or other bleeding disorders
  - • Physical exam: focus on location of bleeding to differentiate posterior from anterior bleeding
  - • Evaluate for hemodynamic stability; evaluate stable patients in upright position
  - • With posterior bleeding, the exact site will rarely be seen, but patient may have significant posterior pharyngeal bleeding

- ■ Differential Diagnosis
  - • Coagulopathy (medications, hemophilia)
  - • Nasopharyngeal malignancy
  - • Sinus or nasal infection
  - • Retained nasal foreign body
  - • Trauma
  - • Dry environmental conditions

- ■ Treatment
  - • Suction out clot or have patient blow nose
  - • Apply local vasoconstrictors directly to bleeding site
  - • Silver nitrate may be used directly on bleeding site
  - • Packing required for persistent bleeding or if specific site cannot be identified
  - • Posterior bleeding may require Foley catheter or specialized epistaxis catheter for bleeding control
  - • ENT consult for posterior bleeding or uncontrollable bleeding
  - • Oral antibiotics (cephalexin or amoxicillin/clavulanate) for anterior epistaxis patients discharged with packing for follow-up

- ■ Pearl

Patients with chronic lung disease may develop hypercarbia with a nasal pack left in place for a prolonged period.

Reference

Pashen D, Stevens M: Management of epistaxis in general practice. Aust Fam Physician 2002;31;717. [PMID: 12189661]

Mastoiditis

■ **Essentials of Diagnosis**

- Relatively rare condition
- Patients usually present with fever, chills, and ear pain; poor feeding and vomiting also common
- Otitis media may develop into mastoiditis because of connection between middle ear and mastoid air cells; otitis media may be seen concurrently
- Hallmark physical sign: tenderness and swelling over mastoid process
- Obtain CT if mastoiditis suspected
- Most common bacteria involved: *Streptococcus pneumoniae, Streptococcus pyogenes,* and *Staphylococcus aureus*

■ **Differential Diagnosis**

- Otitis media
- Mastoid tumor
- Local cutaneous cellulitis

■ **Treatment**

- ENT consult for possible surgical intervention
- Admission for intravenous antibiotics, usually a third-generation cephalosporin such as cefotaxime, 1 g every 4 hours

■ **Pearl**

Check the mastoid process in patients with otitis media because mastoiditis and otitis media generally occur concurrently.

Reference

Tarantino V et al: Acute mastoiditis: a 10 year retrospective study. Int J Pediatr Otolaryngol 2002;66:143. [PMID: 12393248]

Ménière Disease

■ Essentials of Diagnosis

- Acute onset of peripheral vertigo, tinnitus, ear pressure, and hearing loss
- Vertigo commonly lasts 1–2 days during each attack
- Nausea, intense vomiting
- Hearing loss may be unilateral or bilateral, usually paroxysmal with gradual deterioration over time
- Weber and Rinne testing will show sensorineural hearing loss, with air conduction of vibrations longer than bone conduction
- Vertigo is not positional and does not fatigue with the Epley maneuver
- Cause is most likely multifactorial but not well understood

■ Differential Diagnosis

- Acoustic neuroma
- Benign positional vertigo
- Vestibular neuronitis
- Labyrinthitis
- Central causes (eg, cerebrovascular accident, tumor)
- Foreign body lodged next to tympanic membrane

■ Treatment

- Salt restriction
- ENT consult
- Intravenous hydration as needed for severe nausea and vomiting
- Meclizine, diazepam, scopolamine as in benign positional vertigo

■ Pearl

Sometimes Ménière disease is associated with a high salt intake, and these cases may show improvement over time.

Reference

Mancini F et al: History of Ménière's disease and its clinical presentation. Otolaryngol Clin North Am 2002;35:565. [PMID: 12486840]

Nasal Foreign Body

- **Essentials of Diagnosis**
    - Typically seen in infants and small children (eg, child will stuff a colorful piece of plastic or a food item up the nose)
    - Patients often present with purulent rhinitis or foul-smelling breath with organic foreign bodies
    - Clear rhinorrhea or nasal pressure also a common presentation
    - Most patients have acute onset of symptoms
    - Unilateral symptoms most common
    - Foreign body will usually be evident on physical exam using an otoscope or nasal speculum

- **Differential Diagnosis**
    - Viral syndrome
    - Sinusitis
    - Nasopharyngeal tumors, polyps, abscess, or hematomas
    - Choanal atresia
    - Trauma
    - Deviated septum

- **Treatment**
    - Remove foreign body with forceps, suction devices, or balloon catheter (No. 4 or 5 vascular Fogarty or 12 French Foley); removal may be accomplished by having parent occlude unaffected nostril while blowing forcefully into child's mouth
    - Sedation is occasionally needed
    - Consider outpatient treatment by ENT if foreign body cannot be removed easily in emergency department

- **Pearl**

Airway compromise is not a factor in the vast majority of these cases because they are unilateral; thus, outpatient treatment by an ENT may be preferable.

Reference

Kadish HA, Corneli HM: Removal of nasal foreign bodies in the pediatric population. Am J Emerg Med 1997;15:54. [PMID: 9002571]

Otitis Externa

- **Essentials of Diagnosis**
  - Common in swimmers
  - Patients usually present with ear pain, itching, and sometimes purulent discharge
  - Traction on pinna and palpation of tragus is extremely painful
  - External auditory canal will have significant edema and frequently exudates
  - Bacteria involved is frequently *Pseudomonas*
  - Elderly, diabetic, or immunocompromised patients may develop malignant otitis externa; presentation with rapidly progressive necrotizing disease of ear and other local structures
  - Otitis externa may be caused by perforation of suppurative otitis media

- **Differential Diagnosis**
  - Otitis media (especially suppurative with perforation)
  - Foreign body in the ear
  - Sebaceous cyst
  - Bullous myringitis
  - Mastoiditis

- **Treatment**
  - If canal is not obstructed completely, place a cotton wick in canal and place topical steroid and antibiotic combination preparations such as Cortisporin otic suspension or Cipro HC suspension on wick to allow tissues to come in contact with the medication
  - Treat for 3–5 days with outpatient follow-up
  - If malignant otitis externa is suspected, ENT consult for possible admission and intravenous antibiotics (broad-spectrum antipseudomonal agents)

- **Pearl**

Avoid topical steroid and antibiotic solutions if tympanic membrane perforation is suspected, because these solutions contain alcohol and will cause intense pain.

Reference

Schapowal A: Otitis externa: a clinical overview. Ear Nose Throat J 2002; 81(8 Suppl 1):21. [PMID: 12199185]

Otitis Media

- ■ Essentials of Diagnosis
  - • Two forms: serous or suppurative; both forms common in children
  - • Patients usually present with preceding upper respiratory infection, ear pain, bubbling sensation in the ear, and sometimes hearing loss
  - • Serous otitis media: tympanic membrane with decreased motility and light reflex; landmarks visible; air-fluid level frequently seen; viral or allergic cause, relating to eustachian tube dysfunction
  - • Suppurative otitis media: loss or dulling of light reflex with an erythematous tympanic membrane, which may lead to perforation: most commonly caused by *Streptococcus pneumoniae* or *Haemophilus influenzae*

- ■ Differential Diagnosis
  - • Otitis externa
  - • Infected sebaceous cyst
  - • Bullous myringitis
  - • Foreign body
  - • Mastoiditis

- ■ Treatment
  - • Decongestants
  - • Observation may be appropriate if follow-up is certain and diagnosis questionable
  - • Antibiotics for 10 days; common choices are amoxicillin, trimethoprim-sulfamethoxazole, amoxicillin/clavulanate, azithromycin, or cefuroxime
  - • Intramuscular ceftriaxone may be used in selected children
  - • For perforated tympanic membrane: follow-up in 2 weeks with no head immersion in water until follow up

- ■ Pearl

Compare the unaffected ear when in doubt. Simple fever without infection will cause the tympanic membrane to look slightly red.

Reference

Rovers MM et al: Otitis media. Lancet 2004;363:465. [PMID: 14962529]

Peritonsillar Abscess (PTA)

■ Essentials of Diagnosis

- Typical presentation: severe sore throat, fever, and a "hot potato" voice, along with dehydration from poor fluid intake
- Physical findings: asymmetry of the tonsillar pillars and trismus
- PTA and cellulitis are a continuum of the same disease
- PTA will generally feel fluctuant; sometimes difference is hard to feel
- Differentiation between abscess and cellulitis is frequently made with CT or attempted incision and drainage
- Etiologic agents: mixed flora, but *Streptococcus pyogenes* is common

■ Differential Diagnosis

- Peritonsillar abscess
- Retropharyngeal abscess
- Epiglottitis
- Exudative pharyngitis
- Pharyngeal tumor
- Carotid artery aneurysm
- Ludwig angina

■ Treatment

- Needle aspiration or open incision and drainage
- Aspiration or incision and drainage should be performed only by a physician experienced with these techniques because the carotid artery is anatomically close to the peritonsillar space
- ENT consult in the emergency department if emergency medicine physician is not comfortable performing the procedure
- Intravenous fluid resuscitation as needed, sedation for procedures, intravenous antibiotics (penicillin or cefazolin) followed by oral antibiotics
- Admit toxic-appearing patients; for others, outpatient ENT follow-up

■ Pearl

It is uncommon for PTAs to obstruct the airway because they are unilateral and usually occur in adults. Airway compromise is more common in children.

Reference

Rotta AT, Wiryawan B: Respiratory emergencies in children. Respir Care 2003;48:248. [PMID: 12667275]

Pharyngitis

■ Essentials of Diagnosis

- Infection of the pharynx with a variety of causative organisms
- Causative agent difficult to differentiate on purely clinical grounds
- Bacterial agents: *Streptococcus pyogenes, Chlamydia, Mycoplasma, Diphtheria,* or gonococcus
- Other agents: adenovirus, herpes, or mononucleosis (Ebstein-Barr virus or cytomegalovirus)
- Usual presentation with fever, sore throat, pharyngeal exudates, pharyngeal tonsillar and mucosal swelling, and tender anterior cervical adenopathy; occasionally with dehydration secondary to poor oral fluid intake
- Streptococcal pharyngitis more likely in presence of fever to 38°C, tender anterior lymphadenopathy, lack of upper respiratory symptoms, and exudates
- Rapid strep assays can aid in diagnosis, but culture is necessary if rapid test is negative
- Streptococcal pharyngitis uncommon in children younger than 3 years

■ Differential Diagnosis

- Epiglottitis
- Ludwig angina
- Peritonsillar or retropharyngeal abscess
- Allergic reaction
- Vincent angina (anaerobic pharyngitis)
- Foreign body

■ Treatment

- Antimicrobial treatment aimed at likely cause, to include penicillin, cephalosporin, or macrolides for streptococcal pharyngitis
- Intravenous fluid resuscitation for volume depletion
- Nonsteroidal anti-inflammatory drugs and steroids for symptomatic relief in severe pharyngitis
- Most patients can be treated as outpatients

■ Pearl

Untreated streptococcal pharyngitis is associated with rheumatic fever, which is the primary reason for antibiotic treatment.

Reference

Johnson BC, Alvi A: Cost-effective workup for tonsillitis. Testing, treatment, and potential complications. Postgrad Med 2003;113:115. [PMID: 12647478]

Retropharyngeal Abscess

- ■ Essentials of Diagnosis
  - • Mainly affects children younger than age 6 years
  - • Presentation with fever, sore throat, odynophagia, voice change, and stridor if severe
  - • Presence of trismus is worrisome for extension to parapharyngeal space
  - • Movement of thyroid cartilage is very painful
  - • Lateral neck x-rays show enlarged prevertebral soft tissue space; occasionally an air-fluid level is seen
  - • CT scan of neck provides definitive diagnosis
  - • Causative agents: mixed oral flora and anaerobic organisms

- ■ Differential Diagnosis
  - • Peritonsillitis
  - • Epiglottitis
  - • Pharyngitis
  - • Allergic reaction
  - • Bacterial tracheitis
  - • Tracheal ring

- ■ Treatment
  - • Airway stabilization
  - • ENT consult for possible incision and drainage
  - • Admission for intravenous antibiotics, broad-spectrum for mixed oral and anaerobic coverage: clindamycin, 600–900 mg every 8 hours, or ampicillin/sulbactam, 3 g IV every 6 hours

- ■ Pearl

Retropharyngeal abscess may extend or rupture into the mediastinal space or cause parapharyngeal abscess.

Reference

Rotta AT, Wiryawan B: Respiratory emergencies in children. Respir Care 2003;48:248. [PMID: 12667275]

Sinusitis

- **Essentials of Diagnosis**
  - Occurs in setting of anatomic obstruction of ostia of the paranasal sinuses with impaired drainage resulting in bacterial overgrowth
  - Patients commonly present with facial pain and fever with purulent rhinorrhea
  - Maxillary sinus is most commonly affected
  - Typically follows an upper respiratory infection
  - Patients may complain of headache or upper tooth pain
  - Percussion over affected sinus is very tender
  - Lack of transillumination is clue to acute sinusitis
  - X-rays are specific but not as sensitive as CT scan for the presence of disease
  - Chronic sinusitis: presence of infection for more than 3 months

- **Differential Diagnosis**
  - CNS pathology (subarachnoid hemorrhage, cerebrovascular accident, migraine, meningitis, cavernous sinus thrombosis)
  - Nasopharyngeal tumors
  - Foreign body
  - Periorbital cellulitis or abscess
  - Frontal osteomyelitis

- **Treatment**
  - Relief of mechanical obstruction with decongestants or steroids for severe sinusitis with nasal sprays for no more than 3 days to prevent rhinitis medicamentosa
  - Oral antibiotics not needed except in persistent cases or with significant fever; common choices include trimethoprim-sulfamethoxazole, amoxicillin/clavulanate, or cefuroxime for 10–14 days
  - Follow up with primary care physician in a week to 10 days for evaluation of anatomical obstruction

- **Pearl**

In a large percentage of patients with acute sinusitis, the causative agent is a virus.

Reference

Leggett JE: Acute sinusitis. When—and when not—to prescribe antibiotics. Postgrad Med 2004;115:13. [PMID: 14755871]

Temporomandibular Joint (TMJ) Dislocation

- **Essentials of Diagnosis**
  - Typical presentation: patient yawns and then is unable to close mouth
  - A "click" is commonly felt during dislocation
  - Masseter spasm is common and causes severe pain
  - Unilateral dislocation will cause deviation of mandible to one side

- **Differential Diagnosis**
  - Mandible fracture
  - Parotitis
  - Masseter or deep space infection

- **Treatment**
  - Sedation or muscle relaxation for the masseter spasm followed by reduction
  - Reduction: accomplished by padding clinician's thumbs and providing steady downward force on patient's posterior mandibular molars while gripping underside of the mandibular angle; mandible will snap back into place and patient will have near immediate relief (Beware of a bite injury during reduction.)
  - Soft diet for several days

- **Pearl**

Because TMJ dislocations often recur, patients should avoid opening their mouth very wide.

Reference

Shorey CW, Campbell JH: Dislocation of the temporomandibular joint. Oral Surg Oral Med Oral Pathol Oral Radiol Endod 2000;89:662. [PMID: 10846117]

Temporomandibular Joint (TMJ) Syndrome

- **Essentials of Diagnosis**
  - Patients usually present with unilateral or bilateral jaw pain
  - Related to overuse, trauma, or systemic arthritis
  - TMJ will be tender to palpation
  - Moving the mandible or having patient bite down on a tongue blade will reproduce symptoms
  - X-rays not indicated unless acute trauma with fracture is suspected

- **Differential Diagnosis**
  - Mandibular fracture
  - Referred pain (myocardial infarction)
  - Dental pathology (abscess, gingivitis, local trauma)
  - Ear pathology (otitis media or externa)
  - Parotitis or parotid sialadenitis

- **Treatment**
  - Soft diet and nonsteroidal anti-inflammatory drugs for 1–2 weeks
  - Follow up with a dentist if pain persists
  - Occasionally appliances are used to decrease stress on and inflammation of TMJ

- **Pearl**

The TMJ should be tender to palpation internally and externally; otherwise, consider another diagnosis.

Reference

Scrivani SJ, Keith DA: Temporomandibular disorders. Dent Today 2000;19:78. [PMID: 12524823]

16

Head Trauma

Cerebral Contusion

■ Essentials of Diagnosis

- Non-space-occupying discrete blood collection within the brain matter
- Less likely to lead to herniation than other intracranial lesions
- Significant edema can occur resulting in increased intracranial pressure (ICP)
- Diagnosis made by noncontrast CT scan of the head

■ Differential Diagnosis

- Subdural hematoma
- Epidural hematoma
- Subarachnoid hemorrhage

■ Treatment

- Neurosurgical consult
- ICU admission if altered mental status is present; otherwise, admission to a floor bed for observation
- Surgical intervention usually not required; if large contusion with significant shift is present, ICP monitoring may be necessary

■ Pearl

Cerebral contusions with associated edema may require intervention.

Reference

Stieg PE et al: Intracranial hemorrhage: diagnosis and emergency management. Neurol Clin 1998;16:373. [PMID: 9537967]

Diffuse Axonal Injury

- ■ Essentials of Diagnosis
  - • Common cause of posttraumatic coma
  - • Noncontrast CT scan of the head may reveal blurring of the gray and white matter, punctuate hemorrhages in the internal capsule or brain stem, and cerebral edema

- ■ Differential Diagnosis
  - • Cerebral contusion
  - • Traumatic subarachnoid hemorrhage
  - • Epidural hematoma
  - • Subdural hematoma

- ■ Treatment
  - • Neurosurgical consult
  - • May or may not require intracranial pressure (ICP) monitoring and cerebrospinal fluid drainage
  - • Reverse Trendelenburg position to reduce ICP and increase venous drainage; if the possibility of spinal injury is eliminated, elevate the head of the bed by 30 degrees
  - • If signs and symptoms of herniation are present: rapid-sequence intubation; hyperventilation carbon dioxide (pCO_2) of about 30 mm Hg; mannitol, 0.5–1.0 g/kg IV (after consulting a neurosurgeon) if systolic blood pressure >90 mm Hg
  - • Patients with mean arterial pressure (MAP) >125 mm Hg: labetalol to maintain MAP of 100–125 mm Hg (or systolic blood pressure of 140–160 mm Hg); second-line drug is sodium nitroprusside

- ■ Pearl

The mechanism of injury is from shearing forces related to sudden deceleration, causing severe intracranial injury.

Reference

Hammoud DA et al: Diffuse axonal injuries: pathophysiology and imaging. Neuroimaging Clin North Am 2002;12:205. [PMID: 12391632]

Hematoma, Epidural

- **Essentials of Diagnosis**
  - Brief loss of consciousness followed by transient lucid interval is a classic yet rare presentation
  - Collection of blood and clot between the dura mater and the skull bones
  - Usually arterial bleeding source (often the middle meningeal artery)
  - Noncontrast CT scan shows a biconvex hematoma
  - Epidural hematomas can expand rapidly, leading to clinical deterioration

- **Differential Diagnosis**
  - Subdural hematoma
  - Cerebral contusion
  - Subarachnoid hemorrhage

- **Treatment**
  - Neurosurgical emergency
  - Often requires immediate decompression of the space-occupying lesion; if a neurosurgeon is unavailable or the patient requires transport and the clinical condition is deteriorating quickly, emergent decompression via burr hole may be life saving
  - Maintenance of adequate oxygenation, ventilation, and perfusion to prevent secondary brain injury
  - Reverse Trendelenburg position to reduce intracranial pressure and increase venous drainage; if no spinal injury exists, elevate the head of the bed by 30 degrees
  - If signs and symptoms of herniation are present: rapid-sequence intubation; hyperventilation carbon dioxide (pCO_2) of about 30 mm Hg; mannitol, 0.5–1.0 g/kg IV (after consulting a neurosurgeon) if systolic blood pressure >90 mm Hg
  - Patients with mean arterial pressure (MAP) >125 mm Hg: labetalol to maintain MAP of 100–125 mm Hg (or systolic blood pressure of 140–160 mm Hg); second-line drug is sodium nitroprusside

- **Pearl**

Patients with epidural hematomas can deteriorate rapidly; early diagnosis and treatment in a deteriorating patient is important to decrease morbidity and mortality.

Reference

Stieg PE et al: Intracranial hemorrhage: diagnosis and emergency management. Neurol Clin 1998;16:373. [PMID: 9537967]

Hematoma, Scalp

- **Essentials of Diagnosis**
  - Diagnosed by visual inspection and palpitation of the scalp
  - Tenderness, swelling, and redness over the site of the hematoma
  - Evidence of trauma that can be associated with a serious intracranial abnormality
  - Consider imaging if patient has lost consciousness, if history suggests a significant mechanism of injury, or in the extremes of age (eg, infants or elderly patients)

- **Differential Diagnosis**
  - Skull fracture with associated hematoma
  - Intracranial hemorrhage

- **Treatment**
  - Ice, elevation of the head, and nonsteroidal anti-inflammatory drugs
  - Aspiration of scalp hematoma has little benefit and should not be attempted

- **Pearl**

Scalp hematomas alone have little clinical significance but may indicate a more serious intracranial injury.

Reference

Haydel MJ et al: Indications for computed tomography in patients with minor head injury. N Engl J Med 2000;343:100. [PMID: 10891517]

Hematoma, Subdural

■ Essentials of Diagnosis

- Brief loss of consciousness followed by transient lucid interval is a classic yet rare presentation
- Collection of blood and clot between the dura mater and the arachnoid mater
- Usually venous bleeding source (often bridging veins)
- Likely to occur in patients with significant brain atrophy (eg, elderly or alcoholic patients) or in those with coagulopathy (eg, anticoagulated on Coumadin) even after minor head trauma
- Noncontrast CT scan shows a concave hematoma that follows the contour of the brain or develops along dural reflections such as the falx or tentorium
- May be chronic, acute, or acute on chronic
- Patient may or may not have neurologic deficit

■ Differential Diagnosis

- Epidural hematoma
- Cerebral contusion
- Subarachnoid hemorrhage

■ Treatment

- Neurosurgical consult
- May or may not require surgical drainage
- Reverse Trendelenburg position to reduce intracranial pressure and increase venous drainage; if the possibility of spinal injury is excluded, elevate the head of the bed by 30 degrees
- Maintain adequate oxygenation, ventilation, and perfusion to prevent secondary brain injury
- If signs and symptoms of herniation are present: rapid-sequence intubation; hyperventilation carbon dioxide (pCO_2) of about 30 mm Hg; mannitol, 0.5–1.0 g/kg IV (after consulting a neurosurgeon) if systolic blood pressure >90 mm Hg
- Patients with mean arterial pressure (MAP) >125 mm Hg: labetalol to maintain MAP of 100–125 mm Hg (or systolic blood pressure of 140–160 mm Hg); second-line drug is sodium nitroprusside

■ Pearl

Early diagnosis and treatment in the deteriorating patient is important to decrease morbidity and mortality.

Reference

Stieg PE et al: Intracranial hemorrhage: diagnosis and emergency management. Neurol Clin 1998;16:373. [PMID: 9537967]

Minor Head Injury

- **Essentials of Diagnosis**
  - Accounts for the majority of head injuries seen in the emergency department
  - Significant intracranial injury can be ruled out by noting the absence of *all* of the following findings (negative predictive value of the absence of these clinical variables was 100%): headache, vomiting, age >60 years, intoxication, deficits in short-term memory (anterograde amnesia), physical evidence of trauma above the clavicles, seizure
  - A concussion is a traumatic brain injury in which the patient experiences altered mental status ranging from transient confusion to loss of consciousness after a head injury
  - If any of the above signs or symptoms are present or physical exam indicates a significant injury, obtain a noncontrast CT scan of the head to rule out significant intracranial injury

- **Differential Diagnosis**
  - Cerebral contusion
  - Traumatic subarachnoid hemorrhage
  - Epidural hematoma
  - Subdural hematoma

- **Treatment**
  - Discharge home with minor head injury/postconcussion syndrome instructions

- **Pearl**

Athletes who sustain a concussion are at significant risk for compounding the degree of brain injury if another head injury occurs within 2 weeks after the initial injury. Adhere to guidelines (such as those from the American Academy of Neurology) regarding return to competition for patients experiencing sports-related head injuries.

Reference

Jogoda AS et al: Clinical policy: neuroimaging and decision-making in adult mild traumatic brain injury in the acute setting. Ann Emerg Med 2002;40:231. [PMID: 12140504]

Skull Fracture, Basilar

■ Essentials of Diagnosis
  - Skull fracture at base of the skull
  - Clinical signs: hemotympanum, Battle sign, "raccoon" eyes, cerebrospinal fluid leaking from nose or ear, hearing loss
  - Noncontrast CT scan of the head

■ Differential Diagnosis
  - Can be associated with more serious intracranial abnormalities
  - Scalp hematoma
  - Open skull fracture
  - Facial fractures

■ Treatment
  - Admission
  - Neurosurgical consult
  - Intravenous antibiotics (eg, cefazolin) for prophylaxis against meningitis is controversial; prior to administration, discuss the decision to use antibiotics with the neurosurgeon who will be admitting the patient

■ Pearl

When a patient with a basilar skull fracture returns to the emergency department with fever or mental status changes, obtain a CT scan of the head and strongly consider meningitis associated with a dural leak.

Reference

Jogoda AS et al: Clinical policy: neuroimaging and decision-making in adult mild traumatic brain injury in the acute setting. Ann Emerg Med 2002;40:231. [PMID: 12140504]

Skull Fracture, Closed

- ■ Essentials of Diagnosis
    - • Headache, possible loss of consciousness; nausea or vomiting commonly occur
    - • Close visual inspection and palpation of the skull looking for tenderness, swelling, and deformity
    - • Caused by direct trauma to the skull; generally classified as linear, depressed, or comminuted
    - • Noncontrast CT scan of the head with brain and bone windows is the study of choice to look for associated injuries and to better define the fracture
    - • Skull x-rays can identify skull fractures but usefulness is limited because they provide no information about the extent of commonly associated intracranial injuries

- ■ Differential Diagnosis
    - • Often associated with more serious intracranial abnormalities
    - • Scalp hematoma
    - • Open skull fracture

- ■ Treatment
    - • Generally require no specific treatment other than supportive care
    - • Isolated closed skull fractures with no evidence of brain injury generally require admission for a minimum of 24 hours of observation watching for complications such as the development of an epidural hematoma

- ■ Pearl

The significance of a closed nondisplaced skull fracture is generally not related to the fracture itself but rather to the frequently associated injuries such as intracranial bleeding.

Reference

Jogoda AS et al: Clinical policy: neuroimaging and decision-making in adult mild traumatic brain injury in the acute setting. Ann Emerg Med 2002;40:231. [PMID: 12140504]

Skull Fracture, Depressed

- **Essentials of Diagnosis**
  - Headache, possible loss of consciousness; nausea or vomiting commonly occur
  - Close visual inspection and palpation of the skull looking for tenderness, swelling, ecchymosis, bleeding, or other deformity
  - Skull fractures are caused by direct trauma to the skull and are generally classified as linear, depressed, or comminuted
  - Noncontrast CT scan of the head including bone windows is the study of choice to look for skull fractures and associated injuries
  - Open fractures are more common when the skull fracture is depressed; associated findings with open fractures can include pneumocephalus, parenchymal edema, or intracranial bleeding
  - Skull x-rays can identify skull fractures but are of limited value because they provide no information about the extent of commonly associated intracranial injuries

- **Differential Diagnosis**
  - Open or closed skull fracture that is not depressed
  - Scalp contusion

- **Treatment**
  - Some neurosurgeons advocate prophylactic intravenous antibiotics for open skull fractures; because this is controversial, discuss the decision with the neurosurgeon who will be admitting the patient
  - Manage any underlying brain injury and prevent secondary brain injury by ensuring adequate oxygenation, ventilation, and perfusion
  - Neurosurgical consult
  - Hospital admission
  - Often need surgical repair and debridement

- **Pearl**

Surgical correction with elevation of the depressed skull fracture is generally performed when the inner table is displaced.

Reference

Jogoda AS et al: Clinical policy: neuroimaging and decision-making in adult mild traumatic brain injury in the acute setting. Ann Emerg Med 2002;40:231. [PMID: 12140504]

Skull Fracture, Open

- **Essentials of Diagnosis**
  - Visual inspection and palpation of the skull underlying a scalp laceration
  - Noncontrast CT scan
  - Open skull fracture is likely if pneumocephalus is noted on CT scan

- **Differential Diagnosis**
  - Scalp laceration
  - Closed skull fracture
  - Depressed skull fracture

- **Treatment**
  - Some neurosurgeons advocate prophylactic intravenous antibiotics for open skull fractures; because this is controversial, discuss the decision with the neurosurgeon who will be admitting the patient
  - Manage any underlying brain injury and prevent secondary brain injury by ensuring adequate oxygenation, ventilation, and perfusion
  - Neurosurgical consult
  - Hospital admission
  - Requires surgical repair and debridement

- **Pearl**

CT scan is superior to plain radiographs of the skull for diagnosis because it shows fractures and other associated intracranial injuries.

Reference

Jogoda AS et al: Clinical policy: neuroimaging and decision-making in adult mild traumatic brain injury in the acute setting. Ann Emerg Med 2002;40:231. [PMID: 12140504]

Subarachnoid Hemorrhage, Traumatic

- ■ Essentials of Diagnosis
  - • More common than previously believed
  - • Not a space-occupying lesion but can lead to increased intracranial pressure (ICP)
  - • Can block the outflow of cerebrospinal fluid (CSF) from the 3rd and 4th ventricles in the brain
  - • Noncontrast CT scan of head is diagnostic in most cases

- ■ Differential Diagnosis
  - • Cerebral contusion
  - • Subdural hematoma
  - • Epidural hematoma

- ■ Treatment
  - • Neurosurgical consult
  - • May or may not require ICP monitoring or CSF drainage
  - • Reverse Trendelenburg position to reduce ICP and increase venous drainage; if the possibility of spinal injury is excluded, elevate the head of the bed by 30 degrees
  - • If signs and symptoms of herniation are present: rapid-sequence intubation; hyperventilation carbon dioxide (pCO_2) of about 30 mm Hg; mannitol, 0.5–1.0 g/kg IV (after consulting a neurosurgeon) if systolic blood pressure >90 mm Hg
  - • Patients with mean arterial pressure (MAP) >125 mm Hg: labetalol to maintain MAP of 100–125 mm Hg (or systolic blood pressure of 140–160 mm Hg); second-line drug is sodium nitroprusside

- ■ Pearl

Traumatic subarachnoid hemorrhage can lead to increased ICP and acute hydrocephalus.

Reference

Stieg PE et al: Intracranial hemorrhage: diagnosis and emergency management. Neurol Clin 1998;16:373. [PMID: 9537967]

17

Maxillofacial & Neck Trauma

Blunt Neck Trauma

- **Essentials of Diagnosis**
  - History of blunt trauma between base of skull and suprasternal notch or clavicles
  - Identification of airway injury (dysphonia, air leak, subcutaneous emphysema)
  - Cervical spine injury common
  - Vascular injuries suggested when expanding hematoma or bruits are present
  - Esophageal injuries can cause pneumomediastinum or hematemesis

- **Differential Diagnosis**
  - Penetrating neck trauma
  - Mandible or hyoid fracture
  - Neck contusion
  - Laryngeal fracture

- **Treatment**
  - Surgical exploration necessary only in cases of suspected airway injury or the rare case of suspected vascular injury
  - Airway control
  - Never place nasogastric tube due to risk of rupturing pharyngeal hematoma
  - Disposition determined by emergency department physician; consultation with trauma surgeon not always necessary

- **Pearl**

Air leak, subcutaneous emphysema, stridor, hoarseness, painful phonation, or hemoptysis in the setting of blunt neck trauma necessitates direct or indirect laryngoscopy for evaluation of the airway.

Reference

Park SS: Blunt trauma to the face & neck: initial management. Compr Ther 1997;23:730. [PMID: 9360801]

External Ear Trauma

- Essentials of Diagnosis
  - History of trauma to ear outside of tympanic membrane
  - Pain at injury site
  - Identification of tympanic membrane injury or hearing loss

- Differential Diagnosis
  - Otohematoma
  - Contusion
  - Laceration
  - External ear chondritis or abscess

- Treatment
  - Drainage of hematoma
  - Closure of laceration
  - Oral antibiotics for concomitant early lobe inflammation (ciprofloxacin, cephalexin, dicloxacillin)
  - Intravenous antibiotics for severe infection after delayed presentation from trauma
  - Otolaryngology or other facial surgeon referral within 1–2 days for any significant trauma including otohematoma, laceration, or chondritis

- Pearl

Blunt trauma to the external ear (eg, a ball striking the ear) often is associated with tympanic membrane rupture or skull fracture.

Reference

Lee D, Sperling N: Initial management of auricular trauma. Am Fam Physician 1996;53:2339. [PMID: 8638510]

Frontal Sinus Fracture

- **Essentials of Diagnosis**
  - Contusion, swelling, ecchymosis, or laceration on forehead
  - Crepitus over frontal sinus
  - High-energy mechanism
  - Epistaxis common
  - Cerebrospinal fluid rhinorrhea common due to frequency of posterior wall fractures
  - Detailed examination of cervical spine, head, and neurologic function required
  - Axial and coronal facial CT and head CT without contrast

- **Differential Diagnosis**
  - Nasofrontoethmoidal fracture
  - Orbital fracture
  - Cribriform plate fracture
  - Frontal bone fracture not involving the frontal sinus
  - Forehead contusion

- **Treatment**
  - Consultation with maxillofacial surgeon and neurosurgeon at time of emergency department visit
  - Epistaxis control with half-inch iodoform gauze packed tightly in nares
  - For open skull fractures (eg, frontal bone fractures in which posterior table also is fractured), some neurosurgeons advocate prophylactic intravenous antibiotics; because this is controversial, discuss decision with neurosurgeon who will be caring for patient
  - Cover open fractures with saline-soaked gauze

- **Pearl**

Massive force (800–2,200 pounds of force) is required to break the frontal bone (twice the force required for any other facial bone); therefore, the majority of patients with frontal bone fractures have concomitant injuries. Radiographic evaluation of the cervical spine should be considered.

Reference

McGraw-Wall B: Frontal sinus fractures. Facial Plast Surg 1998;14:59. [PMID: 10371894]

Lacerations of the Auricle

- **Essentials of Diagnosis**
    - History of trauma, usually penetrating, to the auricle
    - Integrity of skin compromised and cartilage involved
    - Bleeding

- **Differential Diagnosis**
    - Otohematoma
    - Simple skin laceration

- **Treatment**
    - Tetanus prophylaxis
    - Debridement of devitalized tissue
    - Approximation of lacerated cartilage and perichondrium with absorbable sutures
    - Repair of skin with 6-0 nylon sutures or Steri-Strips
    - Petroleum gauze dressing under light pressure
    - Antibiotic ointment over skin sutures
    - Referral to facial surgeon in 1–2 days
    - For patients with extensive lacerations or those with cartilage loss: immediate specialty surgeon consult and possible hospitalization for surgical repair
    - Reserve prophylactic antibiotics for immunocompromised patients

- **Pearl**

Meticulous cartilage approximation is essential and should be performed with a single layer of suture to prevent scarring and cosmetic deformity.

Reference

Lee D, Sperling N: Initial management of auricular trauma. Am Fam Physician 1996;53:2339. [PMID: 8638510]

Le Fort Fracture

- **Essentials of Diagnosis**
  - Local maxillary tenderness
  - Malocclusion
  - Midface mobility, swelling, and ecchymosis
  - High-energy mechanism
  - Facial CT scan: test of choice
  - Complications: airway obstruction, dyspnea, diplopia, facial emphysema, and cerebrospinal fluid rhinorrhea
  - Multisystem injury frequently present

- **Differential Diagnosis**
  - Le Fort I: fracture line parallel to alveolar process and hard palate of the maxilla
  - Le Fort II: pyramidal fracture involving bony nasal skeleton and middle third of face (includes fracture lines of a Le Fort I injury)
  - Le Fort III: craniofacial dysjunction involving separation of all facial bones; fracture lines extend through ethmoid bones and orbits and into sphenopalatine fossa, passing medially across glabellar region
  - Le Fort IV: involves frontal bone in addition to fracture lines of a Le Fort III injury
  - Zygomaticomaxillary complex fracture
  - Facial contusion

- **Treatment**
  - Aggressive airway management
  - Consider radiographic clearance of cervical spine
  - Nasotracheal intubation and placement of nasogastric tubes absolutely contraindicated
  - Provision of adequate analgesia
  - Consultation with a maxillofacial surgeon at time of emergency department visit

- **Pearl**

Le Fort fractures may occur in any combination (eg, a left hemi–Le Fort II fracture and a right hemi–Le Fort III fracture) and may exist simultaneously in the same patient.

Reference

Katzen JT et al: Craniofacial and skull base trauma. J Trauma 2003;54:1026. [PMID: 12777923]

Mandible Fracture

■ Essentials of Diagnosis

- Mandibular pain
- Dysphagia
- Trismus
- Presence of gross facial asymmetry on inspection
- Malocclusion
- Decreased range of motion at the temporomandibular (TMJ) joint
- Grinding sound in ear with manipulation from bony conduction
- Tongue blade test is 95% sensitive in ruling out mandible fractures: have patient bite down on tongue blade between the molars; twist the stick until it breaks; if the patient can stabilize the stick enough to break it on each side of the mouth, there is no fracture
- Fracture on Panorex examination: if Panorex is negative or unavailable, facial CT can confirm diagnosis and more effectively visualize condylar processes and symphysial area

■ Differential Diagnosis

- Contusion
- Mandible dislocation (deviates away from dislocations and toward fractures)
- Isolated dental trauma

■ Treatment

- All mandible fractures with mucosal, gingival, or tooth socket disruption should be considered open
- Tetanus prophylaxis for open fractures: penicillin, 2–4 million units IV; clindamycin, 600–900 mg IV; or erythromycin, 500–1,000 mg IV
- Relocation if TMJ dislocation involved
- Simple and nondisplaced fractures: consultation with maxillofacial surgeon to arrange outpatient follow-up
- Complex fractures with associated dislocation or potential airway compromise: admission

■ Pearl

The mandible is a ringlike structure that is unlikely to fracture in a single location. Be diligent in looking for other fractures of the mandible when one fracture is identified.

Reference

Schwab RA, Genners K, Robinson W: Clinical predictors of mandibular fractures. Am J Emerg Med 1998;16:304. [PMID: 9596439]

Nasal Fracture

■ Essentials of Diagnosis

- Blunt trauma to nose
- Tenderness, crepitation, or movement of nasal bones
- Nasal swelling and ecchymosis
- Epistaxis common
- Septal hematoma is common and *must* be detected if present
- Abnormal tearing from lacrimal duct injury is not uncommon
- Concomitant ocular injury often present, including retinal detachment, hyphema, and subconjunctival hemorrhage
- Facial CT scan for assessment of concomitant injury

■ Differential Diagnosis

- Orbital, frontal sinus, maxillary sinus, or cribriform plate fracture
- Telecanthus indicates nasoethmoidal fracture
- Nasal contusion
- Isolated epistaxis

■ Treatment

- Control of epistaxis with nasal packing or cautery if necessary (usually stops spontaneously)
- Reduction of fracture *after* consultation with maxillofacial surgeon
- Anesthesia: topical intranasal anesthesia often adequate
- Fracture reduction: laterally displaced fractures need simple thumb pressure opposite direction of displacement; impacted or comminuted fractures need septal traction and lateral manipulation with a Kelly clamp or Asch septal forceps secured to the septum intranasally
- Drain any septal hematomas by aspiration with an 18- to 20-gauge needle or by incising the anterior nasal mucosa; abscess formation is common in persistent hematomas, threatening all septal cartilage
- Antimicrobial prophylaxis is recommended (amoxicillin/clavulanate, sulfa, cephalexin, erythromycin)

■ Pearl

Isolated nasal fracture without airway compromise is not an emergency. Reduction and definitive management by a maxillofacial surgeon in 3–5 days is acceptable.

Reference

Rohrich RJ, Adams WP: Nasal fracture management: minimizing secondary nasal deformities. Plast Reconstr Surg 2000;106:266. [PMID: 10946923]

Orbital Floor (Blowout) Fracture

■ Essentials of Diagnosis

- Periorbital swelling, ecchymosis, and usually but not always tenderness
- Impaired ocular mobility resulting in diplopia is common: inferior rectus entrapment results in impaired upward gaze; medial rectus entrapment results in impaired lateral gaze
- Decreased sensation of infraorbital nerve distribution
- Epistaxis common
- Exophthalmos from periorbital fat herniation common
- Pure blowout fracture: anteroposterior force on globe causes an increase in orbital pressure, forcing the contents of the orbit through the weakest point, the floor
- Impure blowout fracture: anteroposterior force is partially exerted against infraorbital rim, producing the same fracture (lower incidence of ocular injury than in a pure blowout)
- Orbital CT scan

■ Differential Diagnosis

- Orbital contusion
- Retrobulbar hemorrhage
- Ruptured globe
- Zygomaticomaxillary complex fracture
- Periorbital or orbital cellulitis
- Cranial nerve palsy

■ Treatment

- Consultation with maxillofacial surgeon and ophthalmologist at time of emergency department visit
- Provision of adequate analgesia
- Prophylactic antibiotics (amoxicillin, cephalexin, erythromycin) often recommended; discuss with consultant
- Tetanus prophylaxis in all patients
- Avoid any Valsalva maneuvers, especially nose blowing
- Nasal decongestants recommended

■ Pearl

Orbital blowout fractures do not affect visual acuity. If visual acuity is impaired, consider it an ophthalmologic emergency (ruptured globe incidence with blowouts is 5–10%).

Reference

Brady SM: The diagnosis and management of orbital blowout fractures: update 2001. Am J Emerg Med 2001;19:147. [PMID: 11239261]

Otohematoma

- **Essentials of Diagnosis**
  - History of trauma, usually blunt, to the external ear
  - Bleeding between the auricular cartilage and the perichondrium
  - Swelling and ecchymosis

- **Differential Diagnosis**
  - Laceration of the auricle
  - Simple bruised auricle

- **Treatment**
  - Aspiration or incision and drainage of the auricle to completely evacuate any subperichondrial hematoma
  - Application of dental pledget bolsters sutured in place on each side of the auricle that conform to the auricular formation
  - Antibiotic ointment covering wounds
  - Application of firm conforming dressing to prevent further hematoma formation

- **Pearl**

Untreated otohematomas result in disorganized new cartilage formation and chronic ear deformity known as cauliflower ear.

Reference

Lee D, Sperling N: Initial management of auricular trauma. Am Fam Physician 1996;53:2339. [PMID: 8638510]

Penetrating Neck Trauma

- **Essentials of Diagnosis**
  - History of penetrating trauma between the base of the skull and the suprasternal notch or clavicles
  - Determination of whether wound penetrates platysma
  - Identification of airway injury (air leak, subcutaneous emphysema, pneumomediastinum, pneumothorax)
  - Identification of esophageal injury (dysphagia, odynophagia, drooling, soft tissue crepitus)
  - Identification of nerve injury: vagus (voice abnormalities, vocal cord asymmetry), spinal accessory (sternocleidomastoid and trapezius weakness), hypoglossal (deviation of protruded tongue to side of injury), phrenic (use of respiratory accessory muscles, asymmetric diaphragm on chest x-ray)
  - Soft tissue x-rays of the neck, two-dimensional Doppler, angiography, and esophagogram or esophagoscopy may all be necessary depending on location and symptoms

- **Differential Diagnosis**
  - Zone I injury (between suprasternal notch or clavicles and inferior aspect of the cricoid cartilage
  - Zone II injury (between inferior cricoid cartilage and angle of the mandible)
  - Zone III injury (between angle of the mandible and base of the skull)
  - Open mandible or hyoid fracture

- **Treatment**
  - Airway control with low threshold for intubation
  - Direct pressure to control hemorrhage
  - Urgent consult with trauma surgeon immediately after identification of platysma-penetrating injury
  - Never place nasogastric tube due to risk of rupturing a contained pharyngeal hematoma
  - Selective exploration of zone II injuries has become more common
  - Tetanus prophylaxis

- **Pearl**

Never remove impaled foreign bodies from the neck; they may be preventing massive hemorrhage.

Reference

Thompson EC, Porter JM, Fernandez LG: Penetrating neck trauma: an overview of management. J Oral Maxillofac Surg 2002;60:918. [PMID: 12149739]

Tooth Avulsion

- **Essentials of Diagnosis**
  - History of facial trauma
  - Tooth, jaw, or ear pain
  - Pain exacerbated by chewing, drinking, and extremes of temperature
  - Missing tooth
  - Tooth avulsion with concomitant mandible fracture is an open fracture
  - Rule out tooth aspiration by chest x-ray if tooth is not recovered in the field
  - Permanent teeth are numbered sequentially starting at the right maxillary third molar (#1) and going across to the left maxillary third molar (#16); #17 is the left mandibular third molar and the right mandibular third molar is #32
  - Deciduous teeth are lettered sequentially starting with the right maxillary second molar as A and the right mandibular second molar as T

- **Differential Diagnosis**
  - Tooth fracture or subluxation
  - Open mandible fracture

- **Treatment**
  - Rinse tooth gently with saline
  - Administer anesthesia; regional intraoral nerve block is ideal
  - Replace tooth in socket
  - If tooth cannot be immediately replaced in the socket, put it in an isotonic media such as Hank's solution; other options include milk, saline, or saliva (the patient's mouth unless the patient is at risk for aspiration of the tooth)
  - Consult with dentist or oral surgeon at time of emergency department visit to splint tooth and maintain relocation
  - Administer prophylactic antibiotics (penicillin, 500 mg every 6 hours, or clindamycin, 450 mg every 6 hours)

- **Pearl**

Rapid reimplantation of permanent teeth is critical because 1% of the success rate of reimplantation is lost every minute the tooth is out of the socket. Primary teeth should not be reimplanted because of complications that may develop including dentoalveolar ankylosis with resultant facial deformities.

Reference

Dale RA: Dentoalveolar trauma. Emerg Med Clin North Am 2000;18:521. [PMID: 10967737]

Tooth Fracture

■ Essentials of Diagnosis

- History of facial trauma
- Tooth, jaw, or ear pain
- Pain exacerbated by chewing, drinking, and extremes of temperature
- At a minimum, integrity of enamel compromised
- Identification of possibility of tooth fragment aspiration
- Permanent teeth are numbered sequentially starting at the right maxillary third molar (#1) and going across to the left maxillary third molar (#16); #17 is the left mandibular third molar and the right mandibular third molar is #32
- Deciduous teeth are lettered sequentially starting with the right maxillary second molar as A and the right mandibular second molar as T

■ Differential Diagnosis

- Ellis I fracture: involves enamel only
- Ellis II fracture: involves enamel and dentin
- Ellis III fracture: involves enamel, dentin, and pulp
- Tooth avulsion
- Tooth subluxation

■ Treatment

- Ellis I: smooth sharp tooth edges with an emery board and refer to dentist for repair
- Ellis II: dress tooth with calcium hydroxide paste covered with foil or enamel-bonded plastic; consult dentist in emergency department or refer within 24 hours
- Ellis III: consult dentist immediately; cover tooth with moist cotton and dry foil

■ Pearl

If blood is visible within the tooth, the pulp is exposed and an emergent consultation is needed.

Reference

Dale RA: Dentoalveolar trauma. Emerg Med Clin North Am 2000;18:521. [PMID: 10967737]

Tooth Subluxation

- **Essentials of Diagnosis**
  - History of facial trauma
  - Tooth, jaw, or ear pain
  - Pain exacerbated by palpation of tooth, chewing, drinking, and extremes of temperature
  - Tooth subluxation with concomitant mandible fracture is an open fracture
  - Permanent teeth are numbered sequentially starting at the right maxillary third molar (#1) and going across to the left maxillary third molar (#16); #17 is the left mandibular third molar and the right mandibular third molar is #32
  - Deciduous teeth are lettered sequentially starting with the right maxillary second molar as A and the right mandibular second molar as T

- **Differential Diagnosis**
  - Tooth fracture
  - Open mandible fracture

- **Treatment**
  - Gently manipulate the tooth into its proper position
  - Consult with a dentist or oral surgeon at time of emergency department visit for possible splinting if the tooth is loose

- **Pearl**

Children tend to subluxate rather than fracture their primary teeth. Don't forget the possibility of child abuse in children presenting with tooth subluxation.

Reference

Dale RA: Dentoalveolar trauma. Emerg Med Clin North Am 2000;18:521. [PMID: 10967737]

Zygomaticomaxillary Complex (ZMC) Fracture

■ Essentials of Diagnosis
- Local maxillary or "cheek bone" tenderness
- Malocclusion
- Midface mobility, swelling, ecchymosis, or asymmetric deformity
- Often high-energy mechanism
- Facial CT scan
- May include airway obstruction, dyspnea, diplopia, facial emphysema, or cerebrospinal fluid rhinorrhea
- May have injury to the infraorbital nerve with associated numbness of the cheek
- Multisystem injuries frequently present

■ Differential Diagnosis
- Le Fort fracture
- Facial contusion
- Orbital floor (blowout) fracture

■ Treatment
- Evaluation for concomitant cervical spine injury; consider x-ray evaluation of cervical spine
- Adequate analgesia
- Epistaxis control with nasal packing or cautery
- Prophylaxis with antibiotics if fracture extends into sinuses (penicillin, amoxicillin or a fluoroquinolone, doxycycline, clindamycin in the penicillin allergic)
- Consultation with a maxillofacial surgeon at time of emergency department visit to arrange outpatient follow-up or admission for definitive repair depending on severity of injury and any associated complications of ZMC fracture
- Ophthalmologic consultation if patient also has an abnormal eye exam

■ Pearl

ZMC fractures are more commonly called tripod fractures in reference to the three anatomic attachments of the zygoma to the frontal, maxillary, and temporal bones.

Reference

Katzen JT et al: Craniofacial and skull base trauma. J Trauma 2003;54:1026. [PMID: 12777923]

18

Chest Trauma

Aortic Disruption

- **Essentials of Diagnosis**
  - Have a high index suspicion for the diagnosis in all patients with rapid deceleration injuries (eg, motor vehicle accidents, falls from heights)
  - Symptoms and signs: chest pain, back pain, dyspnea, unexplained hypotension, intrascapular murmur, extremity pain consistent with ischemia
  - Chest x-ray: excellent screening tool; look for mediastinal widening, indistinct aortic knob, left mainstem bronchus depression, tracheal deviation, apical caps, and widening of the peritracheal stripe
  - Aortography: considered gold standard but is being replaced by CT aortography

- **Differential Diagnosis**
  - Blunt abdominal injury
  - Hemothorax
  - Tension pneumothorax
  - Cardiac tamponade

- **Treatment**
  - Management of blood pressure by pharmacological methods or permissive hypotension
  - Prompt surgical intervention; mortality increases significantly if definitive operative treatment is delayed

- **Pearl**

Maintain a high index of suspicion in light of the mechanism of injury because delay in diagnosis is associated with a high mortality rate.

Reference

Nagy K et al: Guidelines for the diagnosis and management of blunt aortic injury: an EAST Practice Management Guidelines Work Group. J Trauma 2000;48:1128. [PMID: 10866262]

Chest Trauma, Penetrating

- ■ Essentials of Diagnosis
  - • Mechanism of injury usually stabbing or gunshot
  - • Rapid assessment of ABCs
  - • Decreased breath sounds, muffled heart sounds, or deviation of the trachea are important clinical clues to life-threatening diagnoses such as hemothorax, simple or tension pneumothorax, and hemopericardium
  - • Chest x-ray to assess for pneumothorax or hemothorax

- ■ Differential Diagnosis
  - • Pneumothorax
  - • Hemothorax
  - • Pericardial tamponade
  - • Great vessel injury
  - • Tracheobronchial injury
  - • Esophageal injury

- ■ Treatment
  - • Rapid assessment and management of ABCs
  - • Isotonic intravenous fluids initially for resuscitation; if needed, blood transfusion to treat persistent hypotension
  - • Thoracostomy tube
  - • Emergency department thoracotomy in selected cases
  - • Operative intervention to control severe hemorrhage and repair cardiac, esophageal, or diaphragmatic injuries

- ■ Pearl

In patients with lower chest injuries (eg, wounds below the nipple line) consider and evaluate for abdominal and retroperitoneal injuries.

Reference

von Oppell UO, Bautz P, De Groot M: Penetrating thoracic injuries: what we have learned. Thorac Cardiovasc Surg 2000;48:55. [PMID: 10757162]

Esophageal Disruption

- **Essentials of Diagnosis**
  - An infrequent injury with blunt and penetrating injuries; mortality rate is high if undiagnosed secondary to complications of mediastinitis
  - Have a high index of suspicion for the diagnosis in patients with significant chest, abdominal, and possibly back injuries
  - Symptoms and signs: throat pain, dysphasia, hoarseness, chest pain, hematemesis, neck swelling, subcutaneous emphysema, dyspnea
  - Chest x-ray findings suggestive of esophageal injury: pneumomediastinum, widened mediastinum, left pleural effusion
  - Gastrografin swallow and esophagoscopy best diagnostic tools available other than direct surgical exploration

- **Differential Diagnosis**
  - Blunt diaphragmatic injuries
  - Hemothorax

- **Treatment**
  - Surgical versus nonsurgical (eg, drainage, antibiotics, nutritional support) depending on location

- **Pearl**

Strongly consider the diagnosis in patients with pneumomediastinum and blunt trauma. Maintain a high index of suspicion for the injury in light of the mechanism of injury, due to its low incidence but high associated mortality rate.

Reference

Monzon JR, Ryan B: Thoracic esophageal perforation secondary to blunt trauma. J Trauma 2000;49:1129. [PMID: 11843720]

Flail Chest

■ Essentials of Diagnosis

- Associated with significant force to the chest
- Local and diffuse tenderness of the chest wall
- Three or more contiguous ribs fractured in two or more sites
- Symptoms and signs: chest pain, shortness of breath leading to respiratory distress, crepitus; paradoxical chest wall movement may not be present secondary to muscular splinting in the conscious patient
- Chest x-ray may assist with the diagnosis and reveal underlying pulmonary injuries

■ Differential Diagnosis

- Rib fracture
- Pulmonary contusion
- Hemothorax
- Pneumothorax
- Tension pneumothorax

■ Treatment

- Supplemental oxygen
- Adequate pain management using narcotic analgesia and epidural or intercostal nerve blocks
- Consider early intubation and mechanical ventilation; 50% of patients will need to be intubated
- External chest support (sand bags or taping) will reduce pain but also decrease the vital capacity, worsening ventilation

■ Pearl

Adequate pain management and ventilatory support, including early intubation, should always be a part of the management of flail chest.

Reference

Sivaloganathan M, Stephens R, Grocott M: Management of flail chest. Hosp Med 2000;61:811. [PMID: 11198758]

Hemopericardium

- ■ Essentials of Diagnosis
  - • Even a small amount of blood in the pericardium can be clinically significant in the traumatized patient; the pericardium is not very distensible acutely
  - • Problems result from an increased intrapericardial pressure compressing the heart resulting in decreased preload, which results in a decreased afterload
  - • Symptoms and signs: dyspnea, tachycardia, hypotension, muffled heart tones, narrow pulse pressure; increased jugular venous distention may or may not be present depending on the patient's volume status
  - • Focused assessment with sonography for trauma (FAST) can be rapidly diagnostic

- ■ Differential Diagnosis
  - • Hypovolemia
  - • Aortic disruption
  - • Tension pneumothorax

- ■ Treatment
  - • Volume to increase the preload
  - • Pericardiocentesis may only temporize, may be falsely negative, or may cause damage to the heart and associated vessels
  - • Patients with traumatic hemopericardium: emergent pericardial window or thoracotomy and repair

- ■ Pearl

Early evaluation with the FAST examination has replaced blind aspiration of the pericardium in patients with distended neck veins and hypotension.

Reference

Spodick DH: Acute cardiac tamponade. N Engl J Med 2003;349:684. [PMID: 12917306]

Hemothorax

- ■ Essentials of Diagnosis
  - Decreased breath sounds
  - Dullness to percussion on affected side
  - Respiratory distress
  - Hypotension
  - Diagnosis by chest x-ray: "white out" of the hemithorax
  - Diagnosis by focused assessment with sonography for trauma (FAST) when fluid is noted acutely in the chest after trauma

- ■ Differential Diagnosis
  - Tension pneumothorax
  - Chylothorax
  - Simple pneumothorax
  - Aortic disruption

- ■ Treatment
  - Oxygen
  - Management of hypotension
  - Tube thoracostomy
  - Emergent thoracotomy if hemorrhage is massive

- ■ Pearl

Initial blood loss of more than 1.0–1.5 liters or ongoing blood loss greater than 250 cc/hour requires surgery.

Reference

Parry GW, Morgan WE, Salama FD: Management of haemothorax. Ann R Coll Surg Engl 1996;78:325. [PMID: 8712643]

Myocardial Contusion

- **Essentials of Diagnosis**
  - Motor vehicular accidents most frequent cause
  - Electrocardiogram (ECG) is the best screening tool: sinus tachycardia and nonspecific ST-T changes most common findings but entire range of dysrhythmias, conduction disturbances, and ischemic ST-T wave changes are found
  - Biochemical markers not sensitive or specific
  - Echocardiography not to be used as a screening tool but important for evaluation of patients with hemodynamic instability and risk for myocardial contusion

- **Differential Diagnosis**
  - Tension pneumothorax
  - Hypovolemia
  - Pericardial tamponade
  - Myocardial disease

- **Treatment**
  - Observation on telemetry or, if patient is poorly perfused or arrhythmias develop, in the ICU
  - Treatment of dysrhythmias

- **Pearl**

The ECG is the most important tool available to evaluate the potential for a cardiac contusion. An abnormal ECG in a patient at risk should prompt observation. A normal ECG in a normotensive patient virtually rules out the diagnosis of clinically significant myocardial contusion.

Reference

Sybrandy KC, Cramer MJ, Burgersdijk C: Diagnosing cardiac contusion: old wisdom and new insights. Heart 2003;89:485. [PMID: 1269544]

Pneumothorax

- **■ Essentials of Diagnosis**
  - Tachypnea, tachycardia, chest pain
  - Distant or absent breath sounds
  - Hyperresonance to percussion on affected side
  - Index of suspicion based on mechanism of injury
  - Chest x-ray may demonstrate lung collapse with no vascular marking outside of the lung line
  - In supine patients, evidence of lung collapse may be subtle; air collects anteriorly and laterally; look on chest x-ray for a "deep sulcus sign," which is produced by air separating the lateral diaphragm from the chest wall

- **■ Differential Diagnosis**
  - Rib fracture
  - Sternal fracture
  - Tension pneumothorax
  - Esophageal disruption
  - Pulmonary contusion

- **■ Treatment**
  - Oxygen (supplemental oxygen will help the pneumothorax resolve more rapidly)
  - Observation for small pneumothorax
  - Thoracostomy tube for larger ones or for patients on positive-pressure ventilation
  - Possible outpatient observation if the pneumothorax is small and stable after several hours of observation

- **■ Pearl**

Maintain close observation for development of a tension pneumothorax.

Reference

Ulman EA, Donley LP, Brady WJ: Pulmonary trauma emergency department evaluation and management. Emerg Med Clin North Am 2003;21:291. [PMID: 12793615]

Pneumothorax, Open

- **Essentials of Diagnosis**
  - Usually due to large (2/3 the size of the trachea) penetrating wounds
  - Tachypnea, tachycardia, chest pain, and potentially hypotension
  - Distant or absent breath sounds
  - Sucking chest wound

- **Differential Diagnosis**
  - Obvious diagnosis
  - Tracheobronchial disruption

- **Treatment**
  - Cover the wound with an occlusive dressing sealed on three sides
  - Large chest tube
  - Surgical repair

- **Pearl**

If treated inappropriately, an open pneumothorax can be converted to a tension pneumothorax.

Reference

Ullman EA, Donley LP, Brady WJ: Pulmonary trauma emergency department evaluation and management. Emerg Med Clin North Am 2003;21:291. [PMID: 12793615]

Pneumothorax, Tension

- **Essentials of Diagnosis**
  - Absent or decreased breath sounds
  - Hyperresonance to chest wall percussion
  - Tracheal deviation (away from the side of the pneumothorax) in the setting of respiratory distress and hypotension
  - Respiratory distress, tachypnea, hypotension, hypoxia
  - Should be a clinical diagnosis, not a radiographic diagnosis
  - Will result in hemodynamic instability and death unless treated promptly

- **Differential Diagnosis**
  - Simple pneumothorax
  - Hemothorax
  - Pericardial tamponade
  - Aortic disruption
  - Esophageal disruption

- **Treatment**
  - Oxygen
  - Rapid decompression with 12- to 14-gauge over-the-needle catheter in the second intercostal space midclavicular line
  - Prompt thoracostomy

- **Pearl**

Distention of neck veins may be absent in the presence of hypovolemia.

Reference

Barton ED: Tension pneumothorax. Curr Opin Pulm Med 1999;5:269. [PMID: 10407699]

Pulmonary Contusion

- **Essentials of Diagnosis**
  - Dyspnea, hemoptysis, tachycardia, rib fracture, decreased breath sounds
  - Initial chest x-ray may not visualize the contusion well, although the contusion generally worsens over time
  - Most common intrathoracic injury in blunt injuries
  - Progressive dyspnea and hypoxia

- **Differential Diagnosis**
  - Pneumothorax
  - Hemothorax
  - Rib fracture
  - Flail chest

- **Treatment**
  - Close observation
  - Oxygen
  - Ventilatory support
  - Pain management

- **Pearl**

With compliant chest walls, pediatric patients may suffer significant pulmonary contusions without any evidence of external injury to the chest.

Reference

Keough V, Pudelek B: Blunt chest trauma: review of selected pulmonary injuries focusing on pulmonary contusion. AACN Clin Issues 2001;12:270. [PMID: 11759554]

Rib Fracture

■ Essentials of Diagnosis
- Most common injury sustained with blunt chest trauma
- Localized pain and crepitus
- Associated with pneumothorax and hemothorax
- Chest x-ray may demonstrate rib fracture(s) but in general is helpful only to identify associated injuries

■ Differential Diagnosis
- Contusion
- Flail chest
- Sternal fracture
- Pulmonary contusion
- Pneumothorax

■ Treatment
- Adequate pain management with oral narcotics for outpatient treatment or intercostal nerve blocks or epidural anesthesia if severe
- Treatment of underlying injuries
- No role for splinting or taping the chest wall

■ Pearl

Use chest x-rays to evaluate for pulmonary injuries; rib films in general add little to the management of rib fractures.

Reference

Middleton C et al: Management and treatment of patients with fractured ribs. Nursing Times 2003;99:30. [PMID: 12640789]

Sternal Fracture

- **Essentials of Diagnosis**
  - Blunt injury directly to the anterior chest
  - Tenderness and occasionally crepitus directly over sternum
  - Consider intrathoracic injuries

- **Differential Diagnosis**
  - Contusion
  - Rib fracture

- **Treatment**
  - Pain management
  - Evaluation for intrathoracic injury

- **Pearl**

Pericardial tamponade and other significant intrathoracic injury must be considered.

Reference

Sadaba JR, Oswal D, Munsch CM: Management of isolated sternal fractures: determining risk of blunt cardiac injury. Ann R Coll Surg Engl 2000;82:162. [PMID: 10858676]

19

Abdominal Trauma

Diaphragmatic Injury

- **Essentials of Diagnosis**
  - May be caused by penetrating injury; majority are caused by blunt trauma
  - Diagnosis may be difficult and is often delayed
  - Right-sided rupture leads to more significant hemodynamic instability
  - Left hemidiaphragm ruptures more commonly than the right
  - A nasogastric tube or abdominal contents such as loops of bowel noted above the diaphragm on chest x-ray is pathognomonic for diaphragmatic rupture
  - CT or diagnostic laparoscopy increases sensitivity
  - Patients with diaphragmatic injury are at risk for significant concomitant injuries such as splenic rupture or pulmonary contusion

- **Differential Diagnosis**
  - Hemothorax or pneumothorax
  - Liver or splenic injury
  - Preexisting phrenic nerve injury
  - Preexisting elevated hemidiaphragm
  - Pulmonary contusion

- **Treatment**
  - Primary and secondary survey per ATLS guidelines
  - Operative intervention required as soon as diagnosis of diaphragmatic injury is made; incarceration and strangulation of abdominal organs can occur
  - Laparoscopy versus laparotomy

- **Pearl**

Diaphragmatic injuries never heal spontaneously because of the pressure differential between the abdominal and chest cavities.

Reference

Rubikas R: Diaphragmatic injuries. Eur J Cardiothorac Surg 2001;20:53. [PMID: 11423274]

Duodenal Injury

- ■ Essentials of Diagnosis
  - Usually occurs in the second or third portion of the duodenum secondary to compression against spine
  - Also occurs near fixed points (ligament of Treitz)
  - Occurs more commonly in pediatric patients
  - Associated with chance or transverse vertebral body fractures
  - CT with contrast is a sensitive and noninvasive imaging modality
  - Isolated bowel injury rarely occurs
  - Duodenal hematomas may cause intestinal obstruction with vomiting

- ■ Differential Diagnosis
  - Liver injury
  - Splenic injury
  - Diaphragmatic injury
  - Pancreatic injury
  - Great vessel injury
  - Vertebral fracture

- ■ Treatment
  - Primary and secondary survey per ATLS guidelines
  - Close observation with serial CT scan versus operative intervention
  - Hematomas can be observed
  - Duodenal wall rupture requires surgical intervention

- ■ Pearl

Patients with duodenal injury may be asymptomatic initially and present later with abdominal pain, nausea, and vomiting.

Reference

Hollands M: Duodenal injuries. Injury 2003;34:167. [PMID: 12623244]

Intestinal Injury

■ Essentials of Diagnosis

- May be caused by blunt or penetrating injury
- Blunt trauma occurs due to compressive or decelerative forces
- Injury typically occurs at points of fixation (ligament of Treitz or ileocecal valve)
- Peritoneal signs may be delayed, making clinical exam unreliable
- Initial imaging with x-ray or CT may be negative

■ Differential Diagnosis

- Liver or splenic injury
- Hemothorax or pneumothorax
- Diaphragmatic injury
- Vertebral fracture
- Urogenital injury

■ Treatment

- Primary and secondary survey per ATLS guidelines
- Appropriate crystalloid and colloid resuscitation
- Consultation with trauma surgeon
- Admission for operative versus nonoperative management

■ Pearl

Consider intestinal injury in patients with free intraperitoneal fluid without evidence of solid organ injury noted on abdominal CT.

Reference

Livingston DH: Free fluid on abdominal computed tomography without solid organ injury after blunt abdominal injury does not mandate celiotomy. Am J Surg 2001;182:6. [PMID: 11532406]

Liver Injury

- **Essentials of Diagnosis**
  - More common in blunt trauma than penetrating trauma
  - Alone can be the cause of hemodynamic instability
  - Right upper quadrant pain with possible radiation to right shoulder (Boas sign)
  - Unstable patients evaluated by focused assessment with sonography for trauma (FAST) exam, diagnostic peritoneal lavage, or diagnostic laparotomy
  - Stable patients evaluated by CT scan with contrast
  - Gradation of liver injury has no predictive value regarding need for operative intervention

- **Differential Diagnosis**
  - Diaphragmatic rupture
  - Hemothorax or pneumothorax
  - Biliary tree injury
  - Urogenital injury
  - Mesenteric or intestinal injury

- **Treatment**
  - Primary and secondary survey per ATLS guidelines
  - Appropriate crystalloid and colloid resuscitation
  - Mandatory consultation with a trauma surgeon
  - Unstable patients require operative intervention; stable patients may be observed
  - Avoidance of contact sports in nonoperative management

- **Pearl**

Liver injury must be considered in thoracoabdominal penetrating injuries below the level of the nipple.

Reference

Brasel KJ et al: Incidence and significance of free fluid on abdominal computed tomographic scan in blunt trauma. J Trauma 1998;44:889. [PMID: 9603094]

Pancreatic Injury

- ■ Essentials of Diagnosis
  - • Rare injury, most likely to occur in the setting of blunt trauma
  - • May cause epigastric or flank pain
  - • Unlikely to occur without other thoracoabdominal pathology
  - • May cause retroperitoneal hematoma with tracking to flanks (Grey Turner sign), periumbilical region (Cullen sign), or groin (Fox sign)
  - • Pancreatic enzymes unreliable for diagnosis
  - • Pediatric population at risk owing to improperly positioned lap belts
  - • CT scan with contrast is a sensitive and noninvasive imaging modality
  - • Can be difficult to diagnose initially; delayed presentation 24–48 hours after injury occurs occasionally
  - • Endoscopic retrograde cholangiopancreatography may detect ductal injuries

- ■ Differential Diagnosis
  - • Liver or splenic injury
  - • Vertebral fracture
  - • Duodenal injury
  - • Diaphragmatic injury
  - • Hemothorax or pneumothorax

- ■ Treatment
  - • Primary and secondary survey per ATLS guidelines
  - • Consultation with a trauma surgeon
  - • Admission for operative versus nonoperative management

- ■ Pearl

Pancreatitis, pseudocysts, and phlegmon are common complications of pancreatic injury.

Reference

Cirillo RL: Detecting blunt pancreatic injuries. J Gastrointest Surg 2002;6:587. [PMID: 12127126]

Splenic Injury

- **Essentials of Diagnosis**
  - More common in blunt trauma than penetrating trauma
  - Alone can be the cause of hemodynamic instability
  - Left upper quadrant pain with possible radiation to left shoulder (Kehr sign)
  - Unstable patients evaluated by focused assessment with sonography for trauma (FAST) exam, diagnostic peritoneal lavage, or diagnostic laparotomy
  - Stable patients evaluated by CT scan with contrast
  - Delayed splenic rupture may occur several weeks postinjury
  - Gradation of splenic injury from Grade I (minor) to Grade V (severe injuries involving the hilum) by CT scan helpful for determining need for operative intervention
  - Must be considered in thoracoabdominal penetrating injuries below the level of the nipple

- **Differential Diagnosis**
  - Diaphragmatic rupture
  - Hemothorax or pneumothorax
  - Biliary tree injury
  - Urogenital injury
  - Mesenteric or intestinal injury

- **Treatment**
  - Primary and secondary survey per ATLS guidelines
  - Appropriate crystalloid and colloid resuscitation
  - Mandatory consultation with a trauma surgeon
  - Unstable patients require operative intervention
  - Stable patients with grade I–III injuries typically do not require operative intervention
  - After splenectomy, patients should receive pneumococcal vaccine

- **Pearl**

Splenectomized patients are at risk for infection by encapsulated organisms with progression to sepsis.

Reference

Myers JG, Dent DL, Stewart RM: Blunt splenic injuries: dedicated trauma surgeons can achieve a high rate of nonoperative success in patients of all ages. J Trauma 2000;48:801. [PMID: 10823522]

20

Genitourinary Trauma

Bladder Injury

- **Essentials of Diagnosis**
    - Commonly associated with blunt trauma and pelvic fracture
    - Common findings: gross hematuria, abdominal pain, inability to void
    - Types of injury: bladder wall contusion, bladder rupture (extraperitoneal rupture [85% of all ruptures; usually associated with pelvic fracture] or penetrating trauma to the bladder)
    - Bladder rupture diagnosed by a pelvic CT cystogram or a retrograde cystogram after urethral injury has been ruled out by retrograde urethrogram
    - Cystogram: bladder is distended with 200–400 cc of water-soluble contrast instilled through a Foley catheter, which is then clamped; x-rays also taken with bladder completely drained
    - Simple clamping of the catheter during a contrasted CT scan of the abdomen and pelvis is not adequate to evaluate bladder injuries

- **Differential Diagnosis**
    - Urethral injury
    - Renal injury
    - Pelvic fracture with retroperitoneal hemorrhage

- **Treatment**
    - Intraperitoneal rupture and all penetrating injuries to the bladder: surgical intervention
    - Extraperitoneal injury: nonsurgical management with a Foley catheter, followed by a repeat cystogram in 10–14 days
    - Contusions: Foley catheter drainage and early urologic follow-up

- **Pearl**

The diagnostic study of choice is a CT or conventional cystogram of the bladder.

Reference

Dreitlein DA et al: Genitourinary trauma. Emerg Med Clin North Am 2001;19:569. [PMID: 11554276]

Penile Fracture

- ■ Essentials of Diagnosis
  - Blunt trauma to the erect penis usually during intercourse causing rupture of the corpus cavernosum
  - Diagnosis based on history and physical findings
  - Loud cracking sound as well as immediate onset of severe pain and loss of erection often reported
  - Swollen, ecchymotic, and abnormally shaped penis

- ■ Differential Diagnosis
  - Testicular injury
  - Pelvic fracture with retroperitoneal hemorrhage

- ■ Treatment
  - Immediate urology consult
  - Retrograde urethrogram: to evaluate the possibility of associated urethral injury, if dysuria, inability to void, hematuria, or blood at the meatus is present
  - Surgical repair of the ruptured portion of the corpus cavernosum

- ■ Pearl

Special attention should be given to penile injuries because of their potential for causing impotence and their psychological impact.

Reference

Dreitlein DA et al: Genitourinary trauma. Emerg Med Clin North Am 2001;19:569. [PMID: 11554276]

Renal Injury

- ■ Essentials of Diagnosis
    - • Most common urologic injury
    - • Many can be managed without surgical repair
    - • Hematuria may or may not be present
    - • No specific signs pathognomonic for renal injury, although evidence of potential injury may include localized pain and bruising over flank area
    - • May be associated with lower rib fractures and lumbar vertebral fractures
    - • Extensive blood loss and shock possible due to retroperitoneal bleeding
    - • CT scan of the abdomen and pelvis with intravenous contrast

- ■ Differential Diagnosis
    - • Urethral injury
    - • Bladder injury
    - • Pelvic fracture with retroperitoneal hemorrhage
    - • Liver or splenic injury

- ■ Treatment
    - • Renal contusions (85%) and minor renal lacerations (12%): rarely require operative intervention; outpatient urology follow-up necessary
    - • Major lacerations (3%): may require operative repair
    - • Indications for surgical exploration: uncontrollable renal hemorrhage, shattered kidney, avulsion of the main renal vessels

- ■ Pearl

Renal injuries often (20% of the time) occur with other peritoneal injuries; therefore, CT scan of the abdomen and pelvis with intravenous contrast is the study of choice.

Reference

Dreitlein DA et al: Genitourinary trauma. Emerg Med Clin North Am 2001;19:569. [PMID: 11554276]

Testicular Injury

- **Essentials of Diagnosis**
  - Most commonly due to blunt trauma via direct blow, motor vehicle collisions, or sports-related injuries
  - Scrotal hematoma; tenderness and swelling of the testicle
  - Penetrating injuries also occur and need to be explored to see if only the scrotum is involved or if testicular injury occurred as well
  - Ultrasound with Doppler flow studies has become study of choice

- **Differential Diagnosis**
  - Penile injury
  - Simple scrotal hematoma
  - Pelvic fracture with retroperitoneal hemorrhage

- **Treatment**
  - Urology consult; testicular rupture is a surgical emergency
  - Simple hematomas: scrotal elevation and sitz baths
  - Larger hematomas: may require surgical drainage
  - Testicular rupture and penetrating injuries: surgical repair
  - Surgical repair of testicular injury preserves testicular function in up to 90% of patients (compared with 33% of those managed conservatively)

- **Pearl**

The sensitivity of ultrasound for testicular trauma ranges from 60% to 90%; if there is a high index of suspicion for significant injury, operative exploration should be undertaken.

Reference

Dreitlein DA et al: Genitourinary trauma. Emerg Med Clin North Am 2001;19:569. [PMID: 11554276]

Urethral Injuries, Anterior

- **Essentials of Diagnosis**
  - Common mechanisms of injury: straddle injuries, direct blow to the perineum, instrumentation or improper Foley catheter placement
  - Anterior urethra consists of the bulbous and penile portions
  - In female patients: blood at the urethral meatus and inability to void are most common signs; diagnosis is more difficult because urethrography is not simple; commonly found only during surgical repair of a pelvic fracture
  - Retrograde urethrogram: diagnostic study of choice; tip of Foley catheter placed in urethral orifice and 20–40 cc of water-soluble contrast injected; obtain an oblique x-ray or use fluoroscopy to evaluate urethral continuity

- **Differential Diagnosis**
  - Bladder injury
  - Renal injury
  - Pelvic fracture with retroperitoneal hemorrhage

- **Treatment**
  - Urology consult
  - Long-term catheter drainage to allow healing of the urethra or direct end-to-end reanastomosis

- **Pearl**

Prompt diagnosis and treatment of urethral injuries helps to reduce long-term complications such as urethral strictures and impotence.

Reference

Dreitlein DA et al: Genitourinary trauma. Emerg Med Clin North Am 2001;19:569. [PMID: 11554276]

Urethral Injuries, Posterior

- **Essentials of Diagnosis**
    - Associated with blunt trauma and bony pelvic injuries
    - 35% of patients will also have bladder injuries
    - Posterior urethra consists of the prostatic and membranous urethra
    - Gross hematoma, lower abdominal pain, and inability to void despite sensation of full bladder
    - Classic findings: high-riding or "boggy" prostate noted on rectal exam and blood at the urethral meatus and perineal hematoma
    - Retrograde urethrogram: diagnostic study of choice; tip of Foley catheter placed in urethral orifice and 20–40 cc of water-soluble contrast injected; obtain an oblique x-ray or use fluoroscopy to evaluate urethral continuity

- **Differential Diagnosis**
    - Bladder injury
    - Renal injury
    - Pelvic fracture with retroperitoneal hemorrhage

- **Treatment**
    - Urology consult
    - Suprapubic catheter

- **Pearl**

Maintain a high index of suspicion in any patient with blunt pelvic trauma, especially if pelvic diastasis or fracture is suspected.

Reference

Dreitlein DA et al: Genitourinary trauma. Emerg Med Clin North Am 2001;19:569. [PMID: 11554276]

Vaginal Injury

- **Essentials of Diagnosis**
  - Mechanisms of injury: trauma from sexual intercourse or sexual assault, blunt injury, straddle injury, penetrating injury
  - Vaginal lacerations can result in significant amount of bleeding
  - All vaginal lacerations and penetrating vaginal injuries need exploration to ensure that the pelvic floor has not been penetrated; penetration of the pelvic floor can be associated with significant organ and vascular damage
  - All vaginal bleeding with history of trauma requires speculum examination regardless of whether patient is currently menstruating
  - Concomitant rectal or urologic injuries must be ruled out

- **Differential Diagnosis**
  - Urethral injury
  - Pelvic fracture
  - Rectal injury

- **Treatment**
  - Simple lacerations: repaired with absorbable sutures
  - Operative repair required if unable to obtain hemostasis or when penetration of the pelvic floor has occurred
  - Gynecology referral for all patients with genital injuries

- **Pearl**

The possibility of sexual assault must always be considered during evaluation of a patient with vaginal injuries.

Reference

Dreitlein DA et al: Genitourinary trauma. Emerg Med Clin North Am 2001;19:569. [PMID: 11554276]

21

Vertebral & Spinal Injuries

C1 Fracture

- Essentials of Diagnosis
  - Burst fracture (also known as Jefferson fracture) typically results from axial loading, although hyperextension can fracture the posterior arch
  - Diving is the most frequent cause of injury
  - Associated with odontoid fractures
  - Open mouth odontoid view of cervical spine series most useful image; shows a burst fracture with displaced lateral masses with respect to the axis
  - May be associated with rupture of the transverse ligament

- Differential Diagnosis
  - Hangman or odontoid fracture
  - Herniated disc
  - Osteoarthritis or degenerative disease
  - Atlantoaxial dislocation
  - Occipital condyle fracture

- Treatment
  - Primary and secondary survey per ATLS guidelines
  - Cervical collar and long board immobilization per ATLS guidelines
  - Imaging of entire cervical, thoracic, and lumbar spine
  - Consultation with spine specialist
  - Nonoperative halo immobilization versus operative fixation

- Pearl

Unlike all other vertebrae, C1, also known as the atlas, is a ring-like structure that has no vertebral body. It is composed of a thicker anterior arch and a thinner posterior arch.

Reference

Jackson RS et al: Upper cervical spine injuries. J Am Acad Orthop Surg 2002;10:271. [PMID: 15089076]

Cervical Strain

- **Essentials of Diagnosis**
  - Diagnosis of exclusion; typically results from cervical acceleration-deceleration injury
  - Tenderness to palpation of the trapezius muscles may be evident
  - NEXUS criteria: cervical spine x-rays needed unless patient has no midline tenderness, normal level of alertness, no intoxication, no focal neurologic deficits, and no distracting injury
  - The Canadian c-spine rule suggests that no cervical spine x-rays are required in blunt trauma patients (1) who have no high risk signs or symptoms (age >65 years, high-risk mechanism, or paresthesias in upper extremities), (2) in whom any of the following (low-speed rear-end collision, sitting upright in the emergency department, delayed onset of pain, no midline neck tenderness) suggest that the patient can safely have range of motion tested out of the cervical collar, and (3) who have normal range of motion
  - Range of motion without midline pain helpful in excluding vertebral pathology
  - CT or MRI may be needed if pain persists and x-rays are negative; plain x-rays often miss fractures of C1 and C2

- **Differential Diagnosis**
  - Cervical fracture
  - Herniated disc
  - Osteoarthritis or degenerative disease
  - Carotid artery dissection
  - Epidural hematoma
  - Cardiothoracic injury with referred pain

- **Treatment**
  - Primary and secondary survey per ATLS guidelines
  - Cervical collar and long board immobilization per ATLS guidelines
  - Analgesics, muscle relaxants, ice, and rest

- **Pearl**

When evaluating patients with traumatic neck pain, always assume a fracture is present and protect the spinal column with strict immobilization until the possibility of spinal injury has been excluded.

Reference

Edwards MJ et al: Routine cervical spine radiography for trauma victims: does everybody need it? J Trauma 2001;50:529. [PMID: 11265034]

Clay Shoveler Fracture (Spinous Process Fracture)

- **Essentials of Diagnosis**
    - Typically results from flexion injury resulting in spinous process avulsion or from direct trauma to the posterior neck
    - Usually involves the lower cervical spine, most commonly the C7 spinous process
    - Midline tenderness and crepitus
    - Cervical spine x-rays reveal injury on lateral view
    - Neurologic findings should be absent

- **Differential Diagnosis**
    - Vertebral body fracture
    - Herniated disc
    - Cervical strain

- **Treatment**
    - Primary and secondary survey per ATLS guidelines
    - Cervical collar and long board immobilization per ATLS guidelines
    - Analgesics, muscle relaxants, ice, and rest

- **Pearl**

The clay shoveler fracture is a stable fracture requiring only immobilization and symptomatic management.

Reference

Ivy ME, Cohn SM: Addressing the myths of cervical spine injury management. Am J Emerg Med 1997;15:591. [PMID: 9337369]

Compression Fracture

■ Essentials of Diagnosis

- Typically associated with axial loading or flexion
- Anterior aspect of the vertebral body collapses, although the height of the posterior vertebral body is often preserved
- May be associated with canal compromise and neurologic deficit
- Midline tenderness or stepoff may be evident
- Anteroposterior and lateral x-rays for diagnosis
- CT more sensitive for canal compromise
- Common in the osteoporotic or steroid-dependent patients

■ Differential Diagnosis

- Herniated disc
- Osteoarthritis or degenerative disease
- Epidural hematoma
- Paravertebral spasm

■ Treatment

- Primary and secondary survey per ATLS guidelines
- Cervical collar and long board immobilization per ATLS guidelines
- Imaging of entire cervical, thoracic, and lumbar spine
- Although controversial, steroid administration is generally recommended if spinal cord deficit is found within 8 hours of injury
- Nonoperative management with brace versus operative fixation
- Failure to recognize and brace appropriately may result in permanent kyphotic deformity

■ Pearl

A compression fracture with greater than 40% loss of height along the anterior border of the vertebral body may indicate a burst fracture with retropulsion of the bony fragments and resultant canal compromise.

Reference

Holmes JF: Epidemiology of thoracolumbar spine injury in blunt trauma. Acad Emerg Med 2001;8:866. [PMID: 11535478]

Hangman Fracture

■ **Essentials of Diagnosis**
  • Fracture of lateral masses of C_2
  • Odontoid view may reveal misalignment of lateral masses of C_1 and C_2 vertebrae
  • Typically results from hyperextension and distraction
  • Also may occur with axial loading and lateral flexion
  • Midline tenderness or stepoff may be evident
  • CT may be needed in the setting of persistent pain and negative x-ray findings
  • Extremely unstable fracture

■ **Differential Diagnosis**
  • Jefferson or odontoid fracture
  • Herniated disc
  • Osteoarthritis or degenerative disease
  • Atlantoaxial dislocation

■ **Treatment**
  • Primary and secondary survey per ATLS guidelines
  • Cervical collar and long board immobilization per ATLS guidelines
  • Imaging of entire cervical, thoracic, and lumbar spine when a fracture at one level is identified
  • Consultation with spine specialist
  • Ranges from hard collar immobilization to halo immobilization, cervical traction, or operative intervention, depending on classification of fracture

■ **Pearl**
Apnea may occur with transection of the upper cervical spinal cord.

Reference

Frohna WJ: Emergency department evaluation and treatment of the neck and cervical spine injuries. Emerg Med Clin North Am 1999;17:739. [PMID: 10584102]

Locked Facets, Bilateral

■ Essentials of Diagnosis

- Also known as bilateral interfacetal dislocation; typically results from flexion injury
- Midline tenderness and neurologic deficit may be apparent, but their absence does not exclude this injury
- Cervical spine x-rays aid diagnosis; lateral view reveals anterior prevertebral soft tissue swelling and up to 50% anterior displacement of vertebral body; the facets of the superior vertebra displace anterior to the facets of the inferior vertebra; anteroposterior view shows normal alignment with no rotation of the spinous processes
- Extremely unstable fracture with high likelihood for spinal cord compression

■ Differential Diagnosis

- Vertebral fracture
- Vertebral subluxation
- Herniated disc
- Unilateral locked facet

■ Treatment

- Primary and secondary survey per ATLS guidelines
- Cervical collar and long board immobilization per ATLS guidelines
- Consultation with spine specialist
- Although controversial, steroid administration is generally recommended if spinal cord deficit is found within 8 hours of injury
- Reduction with cervical traction

■ Pearl

Bilateral locked facets is an injury that rarely occurs outside of the cervical spine.

Reference

Mower WR: Use of plain radiography to screen for cervical spine injuries. Ann Emerg Med 2001;38:1. [PMID: 11423803]

Locked Facets, Unilateral (Unilateral Interfacetal Dislocation)

- ■ Essentials of Diagnosis
    - Typically results from flexion and rotation injury
    - Midline tenderness and neurologic deficit may be apparent, but their absence does not exclude this injury
    - Cervical spine x-rays aid diagnosis; anteroposterior view reveals malalignment of spinous processes, whereas lateral view reveals anterior prevertebral soft tissue swelling and up to 25% anterior displacement of vertebral body
    - Plain x-rays may initially be negative
    - Unilateral locked facet injuries are typically more stable than bilateral locked facet injuries
    - Requires high index of suspicion

- ■ Differential Diagnosis
    - Vertebral fracture
    - Vertebral subluxation
    - Herniated disc
    - Bilateral locked facet
    - Cervical strain

- ■ Treatment
    - Primary and secondary survey per ATLS guidelines
    - Cervical collar and long board immobilization per ATLS guidelines
    - Consultation with spine specialist
    - Although controversial, steroid administration is generally recommended if spinal cord deficit is found within 8 hours of injury
    - Reduction with cervical traction

- ■ Pearl

Because the dislocated facet rests in the neuroforaminal canal, nerve impingement signs on the ipsilateral side are often noted with unilateral locked facet injuries.

Reference

Crawford NR: Unilateral cervical facet dislocation: injury mechanism and biomechanical consequences. Spine 2002;7:1858. [PMID: 12221349]

Odontoid Fracture

- ■ Essentials of Diagnosis
  - • Typically results from flexion-extension with rotation
  - • Most common upper cervical spine fracture
  - • Pain or feeling of instability of head on spine
  - • Perform complete neurologic exam to exclude cervical cord or nerve root impingement
  - • Radiography or CT classifies fracture as type I (tip of the dens fracture—rare), II (base of the dens fracture), or III (fracture extends into the body of C2); anterior prevertebral soft tissue swelling often present
  - • Open mouth odontoid view of cervical spine series most useful image; specific findings include misalignment of the lateral masses of the C1 and C2 vertebrae
  - • Type II and III fractures considered unstable and may involve disruption of transverse ligament

- ■ Differential Diagnosis
  - • Jefferson or Hangman fracture
  - • Herniated disc
  - • Osteoarthritis or degenerative disease
  - • Occipital condyle fracture
  - • Atlantoaxial dislocation

- ■ Treatment
  - • Primary and secondary survey per ATLS guidelines
  - • Cervical collar and long board immobilization per ATLS guidelines
  - • Imaging of entire cervical, thoracic, and lumbar spine when a fracture at any level is identified
  - • Consultation with spine specialist
  - • Ranges from hard collar immobilization to halo immobilization to cervical traction to operative intervention, depending on classification of fracture

- ■ Pearl

Neurologic deficits from odontoid fractures can range from quadriplegia to minimal upper extremity deficits secondary to impingement of cervical nerve roots.

Reference

Frohna WJ: Emergency department evaluation and treatment of the neck and cervical spine injuries. Emerg Med Clin North Am 1999;17:739. [PMID: 10584102]

Spinal Cord Injury

- **Essentials of Diagnosis**
  - Typically associated with vertebral fracture but fracture not necessary (SCIWORA: spinal cord injury without radiographic abnormality)
  - Historically patient relates neurologic deficit
  - Requires complete neurologic assessment identifying level of injury based on signs and symptoms
  - Classified as cord contusion, incomplete, or complete injury
  - MRI helpful for diagnosis
  - CT helpful to evaluate fractures and dislocations of the spinal column

- **Differential Diagnosis**
  - Herniated disc
  - Facetal dislocation
  - Spinal hematoma

- **Treatment**
  - Primary and secondary survey per ATLS guidelines
  - Cervical collar and long board immobilization per ATLS guidelines
  - Consultation with spine specialist
  - Although controversial, steroid administration is generally recommended if spinal cord deficit is found within 8 hours of injury

- **Pearl**

Patients with spinal cord injury may develop neurogenic shock from denervation of the sympathetic chain and present with warm, dry skin; hypotension; and paradoxical bradycardia.

Reference

Hendey GW: Spinal cord injury without radiographic abnormality: results of the National Emergency X-Radiography Utilization Study in blunt cervical trauma. J Trauma 2002;53:1. [PMID: 12131380]

Spinal Cord Injury without Radiographic Abnormality (SCIWORA)

- **Essentials of Diagnosis**
    - Plain x-rays and CT scan reveal no evidence of fracture
    - Historically patient relates neurologic deficit (usually weakness or paresthesias) to the time of initial injury; initial symptoms are often transient, but neurologic deficits become more prominent hours to days later
    - Requires complete neurologic assessment identifying level of injury based on signs and symptoms
    - Classified as contusion, incomplete, or complete injury
    - MRI is needed to evaluate the injury
    - Helmet-to-helmet football injuries are a common mechanism

- **Differential Diagnosis**
    - Herniated disc
    - Facetal dislocation
    - Spinal hematoma

- **Treatment**
    - Primary and secondary survey per ATLS guidelines
    - Cervical collar and long board immobilization per ATLS guidelines
    - Consultation with spine specialist
    - Although controversial, steroid administration is generally recommended if a spinal cord deficit is found within 8 hours of injury

- **Pearl**

Previously thought to occur almost exclusively in children, SCIWORA was found only in adults and was very rare (incidence of less than 0.1% of all the patients enrolled) in the recent National Emergency X-Radiography Utilization Study of over 30,000 patients (3,000 of whom were children) evaluated for cervical trauma.

Reference

Hendey GW: Spinal cord injury without radiographic abnormality: results of the National Emergency X-Radiography Utilization Study in blunt cervical trauma. J Trauma 2002;53:1. [PMID: 12131380]

22

Orthopedic Emergencies

Achilles Tendon Rupture

- Essentials of Diagnosis
  - Rupture mechanisms: high-energy injuries, mechanical imbalance, degenerative changes; most commonly secondary to sports, usually from pushing off the forefoot with the knee in extension, or from sudden dorsiflexion
  - Changes in athletic routine and poor footwear can contribute; "weekend warrior"–type athletes tend to be at greater risk
  - Increased rupture rates associated with steroid injection, systemic steroids, fluoroquinolones, and various systemic diseases
  - Sudden onset of pain in acute rupture; ambulation may be difficult
  - Diminished or absent ability to plantar flex the ankle and foot
  - Thompson test to assess integrity of Achilles tendon: patient lies supine with feet over edge of bed, squeeze calf (with intact tendon the foot should plantar flex; always check contralateral side)
  - Ankle swelling, ecchymosis over rupture site; a defect in the tendon may be palpable depending on amount of edema
  - Rupture 2–6 cm proximal to the insertion
  - MRI helpful but not indicated in emergent setting

- Differential Diagnosis
  - Fracture
  - Sprain
  - Contusion

- Treatment
  - Controversial: operative vs. nonoperative
  - Discuss with orthopedist
  - Likely discharge with immobilization in equinus (plantarflexed) position, non-weight-bearing instructions, and early orthopedic follow-up

- Pearl

Conservative (nonsurgical) treatment has a somewhat higher rate of repeat rupture and is generally not recommended for athletes.

Reference

Mazzone MF, McCue T: Common conditions of the Achilles tendon. Am Fam Physician 2002;65:1805. [PMID: 12018803]

Acromioclavicular (AC) Joint Injury

- **Essentials of Diagnosis**
  - Pain, deformity, and tenderness at AC joint
  - Patient examined in dependent position, to maximize any visible deformity
  - Patients often present holding arm in adduction supported by unaffected arm
  - Shoulder series (anteroposterior, scapular Y, and axillary views)
  - Most common mechanism: direct blow or fall on lateral aspect of the shoulder with arm in adduction
  - Most AC joint injuries are sports related; frequent AC joint injuries in players of contact sports

- **Differential Diagnosis**
  - Type I: AC ligament sprain (AC joint tenderness, minimal pain with arm motion)
  - Type II: AC ligament tear with joint separation, coracoclavicular ligaments sprained (distal clavicle slightly superior to acromion and mobile to palpation; x-rays show slight elevation of distal end of clavicle and AC joint widening)
  - Type III: AC and coracoclavicular ligaments torn with AC joint dislocation (deltoid and trapezius muscles usually detached from clavicle; coracoclavicular widening evident)
  - Glenohumeral dislocation or occult fracture
  - Clavicle fracture

- **Treatment**
  - Type I: sling and rest for 7–10 days
  - Type II: sling for 1–2 weeks, start gentle range of motion as soon as possible, refrain from heavy activity for 6 weeks
  - Type III: nonoperative management indicated for inactive, non-laboring, or recreational athletic patients; sling, early range of motion, and strengthening; operative treatment is controversial but may be indicated for competitive athletes or heavy laborers, especially those who do overhead work

- **Pearl**

Type IV, V (clavicle displaces superiorly into trapezius), and VI (clavicle displaces inferiorly) AC injuries involve complete dislocation of the AC joint and must be considered for open reduction and internal fixation.

Reference

Shaffer BS: Painful conditions of the acromioclavicular joint. J Am Acad Orthop Surg 1999;7:176. [PMID: 10346826]

Ankle Dislocation

- **Essentials of Diagnosis**
    - Dislocation of the talus in reference to the tibia
    - Isolated ankle dislocations quite rare; almost always associated with fracture
    - A 1-mm lateral shift decreases surface contact by 40%; 3-mm shift decreases contact by about 60%
    - Mechanism: usually sports related or from high-energy injury such as motor vehicle collision
    - Posterior dislocations are most common; caused by axial loading while foot is in plantarflexion
    - Gross deformity noted; pain, edema, ecchymoses
    - Neurovascular compromise possible

- **Differential Diagnosis**
    - Isolated dislocation
    - Fracture and dislocation
    - Subtalar dislocation
    - Fracture
    - Sprain

- **Treatment**
    - Immediate reduction with longitudinal traction to restore anatomy and diminish neurovascular compromise and long-term sequelae
    - X-rays after reduction
    - Posterior splint and elevation
    - Adequate analgesia
    - Close inspection for open wounds; if present, cover with sterile, saline-soaked gauze
    - Orthopedic consult required

- **Pearl**

Carefully assess neurovascular status before reduction and frequently thereafter; dislocated ankles can be very unstable injuries and may dislocate again.

Reference

Rivera F: Pure dislocation of the ankle: three case reports and literature review. Clin Orthop 2001;382:179. [PMID: 11153985]

Ankle Fracture

■ Essentials of Diagnosis

- Ankle injuries are common; owing to joint mobility and the weight supported by relatively small surface area
- Ankle joint: composed of the tibia (tibial plafond, medial malleolus, and posterior malleolus), fibula (lateral malleolus), talus, calcaneus, and multiple supporting ligaments
- Plantarflexion and dorsiflexion occur at tibiotalar junction; inversion and eversion occur at subtalar joint
- Most fractures and ligamentous injuries are due to inversion
- Mechanism of injury and foot position during incident can help predict fracture pattern and severity
- Examine for deformity, swelling, point tenderness, and ecchymoses; check for open wounds and neurovascular injury
- Examine knee and foot, paying particular attention to the proximal fibula and proximal 5th metatarsal
- Anteroposterior, lateral, and mortise views of ankle if Ottawa ankle rules criteria are met; add knee and foot films based on clinical judgment of associated injury
- Ottawa ankle rules: acute ankle pain associated with bony tenderness at posterior edge or tip of medial malleolus, *or* bony tenderness at posterior edge of lateral malleolus, *or* inability to bear weight both immediately and in the emergency department
- Excluded from Ottawa rules: patients younger than age 18 years; those with underlying neurologic deficit, altered mental status, or multisystem trauma

■ Differential Diagnosis

- Fracture
- Dislocation
- Sprain

■ Treatment

- Open and unstable fractures: orthopedic consult
- Stable, nondisplaced fractures: may be splinted in emergency department; discharge with close orthopedic follow-up
- Rest, ice, elevation, analgesics, and non-weight-bearing instructions

■ Pearl

Post-traumatic arthritis is a common complication with ankle fractures, especially those with an intra-articular component.

Reference

Pijnenburg AC: Radiography in acute ankle injuries: the Ottawa ankle rules vs local diagnostic decision rules. Ann Emerg Med 2002;39:599. [PMID: 12023701]

Calcaneus Fracture

- **Essentials of Diagnosis**
  - Mechanism: requires significant force; injury almost always results from falls from height or motor vehicle collisions
  - High incidence of other injuries (eg, spine fractures and other extremity fractures)
  - Calcaneus is most frequently injured tarsal bone
  - Examine for pain, ecchymoses, deformity, and significant swelling
  - Foot and ankle anteroposterior and lateral x-rays; axial view of the calcaneus (Harris view) is helpful
  - CT may be required to ascertain full extent of fracture and assess for concomitant foot fractures
  - Measurement of Böhler angle can confirm presence of fracture: formed by intersection of a line from the highest point of the anterior process to the highest point of the posterior facet and a line that runs along upper edge of the tuberosity; angle should be about 20–40 degrees, flattening of angle (<20 degrees) indicates fracture; comparison views can be particularly valuable

- **Differential Diagnosis**
  - Fracture
  - Dislocation
  - Subluxation
  - Sprain

- **Treatment**
  - Pain control
  - Nondisplaced and extra-articular fractures: splinting and non-weight-bearing instructions (splint should be very well padded secondary to severe swelling that often occurs with these fractures); advise elevation
  - Displaced and intra-articular fractures: orthopedic consult; usually open reduction and internal fixation

- **Pearl**

Failure to perform a complete trauma evaluation in the face of a calcaneus fracture can lead to significant and life-threatening injuries being missed.

Reference

Juliano P: Fractures of the calcaneus. Orthop Clin North Am 2001;32:35. [PMID: 11465132]

Clavicle Fracture

■ **Essentials of Diagnosis**
- Pain, deformity, or tenderness of clavicle
- Detailed neurovascular exam of affected upper extremity needed to evaluate potential associated brachial plexus or subclavian vessel injuries
- Most heal with conservative management
- Anteroposterior view and anterior and posterior obliques shot at 45 degrees
- Mechanism: approximately 85% due to falls directly onto affected shoulder
- Proximal clavicle fractures often tent the skin; examine skin closely to ensure open fracture is not present

■ **Differential Diagnosis**
- Shoulder dislocation
- Acromioclavicular separation in distal fractures
- Sternoclavicular dislocation

■ **Treatment**
- Closed treatment successful in most cases, with no need for reduction
- Management goal is to brace shoulder girdle with sling immobilization until x-rays demonstrate callus formation (2–4 weeks for children, 4–8 weeks for adolescents or adults)
- Operative indications are rare but consider for open fractures, fracture with associated neurovascular injury, fractures with severe associated injuries such as scapulothoracic dissociation, and for cosmetic reasons; operative scar may be worse than original deformity
- Sling has been shown to give same results as figure-of-eight bandages, while providing more comfort
- Closed fractures: immobilization; primary care or orthopedic follow-up
- Open fractures: often require hospitalization

■ **Pearl**

The medial clavicle protects the brachial plexus, the subclavian and axillary vessels, and the superior lung. Always consider pneumothorax in patients with clavicular fractures and shortness of breath or chest pain.

Reference

Eiff MP: Management of clavicle fractures. Am Fam Physician 1997;55:121. [PMID: 9012272]

Compartment Syndrome

- **Essentials of Diagnosis**
  - Edema within a closed space may result in vascular compromise and decreased blood flow with eventual neurologic compromise
  - The five P's of compartment syndrome: pallor, pulselessness, pain, paresthesias, poikilothermia
  - Pulselessness is a very late and ominous finding
  - Pain with passive range of motion; often out of proportion to exam
  - Compartment pressures may be measured with a Stryker needle or with a needle connected to an arterial line monitor (pressures >30 mm Hg are abnormal)

- **Differential Diagnosis**
  - Occult fracture or dislocation
  - Contusion

- **Treatment**
  - Initial measures: immobilization, elevation, and removal of any constricting bandage or splint
  - Pressures >30 mm Hg: generally require immediate fasciotomy, preferably by a surgeon
  - Pressures <30 mm Hg but with significant clinical findings: often require hospitalization for serial exams and compartment pressure measurements
  - Look for and treat associated complications such as rhabdomyolysis, hypovolemia, renal failure, and hyperkalemia

- **Pearl**

The diagnosis of compartment syndrome is much more difficult in patients with altered consciousness; therefore, clinicians caring for such patients must frequently reexamine injured extremities and maintain a high degree of suspicion for compartment syndrome.

Reference

Malinoski DJ, Slater MS, Mullins RJ: Crush injury and rhabdomyolysis. Crit Care Clin 2004;20:171. [PMID: 14979336]

Distal Femur Fracture

- **Essentials of Diagnosis**
    - Mechanism: direct or indirect forces but more commonly from direct trauma
    - Pain and deformity of femur; shortening due to hamstring and quadriceps muscle groups, with angulation and posterior displacement from gastrocnemius muscle action
    - Anteroposterior and lateral views of femur and knee required for diagnosis; CT utilized occasionally to evaluate intra-articular extension of fracture
    - May still lose large blood volume, though generally less than with femoral shaft fractures
    - Patients with nondisplaced femoral condyle fractures may sometimes be ambulatory

- **Differential Diagnosis**
    - Fracture
    - Knee dislocation
    - Contusion
    - Ligamentous or meniscal injury

- **Treatment**
    - Pain control
    - Close monitoring of neurovascular status
    - Traction
    - Orthopedic consult
    - Most patients admitted for definitive operative management

- **Pearl**

All long bone injuries can result in hemodynamically significant blood loss.

Reference

Emparanza JI: Validation of the Ottawa knee rules. Ann Emerg Med 2001;38:364. [PMID: 11574791]

Elbow Dislocation

- **Essentials of Diagnosis**
  - Most common mechanism: fall onto an outstretched arm or elbow; associated fractures common
  - Elbow is second only to shoulder as most commonly dislocated major joint
  - Patients present guarding affected arm and holding elbow in flexion with variable instability and massive swelling
  - Most common dislocations are posterior
  - Careful neurovascular exam is crucial; should be performed immediately and after any manipulation occurs
  - Most common associated neurovascular injuries occur to the brachial artery and the median nerve

- **Differential Diagnosis**
  - Humerus or forearm fracture
  - Elbow sprain or strain
  - Elbow effusion

- **Treatment**
  - Closed reduction appropriate for most elbow dislocations without associated fracture or neurovascular injury
  - Closed reduction of posterior dislocations: apply longitudinal traction to the forearm as an assistant stabilizes the humerus; while maintaining longitudinal traction, flex the elbow to 90 degrees as the assistant applies posterior pressure to the humerus
  - Ensure neurovascular integrity after reduction and postreduction radiographic evaluation
  - After successful reduction, splint arm with a long arm posterior splint with the elbow at 90 degrees
  - Reduction of anterior dislocations: apply initial longitudinal traction to the flexed forearm, followed by dorsally directed pressure on the volar forearm coupled with anteriorly directed pressure on the distal humerus
  - For most patients: discharge home with splint and sling immobilization and orthopedic follow-up within 48 hours

- **Pearl**

A radial pulse does not rule out brachial artery compromise because there may be collateral supply.

Reference

Villarin LA, Belk KE, Freid R: Emergency department evaluation and treatment of elbow and forearm injuries. Emerg Med Clin North Am 1999;17:843. [PMID: 10584105]

Femoral Shaft Fracture

- **Essentials of Diagnosis**
  - Suggested by thigh pain, deformity, swelling, or shortening
  - Generally requires significant mechanism of injury
  - Thorough neurovascular exam is essential; significant blood loss into the closed space possible, with potential to produce hypotension or a lower extremity compartment syndrome
  - Anteroposterior and lateral views of femur, as well as hip and knee views; associated fractures are common
  - Fractures with minimal trauma should raise suspicion of pathologic fracture
  - Thorough trauma evaluation for serious associated injuries, such as spinal fractures and intra-abdominal hemorrhage

- **Differential Diagnosis**
  - Hip fracture or dislocation
  - Knee fracture or dislocation
  - Thigh contusion or hematoma

- **Treatment**
  - Careful attention to the ABCs of evaluation and resuscitation
  - Early immobilization and adequate analgesia
  - Inline traction to minimize potential volume for blood loss; helps to minimize pain
  - Orthopedic consult required
  - Open fractures: emergent treatment in operating room with irrigation, debridement, and fixation
  - Femur fractures with neurovascular compromise, absent distal pulses, or expanding hematoma: emergent angiography or femoral artery exploration possibly required

- **Pearl**

Knee dislocations and compartment syndrome are two commonly missed associated injuries that may result in significant morbidity; therefore, repetitive neurovascular checks may help limit missed diagnoses and subsequent adverse sequelae.

Reference

Russell GV et al: Complicated femoral shaft fractures. Orthop Clin North Am 2002;33:127. [PMID: 11832317]

Fibula Fracture

- ■ Essentials of Diagnosis
    - • Isolated fibula fractures relatively uncommon
    - • Mechanism: usually a direct blow
    - • High degree of association with tibia fractures owing to transmission of forces along the interosseous membrane
    - • Patients with medial malleolus fractures or medial ankle ligamentous disruption can have associated proximal fibula fractures from transmission of the external rotational forces on the foot through the interosseous membrane (Maisonneuve fracture)
    - • Isolated fibula fractures: patients may be ambulatory; generally heal well secondary to stabilization from the surrounding musculature and the tibia
    - • Fractures of the fibular neck may result in peroneal nerve damage and lead to foot drop
    - • Anteroposterior and lateral views of knee, tibia, fibula, and ankle

- ■ Differential Diagnosis
    - • Fracture
    - • Contusion
    - • Stress fracture
    - • Knee sprain

- ■ Treatment
    - • Pain control
    - • Weight bearing as tolerated (crutches for comfort)
    - • Long leg cast or splint is unnecessary
    - • Orthopedic follow-up

- ■ Pearl

Because isolated fibula fractures are rare, it is important to look closely for associated fractures of the tibia.

Reference

Donatto KC: Ankle fractures and syndesmosis injuries. Orthop Clin North Am 2001;32:79. [PMID: 11465135]

Forearm Fracture

■ **Essentials of Diagnosis**

- Common mechanisms: direct trauma, fall onto an outstretched hand (FOOSH); commonly result from contact sports and motor vehicle collisions
- Hallmarks: forearm pain, deformity, crepitus, decreased range of motion
- X-ray evaluation (anteroposterior and lateral views including the elbow and the wrist) confirms diagnosis
- Careful neurovascular exam to document radial, ulnar, and median nerve function as well as distal pulses; watch for development of compartment syndrome
- Eponyms often used to describe common fracture patterns: Colles fracture (transverse fracture of distal radius with dorsal angulation), Smith fracture (transverse fracture of distal radius with volar displacement), Barton fracture (intra-articular fracture of distal radius, often associated with dislocation of the carpal bones), Hutchinson (chauffeur's) fracture (intra-articular fracture of the radial styloid), Monteggia fracture (proximal ulnar fracture, associated with dislocation of the radial head), Galeazzi fracture (distal radius fracture associated with distal radioulnar joint dislocation)

■ **Differential Diagnosis**

- Forearm contusion, sprain, or strain
- Radial head or other subluxation or dislocation

■ **Treatment**

- Open fractures: intravenous antibiotics and irrigation, debridement, and fixation in the operating room
- Fractures with tenting of the skin or severe displacement: generally reduced and splinted under procedural sedation in the emergency department
- Minimally displaced fractures: sugar-tong splint and prompt orthopedic follow-up

■ **Pearl**

In patients with altered mental status and significant fractures of the forearm, maintain high suspicion for compartment syndrome and associated neurovascular injuries; arrange emergent intervention if present.

Reference

Andersen DJ et al: Classification of distal radius fractures: an analysis of interobserver reliability and intraobserver reproducibility. J Hand Surg [Am] 1996;21:574. [PMID: 8842946]

Hip Fracture

- **Essentials of Diagnosis**
  - Suggested by groin, hip, thigh, or medial knee pain with weight bearing or movement
  - Common in elderly patients, especially women with osteoporosis; often occurs with minimal trauma
  - Patients often present with affected limb abducted, shortened, and externally rotated
  - Anteroposterior and lateral x-rays usually sufficient for initial diagnosis
  - Consider CT scan if x-rays appear negative but clinical suspicion is high; CT useful in further defining the fracture for treatment options
  - Hip fractures are generally described anatomically as femoral neck, intertrochanteric, or subtrochanteric
  - Nondisplaced femoral neck fractures may be difficult to visualize; may be seen as stress fractures in young patients such as runners or military recruits
  - Subtrochanteric fractures are a common site for pathologic fracture

- **Differential Diagnosis**
  - Pelvic fracture
  - Lumbar spine injury
  - Septic joint
  - Hip dislocation
  - Pathologic fracture

- **Treatment**
  - Immobilization and gentle traction: important initial measures to minimize potentially significant blood loss
  - If fracture is closed and no neurologic deficit is present, traction may be achieved with a Hare traction splint
  - Femoral neck fractures are associated with 20% incidence of avascular necrosis; involve orthopedics as soon as possible
  - All hip fractures or dislocations require orthopedic consult, which must occur emergently if neurovascular compromise is present

- **Pearl**

Early immobilization and analgesia are important in all hip fractures and may help limit long-term sequelae and morbidity.

Reference

Brunner LC, Eshilian-Oates L, Kuo TY: Hip fractures in adults. Am Fam Physician 2003;67:537. [PMID: 12588076]

Humerus Fracture

■ Essentials of Diagnosis

- Common fracture in the elderly, especially in women with osteoporosis
- Often seen with falls onto an outstretched hand (FOOSH) injuries
- Suggested by pain, deformity, and difficulty initiating motion at shoulder joint
- Anteroposterior and lateral views of humerus confirm diagnosis; anteroposterior, lateral, and axillary lateral or scapular Y views of the shoulder to exclude possibility of concomitant glenohumeral dislocation
- Assessment of axillary, radial, ulnar, and median nerve function
- Brachial artery is near distal humeral shaft
- Proximal humerus fractures most common

■ Differential Diagnosis

- Traumatic rotator cuff tear
- Dislocation
- Calcific tendonitis
- Acromioclavicular separation
- Tendon rupture
- Pathologic fracture

■ Treatment

- Immediate immobilization with coaptation splint for shaft fractures; sling for proximal fractures to prevent further neurovascular injury
- Orthopedic consult concerning operative vs. nonoperative management: one- or two-part fractures often treated with closed reduction; three- or four-part fractures are unstable and may require open reduction and internal fixation
- Conservative management is generally the rule, especially in the elderly; approximately 90% of humerus fractures heal with nonsurgical management
- Orthopedic follow-up within 3–4 days; for young patients, consider orthopedic consult in emergency department

■ Pearl

Ensure intact neurovascular status before and after any manipulation of humeral shaft fractures such as application of a coaptation splint, because the prevalence of associated radial nerve injury may be as high as 18%.

Reference

Ring D, Jupiter JB: Fractures of the distal humerus. Orthop Clin North Am 2000;31:103. [PMID: 10629336]

Knee Ligamentous Injury

- **Essentials of Diagnosis**
  - Four main ligaments: medial and lateral collateral (MCL, LCL) and anterior and posterior cruciate (ACL, PCL)
  - Collateral ligaments are around the joint; cruciate ligaments are within the joint
  - Isolated LCL injury is rare; generally associated with posterolateral complex injuries, with or without ACL or PCL damage
  - MCL tears are secondary to valgus stress; may be isolated or associated with ACL, PCL, or LCL injuries
  - ACL prevents anterior translation of tibia on femur; PCL prevents posterior translation
  - Patients usually complain of pain and a popping sensation, possibly report knee giving out, especially with ACL rupture
  - Most commonly patients are still able to bear weight but may complain of instability in varying degrees
  - Cruciate injuries associated with joint effusion; collateral injuries may have tenderness on palpation and perhaps ecchymoses
  - Careful exam required of both injured and noninjured limbs to check for stability; may be difficult secondary to an effusion or guarding in the immediate postinjury period
  - Anteroposterior and lateral views if indicated to rule out fracture
  - MRI not an appropriate or necessary emergency department study for these injuries

- **Differential Diagnosis**
  - Contusion
  - Fracture
  - Dislocation
  - Meniscal tear

- **Treatment**
  - Hinged knee brace for immobilization if no fracture
  - Pain control and weight-bearing activity as tolerated; crutches for comfort
  - Early orthopedic follow-up to determine operative vs. nonoperative (strength and mobility rehabilitation) treatment

- **Pearl**

Stiffness or instability can be long-term complications resulting from ligamentous injuries of the knee.

Reference

Perryman JR: The acute management of soft tissue injuries of the knee. Orthop Clin North Am 2002;33:575. [PMID: 12483953]

Knee Dislocation

- ■ Essentials of Diagnosis
  - Traumatic knee dislocation is an uncommon but limb-threatening condition
  - Common mechanism: high-impact or high-velocity injury, but may occur with low-velocity injuries such as in sports
  - Dislocation described in terms of the tibia's displacement relative to the femur: anterior, posterior, lateral, medial, and rotational
  - Look for open fracture or dislocation
  - Neurovascular injuries are commonly related
  - Popliteal artery is essentially tethered proximally and distally; highly susceptible to injury or disruption in knee dislocations
  - Peroneal nerve also particularly susceptible to damage
  - Ligamentous injuries usually associated, especially anterior cruciate and posterior cruciate, then collateral ligaments, with menisci and capsular injuries occurring less frequently
  - Three of the four main ligaments (cruciate and collateral) must be injured to have a dislocation
  - As many as 50% of knee dislocations may reduce spontaneously before presentation
  - Anteroposterior and lateral x-rays before and after reduction; obliques may reveal small fractures otherwise not noted
  - Arteriogram indicated to rule out popliteal arterial injury

- ■ Differential Diagnosis
  - Fracture or contusion
  - Ligamentous injury

- ■ Treatment
  - Close monitoring of neurovascular status throughout visit
  - Pain control and closed reduction if possible; appropriate orthopedic and vascular surgery consults where applicable
  - Immobilization after reduction
  - Monitoring for development of compartment syndrome

- ■ Pearl

Be sure to discuss with patients and their families that knee dislocations are problematic injuries and that a completely functional and pain-free recovery is rare.

Reference

Frykberg ER: Popliteal vascular injuries. Surg Clin North Am 2002;82:67. [PMID: 11905952]

Meniscal Tear

- **Essentials of Diagnosis**
  - Possibly the most common knee injury
  - Medial meniscus is C shaped; lateral meniscus is more rounded, or O shaped, and covers a greater area of the tibial surface
  - Both menisci have some degree of mobility; allows them to conform more readily to the tibial and femoral articular surfaces during motion
  - Menisci made of predominantly avascular fibrocartilaginous tissue
  - Tears may be related to traumatic event but are more commonly due to twisting or positional changes
  - Patients may not be able to determine specific inciting event
  - Pain generally at joint line and may be intermittent
  - Effusion may or may not be present, even with acute injury
  - Patients often report the knee locking, catching, or popping
  - Careful examination to check for joint line tenderness and range of motion
  - Range of motion may be limited secondary to pain or may result from a mechanical block within joint
  - X-rays to rule out fracture and arthritis
  - MRI is a more definitive test, done as an outpatient

- **Differential Diagnosis**
  - Ligamentous injury
  - Fracture
  - Contusion
  - Arthritis
  - Plica

- **Treatment**
  - Conservative, nonoperative trial
  - Nonsteroidal anti-inflammatory drugs
  - Activity modification
  - Crutches if unable to bear weight
  - Orthopedic follow-up and usually physical therapy
  - Operative treatment for athletes or patients with a locked knee or a "bucket handle" tear on MRI

- **Pearl**

A meniscal tear is one of the common causes of an immediate traumatic knee effusion.

Reference

Calmbach WL: Evaluation of patients presenting with knee pain: part I. History, physical examination, radiographs, and laboratory tests. Am Fam Physician 2003;68:907. [PMID: 13678139]

Metatarsal Fracture

- **Essentials of Diagnosis**
  - Fairly common, usually from direct trauma or twisting
  - Look for pain, swelling, ecchymoses; ask about pain on ambulation or inability to ambulate
  - Consider tarsometatarsal joint disruption (Lisfranc injury)
  - Assess neurovascular status and range of motion
  - Compartment syndrome of the foot is not uncommon
  - Check any and all wounds carefully for open fracture
  - 1st metatarsal: least commonly injured but important in ambulation; head of this bone bears about twice as much weight as the other metatarsal heads
  - 2nd–4th metatarsals: fractures fairly common but usually heal well unless associated with Lisfranc injury
  - 5th metatarsal: most commonly fractured, especially the proximal shaft
  - Jones fracture: transverse fracture at the base of the 5th metatarsal occurring at least 15 mm proximal to distal end of metatarsal tuberosity
  - Pseudo-Jones: an avulsion fracture at the proximal tuberosity of the 5th metatarsal
  - Foot x-rays usually sufficient for diagnosis

- **Differential Diagnosis**
  - Other fracture or dislocation of the forefoot
  - Sprain or contusion

- **Treatment**
  - Jones fracture: non-weight-bearing instructions, posterior splint
  - Pseudo-Jones, nondisplaced shaft of 2nd–5th metatarsal: weight bearing as tolerated in cast shoe (hard-sole shoe)
  - 1st metatarsal: non-weight-bearing instructions, often requires open reduction and internal fixation (ORIF)
  - Lisfranc fracture or dislocation: requires ORIF
  - Splint, rest, ice, elevation, analgesia, orthopedic follow-up

- **Pearl**

Lisfranc joint injuries are frequently misdiagnosed and can lead to significant long-term morbidity when missed.

Reference

Perron AD: Evaluation and management of the high-risk orthopaedic emergency. Emerg Med Clin North Am 2003;21:159. [PMID: 12630737]

Olecranon Fracture

- ■ Essentials of Diagnosis
  - Pain and swelling over the olecranon; effusions of the elbow always present because all fractures of the olecranon process have an intra-articular component
  - Bimodal distribution of fractures: younger age peak sustaining olecranon fractures as a result of high-energy trauma, older age peak sustaining olecranon fractures as a result of falls
  - Most common mechanism is direct trauma or less commonly with contraction of the triceps while elbow is flexed
  - Patients usually present with elbow flexed and supported with other arm
  - Inability to extend elbow indicates disruption of triceps mechanism
  - Careful neurovascular exam; associated ulnar nerve injuries are not uncommon
  - Anteroposterior and lateral views; obtain a true lateral to best evaluate for possible radial head fracture

- ■ Differential Diagnosis
  - Distal humerus fracture
  - Radial head fracture
  - Olecranon bursitis
  - Medial or lateral epicondylitis

- ■ Treatment
  - Nondisplaced olecranon fractures: nonoperative
  - Immobilization with a long arm posterior splint with the elbow at 45–90 degrees of flexion
  - If the extensor mechanism is intact, orthopedic follow-up and repeat x-rays within 1 week; union usually not complete until 6–8 weeks
  - Indications for open reduction and internal fixation: disruption of extensor mechanism, fractures with more than 2 mm of displacement, fractures associated with ulnar nerve deficit

- ■ Pearl

Many olecranon fractures have little to no displacement because the surrounding fibrous soft tissue maintains close approximation of the fracture fragments.

Reference

Kuntz DG, Baratz ME: Fractures of the elbow. Orthop Clin North Am 1999;30:37. [PMID: 9882724]

Osgood-Schlatter Disease

- ■ Essentials of Diagnosis
  - • Characterized by pain localized to the tibial tuberosity
  - • Common in adolescent athletes, most often in 10–14 year olds
  - • Results from patellar tendon injury at insertion on tibial tuberosity; avulsion of tendon is rare
  - • Generally a clinical diagnosis; x-rays not required but a lateral view may be useful and an anteroposterior view may help rule out other injury patterns
  - • May see ossification or bony fragments on x-ray
  - • Pain, tenderness, heat, and swelling at the tibial tuberosity are indicators
  - • Usually resolves with skeletal maturity

- ■ Differential Diagnosis
  - • Contusion
  - • Fracture
  - • Accessory ossification site
  - • Infectious apophysitis (rare)
  - • Malignancy (rare)

- ■ Treatment
  - • Conservative
  - • Nonsteroidal anti-inflammatory drugs
  - • Limit activity
  - • Rarely requires operative intervention

- ■ Pearl

Studies show Osgood-Schlatter Disease to be more common in males, but this finding is thought to be due to increased participation in athletics.

Reference

Duri ZA: The immature athlete. Clin Sports Med 2002;21:461. [PMID: 12365238]

Patella Dislocation

- ■ Essentials of Diagnosis
  - The knee is a large synovial joint; the most commonly involved joint in orthopedic injuries seen in the emergency department
  - Patients may report history of feeling their knee go out or a popping or tearing sensation
  - Common in adolescents
  - Most common mechanism: direct blow to anterior or medial aspect of the patella
  - Patella almost always displaced laterally
  - Patients present with obvious deformity, restriction of motion at the knee, often with knee effusion
  - Dislocation often reduces spontaneously before emergency department presentation
  - Fairbanks sign (apprehension test): patients have significant pain or apprehension when the examiner attempts to displace the patella laterally with the knee flexed to 30 degrees
  - Anteroposterior and lateral knee views; postreduction films: patellar sunrise view, evaluation of possible postreduction fracture

- ■ Differential Diagnosis
  - Patella fracture
  - Quadriceps or patella tendon rupture
  - Femur or tibia fracture
  - Traumatic bursitis

- ■ Treatment
  - Reduction achieved by flexing the hip and extending the knee while applying gentle medial force over the patella
  - Postreduction: knee immobilizer, crutches, and non-weight-bearing instructions until orthopedic follow-up
  - Recurrent subluxations or dislocations: surgical repair may be needed

- ■ Pearl

Almost all patients with patella dislocation are predisposed to the injury because of patellofemoral dysplasia.

Reference

O'Shea KJ et al: The diagnostic accuracy of history, physical examination, and radiographs in the evaluation of traumatic knee disorders. Am J Sports Med 1996;24:164. [PMID: 8775114]

Patella Fracture

■ **Essentials of Diagnosis**

- Accounts for 1% of all fractures
- Mechanism: direct trauma or forceful contraction of quadriceps muscle with knee flexed
- Ambulation possible if fracture is nondisplaced
- Check straight leg raise to test extensor mechanism preservation
- With falls or direct trauma, examine abrasions and wounds closely for possibility of open fractures
- In the anteroposterior view, patella is often difficult to visualize; most fractures are identified on lateral views of knee, although an axial, or sunrise, view of the patella is often helpful and should be obtained routinely when evaluating patella injuries

■ **Differential Diagnosis**

- Patella dislocation
- Bipartite patella (normal variant of the patella; may be confused with a fracture; noted by smooth margins of each part of the patella, bilateral in 50% of people)

■ **Treatment**

- Nondisplaced or minimally displaced fractures with intact extensor mechanism: knee immobilizer and orthopedic follow-up, non-weight-bearing instructions for that extremity until orthopedic evaluation, then likely early weight bearing
- Displaced fractures and fractures with loss of extensor retinaculum: usually require open reduction with internal fixation

■ **Pearl**

The patella is the largest sesamoid bone in the body.

Reference

Bharam S: Knee fractures in the athlete. Orthop Clin North Am 2002;33:565. [PMID: 12483953]

| **Pelvic Fracture** |

- **Essentials of Diagnosis**
  - Suggested by localized pain, swelling, or ecchymoses over hips, groin, perineum, or lower back
  - Other physical exam findings suggestive of pelvic fracture: scrotal hematoma, blood at the urethral meatus, boggy or high-riding prostate
  - Pelvic fractures in young patients require a significant mechanism, often motor vehicle collisions; pelvic fractures occur much more frequently in the elderly with minimal force, such as falls from standing
  - Tears of the posterior venous plexus are common; may result in life-threatening hemorrhage
  - If examiner is able to displace the iliac crests with moderate anteroposterior or lateral compression on exam, an unstable fracture may be present
  - Pelvic x-rays including anteroposterior, inlet, and outlet views; CT scans, in stable patients, often necessary to classify the extent of injury and make treatment plans
  - If urethral injury is suspected, do not place a Foley catheter; obtain a retrograde urethrogram to evaluate urethra

- **Differential Diagnosis**
  - Intra-abdominal injury or hemorrhage
  - Lumbar spine injury or fracture
  - Bladder or urethral injury
  - Hip fracture
  - Ligamentous injury

- **Treatment**
  - Open book fractures, those associated with disruption of the symphysis pubis, are frequently associated with massive bleeding
  - A sheet wrapped around the patient's pelvis and tied tightly may be used to temporarily stabilize the fracture, decrease the volume of the pelvis, and help tamponade bleeding
  - Treatment varies greatly based on the type and stability of the fracture

- **Pearl**

Pelvic fractures in the young suggest a high-energy mechanism of injury; therefore, a thorough workup is essential to rule out other potential life-threatening injuries.

Reference

Mirza A, Ellis T: Initial management of pelvic and femoral fractures in the multiply injured patient. Crit Care Clin 2004;20:159. [PMID: 14979335]

Phalangeal Injury of the Foot

- ■ Essentials of Diagnosis
    - Generally results from stub injury or other direct trauma
    - Fractures of the phalanges are relatively common
    - Dislocations of the metatarsophalangeal (MTP) and interphalangeal (IP) joints are less common; usually involve the great, or first, toe
    - Injury to the great toe requires better reduction and more aggressive treatment due to its greater importance in balance and weight bearing
    - MTP and IP joint function of toes 2–5 are not important for proper foot function and ambulation
    - Pain, swelling, deformity, and ecchymoses
    - Clinical exam and foot x-rays usually sufficient for diagnosis

- ■ Differential Diagnosis
    - Fracture
    - Dislocation
    - Sprain
    - Contusion

- ■ Treatment
    - Reduce dislocations and displaced fractures with local anesthesia
    - Buddy-tape toes together for support
    - Orthopedic referral and follow-up for great toe injuries
    - Weight bear as tolerated; may use a cast shoe for protection and comfort

- ■ Pearl

Use caution so as not to miss subtle fractures, particularly intra-articular fractures of the great toe.

Reference

Armagan OE: Injuries to the toes and metatarsals. Orthop Clin North Am 2001;32:1. [PMID: 11465121]

Radial Head Fracture

- **Essentials of Diagnosis**
  - Most common elbow fracture in adults
  - Most common mechanism: fall onto an outstretched hand (FOOSH); may occur with direct trauma
  - Patients usually present with localized pain, particularly with pronation or supination, and limited range of motion at the elbow
  - Elbow joint effusion may be palpable
  - Plain x-rays often do not show a radial head fracture; however, a posterior fat pad sign or an enlarged anterior fat pad should raise clinical suspicion
  - Assessment of wrist and shoulder for associated injury; evaluation of neurovascular status of entire limb

- **Differential Diagnosis**
  - Radial head dislocation
  - Other elbow fracture or dislocation
  - Elbow strain or sprain
  - Olecranon bursitis
  - Medial or lateral epicondylitis

- **Treatment**
  - Nondisplaced radial head fractures: sling immobilization, ice, analgesia, and orthopedic follow-up within 3–5 days
  - Comminuted or displaced fractures: orthopedic consult in the emergency department

- **Pearl**

A small anterior fat pad sign may be normal, but a posterior fat pad is never normal; the physician should immobilize the joint and treat for an occult intra-articular elbow fracture.

Reference

Kandemir U, Fu FH, McMahon PJ: Elbow injuries. Curr Opin Rheumatol 2002;14:160. [PMID: 11845021]

Radial Head Subluxation

- **Essentials of Diagnosis**
  - Also called nursemaid's elbow; common pediatric injury, accounting for as many as 25% of childhood elbow injuries
  - Usually occurs in the 1–3 year olds; rare after age 6
  - Patients usually present with the classic history of a toddler whose arm has been pulled into full extension (as when a child starts to step into the street and is quickly pulled back by parent); parents often report an audible snap
  - The injury occurs due to longitudinal traction on the arm, allowing the annular ligament to become entrapped between the radial head and capitellum
  - X-ray evaluation controversial; most believe x-rays are not needed with appropriate history and injury mechanism
  - Thorough neurovascular exam needed; any deficit after reduction should alert the physician to the possibility of other injury

- **Differential Diagnosis**
  - Radial head or supracondylar fracture
  - Elbow sprain or strain
  - Septic elbow joint

- **Treatment**
  - Closed reduction achieved by supinating the forearm while applying pressure over the radial head with one's thumb; in the final step, the elbow is fully flexed while the forearm is held in supination
  - Patient typically experiences a brief period of pain after reduction, followed by the absence of pain and normal use of the limb within 5–10 minutes
  - Postreduction films generally unnecessary
  - Sling immobilization not indicated in a child able to use the arm without complaint

- **Pearl**

Although radial head subluxation is a common injury, it is important to obtain a thorough history to allay concerns of potential child abuse.

Reference

Macias CG, Bothner J, Wiebe R: A comparison of supination/flexion to hyperpronation in the reduction of radial head subluxations. Pediatrics 1998;102:e10. [PMID: 9651462]

Scapula Fracture

■ **Essentials of Diagnosis**

- Severe shoulder or back pain with decreased range of motion of the ipsilateral upper extremity; signs include swelling, tenderness, crepitus, and ecchymosis in the scapular region
- Detailed exam to identify neurovascular deficits
- Presence of scapula fracture suggests significant trauma
- May be associated with severe intrathoracic injuries; chest x-ray is essential
- Axillary, anteroposterior, and scapular Y views
- CT scan of the scapula can provide additional information, especially if operative therapy is being considered

■ **Differential Diagnosis**

- Type I: fracture of coracoid process, acromion process, or scapular spine
- Type II: fracture of the scapular neck
- Type III: intra-articular fracture involving the glenoid fossa
- Type IV: fracture of the body of the scapula (most common)
- Rib fracture
- Pneumothorax
- Aortic dissection
- Spinal column injury
- Associated brachial plexus injury

■ **Treatment**

- The vast majority of scapula fractures are amenable to nonoperative treatment: sling and early range of motion
- Surgical indications are controversial; operative treatment generally suggested for intra-articular and highly displaced fracture
- Patients may need short course of narcotics for adequate analgesia

■ **Pearl**

The presence of scapula fracture indicates a high-energy mechanism of injury; the physician should maintain a high index of suspicion for associated occult injuries to the chest and abdomen.

Reference

Cole PA: Scapula fractures. Orthop Clin North Am 2002;33:1. [PMID: 11832310]

Shoulder Dislocation, Anterior

- ■ Essentials of Diagnosis
    - • 95% of shoulder dislocations are anterior; suggested by shoulder pain, deformity, and decreased range of motion
    - • Shoulder is often squared off with prominent acromion process and palpable anterior fullness
    - • Thorough neurovascular exam, including testing the axillary nerve (cutaneous sensation over lateral shoulder and motor function of the teres minor and deltoid)
    - • Anteroposterior, axillary, and scapular Y views
    - • Patients usually present with arm held in abduction and external rotation
    - • Mechanism: force applied to abducted and externally rotated arm or direct blow to posterior lateral shoulder
    - • Shoulder is most commonly dislocated major joint in the body
    - • Hill-Sachs deformity: impaction of the posterolateral humeral head that may occur with dislocation
    - • Bankart fracture: fracture of the anterior inferior glenoid rim associated with anterior dislocation

- ■ Differential Diagnosis
    - • Luxatio erecta is an uncommon form of anterior dislocation, in which the humeral head dislocates and becomes lodged inferior to the subglenoid fossa; clinically, the arm will be adjacent to the head with the forearm flexed over the head
    - • Shoulder strain or rotator cuff injury
    - • Fracture of the humeral head or shaft
    - • Acromioclavicular injury
    - • Hemarthrosis
    - • Septic joint

- ■ Treatment
    - • Prompt reduction after x-ray confirmation except in presence of neurovascular compromise
    - • After successful reduction (confirmed by postreduction views): discharge with adequate analgesia, shoulder sling immobilization, and prompt orthopedic follow-up

- ■ Pearl

Any neurologic deficit before or after reduction should prompt an orthopedic consult in the emergency department.

Reference

Wen DY: Current concepts in the treatment of anterior shoulder dislocations. Am J Emerg Med 1999;17:401. [PMID: 10452444]

Shoulder Dislocation, Posterior

- ■ Essentials of Diagnosis
  - • Suggested by pain, deformity, and decreased range of motion
  - • Coracoid process prominent with palpable posterior bulge
  - • Patient usually presents with arm held in slight adduction and internal rotation
  - • Mechanism: force applied to an adducted and internally rotated arm; most common mechanism is seizure and associated sudden muscle contraction (may also be seen with electrocution injuries or electroconvulsive therapy without muscle relaxation)
  - • Reverse Hill-Sachs deformity: from compression fracture of the anterior medial humeral head
  - • Anteroposterior, axillary, and scapular Y views

- ■ Differential Diagnosis
  - • Fracture of humeral head or shaft
  - • Acromioclavicular injury
  - • Hemarthrosis
  - • Septic shoulder

- ■ Treatment
  - • Prompt reduction with x-ray evaluation before and after reduction
  - • Sling immobilization and prompt orthopedic follow-up
  - • Narcotics may be necessary for adequate analgesia
  - • Shoulder should be immobilized 2–3 weeks in young patients; immobilization time should be much less in older patients, who are at increased risk of developing a frozen shoulder

- ■ Pearl

Maintain a high index of suspicion for posterior shoulder dislocation in patients with shoulder pain after a seizure; these injuries can be missed initially.

Reference

Beeson MS: Complications of shoulder dislocation. Am J Emerg Med 1999;17:288. [PMID: 10337892]

Sternoclavicular Dislocation

■ Essentials of Diagnosis

- Chest wall deformity and tenderness present in most cases
- Frequently associated with motor vehicle collisions and sports injuries
- Anterior dislocations are most common
- Posterior dislocations are associated with crush injury to the anterior chest; up to 25% may be associated with mediastinal injuries
- Anteroposterior, oblique, and serendipity views (40-degree cephalic tilt view)
- Chest CT will identify injury and associated structures in the superior mediastinum that may be compressed by posterior dislocations

■ Differential Diagnosis

- Medial clavicle fracture
- Sternoclavicular sprain or subluxation

■ Treatment

- Anterior dislocations: may be reduced in emergency department, procedural sedation may be required for adequate analgesia; place a rolled towel between the supine patient's shoulder blades; apply traction to the ipsilateral arm with the shoulder abducted to 90 degrees; an assistant then applies gentle inward pressure over the medial clavicle
- Immobilization with a figure-of-eight dressing or secure sling after reduction
- Posterior dislocations: require prompt treatment, usually reduced in the operating room
- If patient has serious neurologic, airway, or vascular compromise associated with a posterior dislocation, then emergent reduction in emergency department is attempted using sedation and a sterile towel clamp: make a small incision over the medial clavicle, use a sterile towel clamp to clasp the clavicular head, and apply gentle anterior traction until reduction is achieved
- Orthopedic follow-up

■ Pearl

Posterior dislocations may not be readily apparent because soft tissue swelling at the sternoclavicular joint may mask the appearance of the posterior displacement of the medial clavicle.

Reference

Eiff MP: Management of clavicle fractures. Am Fam Physician 1997;55:121. [PMID: 9012272]

Subtalar Dislocation

■ **Essentials of Diagnosis**

- Uncommon injury
- Dislocation of the talus from the calcaneus and navicular; usually accompanied by ligamentous injuries
- Subtalar joint accounts for approximately 40% of the inversion and eversion of the foot
- Medial dislocation is the most common, followed by lateral
- Dislocations in the anteroposterior plane rare
- Generally due to forceful rotation
- Visible deformity, pain, swelling, likely ecchymosis
- Plain x-rays confirm diagnosis

■ **Differential Diagnosis**

- Ankle dislocation
- Fracture
- Sprain

■ **Treatment**

- Immediate reduction with procedural sedation if possible
- After reduction, posterior splinting with stirrups
- Orthopedic consult and referral
- Pain control
- Non-weight-bearing instructions

■ **Pearl**

Closed subtalar dislocation due to a low-energy injury can be expected to have a good long-term outcome if reduced and immobilized quickly and properly.

Reference

Perugia D: Conservative treatment of subtalar dislocations. Int Orthop 2002; 26:56. [PMID: 11954852]

Supracondylar Fracture

- ■ Essentials of Diagnosis
  - Common mechanism: fall onto an outstretched hand (FOOSH)
  - Suggested by elbow pain, deformity, and decreased range of motion
  - Posterior fat pad on lateral x-ray is highly suggestive of an intra-articular injury such as a supracondylar fracture
  - Most common in children aged 5–10 years; rarely occurs after age 15 years
  - Extension type fractures: 98% of all supracondylar fractures
  - Pediatric elbow has complex anatomy with multiple ossification centers occasionally simulating fracture lines; comparison views of the unaffected elbow often useful
  - Neurovascular exam should note anterior interosseous nerve sensory distribution and any indication of compartment syndrome
  - An anterior fat pad may be normal, but when injury is present the fat pad is larger and more perpendicular to the anterior humeral cortex (sail sign); a posterior fat pad is never normal
  - A line drawn from the anterior border of the humerus on a true lateral film should intersect the middle third of the capitellum; if the line intersects anterior to the middle third, a supracondylar fracture is most likely present

- ■ Differential Diagnosis
  - Elbow sprain, strain, or effusion
  - Medial or lateral epicondylitis
  - Bursitis

- ■ Treatment
  - Orthopedic consult required due to high morbidity and potential complication of Volkmann ischemia; patients with nonoperative fractures may require admission for observation for signs of compartment syndrome
  - After orthopedic consult, posterior splint may be applied with the elbow flexed to 90 degrees

- ■ Pearl

Maintain high index of suspicion for supracondylar fractures in children aged 5–10 years with FOOSH injuries and elbow pain.

Reference

Minkowitz B, Busch MT: Supracondylar humerus fractures. Current trends and controversies. Orthop Clin 1996;25:581. [PMID: 8090472]

Talus Fracture

- **Essentials of Diagnosis**
  - 60% of the talus is covered by articular cartilage
  - Talus is only foot bone with tibia and fibular articulation
  - A tenuous blood supply makes avascular necrosis a significant problem, especially with talar neck fractures
  - Mechanism: usually forceful dorsiflexion as in motor vehicle collisions or falls from height
  - Tibiotalar joint is the site of dorsiflexion and plantarflexion; subtalar joint (talonavicular and talocalcaneal) is responsible for inversion, eversion, and rotation
  - Examine for pain, swelling, deformity, ecchymoses, and neurovascular compromise; assess contralateral side for comparison
  - Look closely for multiple foot fractures (common)
  - Mechanism: usually high-energy injuries; consider complete trauma evaluation
  - Obtain foot and ankle x-rays
  - CT often required to fully delineate specific fracture pattern
  - Acute complications include compartment syndrome of the foot, neurovascular compromise, entrapment of flexor tendons, and skin sloughing

- **Differential Diagnosis**
  - Dislocation
  - Subluxation
  - Sprain

- **Treatment**
  - Pain control
  - Immobilization
  - Emergent orthopedic consult for most fractures
  - Always non-weight-bearing instructions

- **Pearl**

Avascular necrosis is a serious problem, and the faster and more anatomic the reduction of a talus fracture, the better the patient's chance for an acceptable functional outcome.

Reference

Judd DB, Kim DH: Foot fractures frequently misdiagnosed as ankle sprains. Am Fam Physician 2002;66:785. [PMID: 12322769]

Tibial Plateau Fracture

- **Essentials of Diagnosis**
  - Accounts for 1% of all fractures
  - Majority of tibial plateau fractures involve the lateral plateau; up to one-third involve concomitant ligamentous injuries
  - Mechanism: axial loading with valgus or varus stress
  - Deformity, pain, ecchymosis, limb rotation, crepitus
  - Check neurovascular status
  - Open injuries frequently present
  - Patient rarely able to ambulate
  - Ottawa knee rules useful for deciding on knee x-rays; if any of the following are present, obtain x-rays: age ≥55 years, tenderness at fibular head, isolated patella tenderness, inability to flex to 90 degrees, unable to bear weight (four steps) at time of injury and in emergency department
  - Anteroposterior and lateral views of knee

- **Differential Diagnosis**
  - Ligamentous injury
  - Contusion
  - Dislocation

- **Treatment**
  - Pain control
  - Immobilization
  - Close monitoring of neurovascular status
  - Almost always requires operative intervention to restore joint surface
  - CT, or even MRI, can be useful for orthopedist's planning
  - Close monitoring for signs and symptoms of compartment syndrome

- **Pearl**

If a lipohemarthrosis (horizontal straight line below patella) is identified on a lateral x-ray of the knee, an intra-articular fracture is present.

Reference

Steven DG: The long-term functional outcome of operatively treated tibial plateau fractures. J Orthop Trauma 2001;15:312. [PMID: 11433134]

Tibial Shaft Fracture

- **Essentials of Diagnosis**
  - Most common long bone fracture; most common site of fracture nonunion; associated fibula fractures usually present
  - Mechanism: high energy (motor vehicle collision) or low energy (twisting, fall from standing), and occasionally penetrating (gunshot wound)
  - Low-energy injuries usually exhibit spiral fracture pattern with minimal displacement and minimal soft tissue injury
  - High-energy fractures associated with more comminution, displacement, and soft tissue injury; a high-energy mechanism warrants complete trauma evaluation
  - Compartment syndrome is a limb-threatening condition; increased pain and distal sensory loss are generally first signs noted
  - Other complications: neurovascular compromise, infections, malunions, nonunions
  - Examine for pain, deformity, crepitus, and ecchymosis
  - Check any and all wounds for possibility of open fracture
  - Anteroposterior and lateral views of knee, ankle, tibia, and fibula

- **Differential Diagnosis**
  - Dislocation
  - Contusion
  - Stress fracture

- **Treatment**
  - Nondisplaced low-energy fractures: long leg splinting, analgesics, close orthopedic follow-up
  - Most fractures require emergent orthopedic referral and evaluation, often with admission and observation for compartment syndrome
  - Open fractures: nothing-by-mouth status, check tetanus status, anti-staphylococcal antibiotics, emergent orthopedic consult for open reduction and internal fixation
  - Stress fractures: cessation of specific activity, partial weight bearing, orthopedic follow-up

- **Pearl**

Because tibial shaft fractures are often open secondary to the very thin tissue layer over the tibia, careful examination of even tiny wounds is essential.

Reference

French B: High-energy tibial shaft fractures. Orthop Clin North Am 2002;33:211. [PMID: 11832322]

Traumatic Amputation

- **Essentials of Diagnosis**
  - Sharp injuries are best candidates for reimplantation
  - Crush or avulsion injuries have poor prognosis for reimplantation
  - Determine occupation and handedness of patient

- **Differential Diagnosis**
  - X-ray evaluation may help delineate occult fractures or dislocations

- **Treatment**
  - Keep amputated part clean, wrap in sterile gauze, moisten with saline, place in plastic bag, and put on ice (Do not allow part to freeze!)
  - Cooling will increase viability of amputated part up to 12–24 hours
  - Treat as an open fracture with antibiotics and tetanus prophylaxis
  - Majority of amputations require immediate surgical consult; expeditious referral to a surgeon capable of reimplantation is often required and transfer may need to be arranged quickly
  - Small distal digit amputations may be managed in the emergency department with close follow-up

- **Pearl**

Many factors go into the decision to reimplant an amputated part including the patient's handedness, the importance of the part (eg, the thumb is more important than the fifth digit), the level of injury, the anticipated return of function, and the mechanism of injury (eg, crush or sharp injury).

Reference

Soucacos PN: Indications and selection for digital amputation and replantation. J Hand Surg [Br] 2001;26:572. [PMID: 11884116]

Wrist Fracture

- ■ Essentials of Diagnosis
  - • Suggested by localized pain, swelling, or deformity
  - • Most common mechanism: fall onto an outstretched hand (FOOSH)
  - • Diagnosis requires high index of suspicion; x-rays commonly inconclusive
  - • Two hallmarks of scaphoid injury: anatomic snuffbox tenderness and pain with axial loading of the thumb
  - • Consider a dedicated scaphoid view (anteroposterior view with the wrist in slight flexion and ulnar deviation)
  - • The scaphoid is the most commonly fractured carpal bone; missed injuries may have significant sequelae
  - • The lunate is the second most commonly fractured carpal bone, these injuries often go unrecognized until they progress to osteonecrosis, at which time they are diagnosed as Kienböck disease
  - • If fracture is suggested clinically but x-rays are negative, the wrist should be immobilized in a thumb spica splint and films repeated in 1–2 weeks

- ■ Differential Diagnosis
  - • Proximal metacarpal fracture
  - • Distal radius or ulna fracture
  - • Lunate or perilunate dislocation
  - • Avoid the diagnosis of simple "wrist sprain" due to the significant incidence of missed occult injuries such as scaphoid fractures

- ■ Treatment
  - • Confirmed and suspected scaphoid injuries: immobilization with a thumb spica splint with prompt orthopedic follow-up
  - • Other carpal injuries or fractures: volar splint immobilization
  - • If initial x-rays are negative: immobilization and repeat films arranged in 2 weeks

- ■ Pearl

Proper management of any wrist injury entails a very low threshold for splint immobilization even when x-rays do not demonstrate an abnormality.

Reference

Parvizi J et al: Combining the clinical signs improves diagnosis of scaphoid fractures. A prospective study with follow-up. J Hand Surg [Br] 1998;23:324. [PMID: 9665518]

23

Hand Emergencies

Boutonnière Deformity

- **Essentials of Diagnosis**
  - Mechanism is disruption of the central slip tendon: often axial loading or a blow to the dorsal aspect of the proximal interphalangeal (PIP) joint; laceration of the central slip tendon can occur with open injuries
  - Tender, swollen PIP joint often with extensor lag or painful, weak extension at the PIP joint
  - Patients usually present several weeks after closed injury or occasionally acutely with an open laceration or with a closed injury in which the central slip tendon has avulsed the dorsal aspect of the middle phalanx
  - High index of suspicion for this injury needed with any trauma near the PIP joint; significant long-term disability possible
  - Disruption of the central slip tendon leads to unopposed action of the flexor digitorum superficialis; the lateral bands slip into a volar position and act as flexors of the PIP joint

- **Differential Diagnosis**
  - Other phalangeal fracture
  - Other tendon injury
  - Soft tissue injury
  - Sprain

- **Treatment**
  - Urgent referral to hand surgeon
  - Splint PIP joint in hyperextension for 6 weeks
  - Open injury requires repair by hand surgeon

- **Pearl**

The Boutonnière deformity results in volar direction of the middle phalanx, as opposed to Swan neck deformity, which is dorsal angulation of the middle phalanx.

Reference

Harrison BP, Hilliard MW: Emergency department evaluation and treatment of hand injuries. Emerg Med Clin North Am 1999;17:793. [PMID: 10584103]

Carpal Bone Fracture

- **Essentials of Diagnosis**
    - Mechanism: trauma with wrist in hyperextension (eg, falls onto an outstretched hand, or FOOSH) or direct trauma to wrist
    - Scaphoid fractures comprise 60–70%, triquetrum fractures next most common
    - Approximately 15% of scaphoid fractures not seen on initial x-rays; dedicated scaphoid view may help
    - Carpal tunnel view to identify hook of the hamate or pisiform fractures depending on clinical suspicion
    - Clinical identification of scaphoid fracture: pain or tenderness in the anatomic snuffbox, on direct palpation of the bone, or on pronation and supination against resistance
    - Assessment of nerve involvement with injury; of particular concern is ulnar nerve with fractures of pisiform bone
    - Associated injuries of ligaments and blood supply are common

- **Differential Diagnosis**
    - Perilunate or lunate dislocation
    - Scapholunate dissociation
    - Distal radial or ulnar fracture
    - Carpal bone fracture
    - Wrist ligamentous injury

- **Treatment**
    - Suspected carpal injury: splint regardless of x-ray findings
    - Scaphoid fracture: thumb spica splint
    - Triquetral, hamate, and pisiform fracture: may be managed in emergency department with ulnar gutter splints as long as ulnar nerve function is normal
    - For most patients: refer for hand surgeon consult within 1 week
    - Nerve compromise or fractures through regions of tenuous vascular supply (eg, proximal scaphoid): urgent hand surgeon consult

- **Pearl**

Negative x-rays warrant follow-up films, CT or MRI, or bone scan at 1 week. Always splint patient's hand if traumatic wrist pain is reported.

Reference

Ritchie JV, Munter DW: Emergency department evaluation and treatment of wrist injuries. Emerg Med Clin North Am 1999;17:823. [PMID: 10584104]

Cellulitis

- **Essentials of Diagnosis**
    - Usual pathogen is *Staphylococcus aureus,* or *Streptococcus pyogenes* in immunocompetent patients
    - For bite wounds, suspect polymicrobial or contamination with other species
    - Suspect polymicrobial infection with some gram-negative organisms in diabetic patients
    - Suspect mixed anaerobic-aerobics in drug abusers
    - Consider hand x-rays to evaluate for radiopaque foreign bodies or gas-forming infection

- **Differential Diagnosis**
    - Retained foreign body
    - Flexor tenosynovitis
    - Paronychia
    - Lymphangitis
    - Abscess
    - Osteomyelitis
    - Septic arthritis
    - Soft tissue injury
    - Hypersensitivity

- **Treatment**
    - First-generation cephalosporin or antistaphylococcal penicillin such as cefazolin or nafcillin (2 g IV every 4 hours)
    - Consider vancomycin, 1 g every 12 hours, in drug abusers
    - Consider coverage for multiple organisms in appropriate clinical situations
    - May require inpatient intravenous antibiotics unless the patient has a very mild cellulitis and is immunocompetent

- **Pearl**

Patients with cellulitis of the hand must be assessed for serious underlying conditions such as osteomyelitis, retained foreign body, deep space abscess formation, or septic arthritis.

Reference

Harrison BP, Hilliard MW: Emergency department evaluation and treatment of hand injuries. Emerg Med Clin North Am 1999;17:793. [PMID: 10584103]

Extensor Tendon Laceration

- **Essentials of Diagnosis**
  - High index of suspicion for extensor tendon lacerations with open wounds on dorsum of hand
  - Appropriate assessment of tendon function by testing against resistance
  - For open wounds, assessment of whether more than 50% cross-sectional area is involved
  - Management depends on the anatomic area of the hand or forearm involved
  - History: type, direction, and amount of force as well as position of hand at time of injury
  - Assessment of neurovascular status

- **Differential Diagnosis**
  - Phalangeal fracture
  - Other tendon injury
  - Soft tissue injury
  - Infection
  - Sprain

- **Treatment**
  - Tendon injuries proximal to the metacarpals: primary repair by hand surgeon
  - Closed injuries from the proximal interphalangeal joint distally: splint in full extension for 3–6 weeks
  - Open injuries: repair and splint in neutral position for 6 weeks
  - Injuries in the region of the metacarpals: repair and splint with wrist at 30–45 degrees extension and affected metacarpal phalangeal (MCP) joint in neutral position with unaffected MCP joints at 15-degree flexion
  - Referral for urgent follow-up with hand surgeon

- **Pearl**

Open extensor tendon injuries in the region of the MCP joint indicate possible human bite. Cover wound with appropriate antibiotics and consult a hand surgeon for irrigation and repair.

Reference

Harrison BP, Hilliard MW: Emergency department evaluation and treatment of hand injuries. Emerg Med Clin North Am 1999;17:793. [PMID: 10584103]

Fascial Space Infection

- ■ Essentials of Diagnosis
  - • Five distinct deep space infections of the hand
  - • Subfascial web space (bacterial spread from palmar blisters; occurs near base of digits)
  - • Interdigital space or "collar button" abscess (infection spreads dorsally from subfascial web space into interdigital space; pain with digits held in resting adduction)
  - • Subaponeurotic space (swelling of dorsum of hand with pain on passive extension of extensor tendons)
  - • Midpalmar space (deep to flexor tendons located in middle of palm; loss of midpalmar arch due to swelling)
  - • Thenar space (palmar and ulnar to the adductor pollicis; severe pain and swelling with thumb in abduction and slightly flexed position)
  - • Usual pathogens: *Staphylococcus aureus,* streptococci, and coliforms
  - • Hand x-rays to evaluate for radiopaque foreign body and gas-forming infections

- ■ Differential Diagnosis
  - • Retained foreign body
  - • Fracture
  - • Cellulitis
  - • Tendonitis

- ■ Treatment
  - • Initiation of broad-spectrum antibiotic coverage in emergency department
  - • Immediate referral to hand surgeon for operative exploration and drainage

- ■ Pearl

Antibiotics must be started in the emergency department.

Reference

Harrison BP, Hilliard MW: Emergency department evaluation and treatment of hand injuries. Emerg Med Clin North Am 1999;17:793. [PMID: 10584103]

Felon

- **Essentials of Diagnosis**
    - Abscess of distal phalanx pad (pulp space), usually caused by *Staphylococcus aureus*
    - Occurs after penetrating skin break in the region
    - Septae in the finger pad compartmentalize the area from the rest of the hand
    - Patients usually present with severely painful, swollen, tender distal pulp space

- **Differential Diagnosis**
    - Herpetic whitlow
    - Paronychia
    - Cellulitis
    - Soft tissue injury
    - Distal phalangeal fracture
    - Flexor tendon injury

- **Treatment**
    - Incision and drainage at the point of maximal fluctuance after digital block: incision is made on ulnar side of the digit (except for the thumb and fifth digits, in which incision is made on the radial side) just volar to lateral nailbed (avoiding neurovascular bundle) or longitudinally in the midline on the palmar side (avoiding the flexor digitorum profundus insertion); cavity is irrigated and loosely packed
    - Antistaphylococcal antibiotics
    - Follow-up in 24–48 hours for reevaluation

- **Pearl**

Be careful not to disrupt too many septae. It could cause pad instability and long-term disability.

Reference

Harrison BP, Hilliard MW: Emergency department evaluation and treatment of hand injuries. Emerg Med Clin North Am 1999;17:793. [PMID: 10584103]

Fingertip Amputation

■ Essentials of Diagnosis

- Zone I: preservation of proximal two-thirds of nailbed
- Zone II: bone exposed
- Zone III: loss of entire nailbed
- Evaluate perfusion of partial amputations
- X-rays to determine if fracture or foreign body is present

■ Differential Diagnosis

- Usually clear on visual inspection
- Rule out other bony or soft tissue injury

■ Treatment

- Digital block for regional anesthesia of the finger for irrigation, exploration, and repair
- Try to maintain length of thumb and index finger
- Try to keep intact pulp-to-pulp contact points of thumb and index finger
- Consider age, health, handedness, and occupation of patient
- Otherwise, amputations distal to distal interphalangeal joint require only conservative wound management as long as wound diameter is less than 1 cm
- If less than 0.5 cm of phalangeal bone is exposed: may rongeur and allow to heal by secondary intention
- More extensive amputations with extensive tissue loss: hand surgeon consult; treatment options include a V-Y flap, split- or full-thickness skin graft, pedicle, and various other flaps for coverage of bone or soft tissues
- Inform patients that chronic fingernail deformities often occur with injuries to the germinal matrix or more distal parts of the nailbed
- Tetanus, splinting, and antibiotics (if open fracture is present), as appropriate

■ Pearl

Treatment is individualized based on site of injury and patient's occupation.

Reference

Jackson EA: The V-Y plasty in the treatment of fingertip amputations. Am Fam Physician 2001;64:455. [PMID: 11515834]

Flexor Tendon Laceration

■ Essentials of Diagnosis

- Most caused by laceration, thus, an open injury
- Jersey finger is closed, caused by forced extension of a flexed distal interphalangeal (DIP) joint
- Test flexor digitorum superficialis by holding all other fingers in full extension and asking the patient to attempt flexion of the proximal interphalangeal (PIP) joint against resistance
- Test flexor digitorum profundus by holding the PIP joint in extension and asking the patient to flex the DIP joint against resistance

■ Differential Diagnosis

- Phalangeal fracture
- Other tendon injury
- Collateral ligament injury
- Sprain

■ Treatment

- Many hand surgeons will repair these injuries urgently (within 12–24 hours)
- Proper wound care and debridement
- Antibiotic coverage as appropriate
- Prompt referral to a hand surgeon

■ Pearl

Significant disability (eg, synovial adhesions, missed injuries to pulley system, triggering, bow stringing) may result from these injuries. Flexor tendon injuries are not repaired by emergency physicians. Patients with all such injuries should be referred to hand surgeons for definitive care.

Reference

Harrison BP, Hilliard MW: Emergency department evaluation and treatment of hand injuries. Emerg Med Clin North Am 1999;17:793. [PMID: 10584103]

Gamekeeper's Thumb

- ■ Essentials of Diagnosis
    - • Any partial or complete tear of the thumb ulnar collateral ligament (UCL)
    - • Usually occurs as result of ski-pole or football injuries from forcible extension and abduction of the thumb
    - • Exam reveals edema and tenderness at the dorsoulnar aspect of thumb metacarpal phalangeal joint
    - • May have a weak pinch
    - • Laxity from complete tears difficult to assess acutely
    - • Comparison with opposite hand may be unreliable
    - • X-rays to evaluate for underlying avulsions, fractures, and dislocations

- ■ Differential Diagnosis
    - • First metacarpal fracture
    - • Proximal phalangeal fracture of thumb
    - • Other ligamentous injury
    - • Soft tissue injury or sprain

- ■ Treatment
    - • Thumb spica splint for 4 weeks
    - • Refer to hand surgeon for early follow-up
    - • Some hand surgeons routinely treat these injuries intraoperatively with exploration and repair of the UCL
    - • Ice and elevation
    - • Analgesia

- ■ Pearl

The Stener lesion is a complication defined as entrapment of the proximal fragment of the UCL in the adductor pollicis aponeurosis. The soft tissue entrapment leads to improper healing, which makes early referral important.

Reference

Harrison BP, Hilliard MW: Emergency department evaluation and treatment of hand injuries. Emerg Med Clin North Am 1999;17:793. [PMID: 10584103]

Herpetic Whitlow

- ■ Essentials of Diagnosis
  - Appears as grouped vesicles on an erythematous base
  - Pain out of proportion to exam findings
  - Prodromal symptoms of pruritus, burning, or paresthesias possible
  - Caused by herpes simplex virus I or II
  - Seen in health care workers, children with herpetic gingivosto-matitis, or adults with genital herpes
  - Lesions typically contain clear fluid but may turn purulent appearing as they form crust
  - Diagnosis is clinical; may be confirmed with Tzanck smear or viral culture of lesions

- ■ Differential Diagnosis
  - Felon
  - Candidal lesion
  - Cellulitis
  - Hypersensitivity reaction

- ■ Treatment
  - Symptomatic
  - Oral acyclovir for recurrent cases or for immunocompromised patients
  - Cover lesions with a dry gauze dressing to prevent infection transmission
  - May need to unroof nailbed lesions if they cause pain

- ■ Pearl

Herpetic whitlow may be distinguished from a felon by the absence of a tense distal finger pad.

Reference

Harrison BP, Hilliard MW: Emergency department evaluation and treatment of hand injuries. Emerg Med Clin North Am 1999;17:793. [PMID: 10584103]

High-Pressure Injection Injury

- ■ Essentials of Diagnosis
  - Careful history to obtain information about possible injection injury; delay in presentation is not uncommon and complicates treatment
  - Use of high-pressure injection guns, typically grease or paint guns; obtain information on the pounds per square inch and the specific agent involved
  - Digits with high-pressure injection injury often look deceivingly normal; injury may be only a small puncture wound, typically on the finger pad
  - Paints and solvents have much higher potential for severe injury secondary to infection and tissue necrosis
  - Compressive force of injected material leads to soft tissue destruction and vascular ischemia secondary to mechanical tamponade by surrounding tissue
  - Anteroposterior and lateral hand x-rays; some injected materials are radiopaque

- ■ Differential Diagnosis
  - Other puncture wound to hand
  - Cellulitis
  - Fracture
  - Tenosynovitis

- ■ Treatment
  - Updated tetanus
  - Emergent evaluation by hand surgeon
  - Open lavage and debridement in operating room
  - Wound packed open and treated with antibiotics
  - Rest, ice, elevation

- ■ Pearl

Maintain a high index of suspicion for high-pressure injection injury. The initial appearance of the wound and digit may look deceptively benign, although the injury can be devastating to the normal function of the digit and hand.

Reference

Harrison BP, Hilliard MW: Emergency department evaluation and treatment of hand injuries. Emerg Med Clin North Am 1999;17:793. [PMID: 10584103]

Lunate Dislocation

■ Essentials of Diagnosis

- Caused by forceful hyperextension of the wrist
- Occurs after a fall onto an outstretched hand (FOOSH)
- Significant pain and tenderness
- Loss of range of motion
- More severe than perilunate dislocation
- Enters carpal tunnel; median neuropathy may be apparent
- Associated injuries common, including scapholunate ligament or other bony injuries
- X-ray evaluation: on lateral view, lunate is displaced and rotated in a palmar direction while the capitate moves proximally over the distal radius; on posteroanterior view, the normal carpal arcs are disrupted

■ Differential Diagnosis

- Perilunate dislocation
- Scapholunate dissociation
- Wrist fracture
- Distal radial or ulnar fracture
- Metacarpal fracture

■ Treatment

- Prompt reduction required
- Urgent hand surgeon consult
- Long arm splint required if patient transferred for care or after reduction
- Analgesia

■ Pearl

The tipped teacup sign refers to the classic sign used to describe the dislocated position of the lunate in the palmar direction on the lateral view.

Reference

Ritchie JV, Munter DW: Emergency department evaluation and treatment of wrist injuries. Emerg Med Clin North Am 1999;17:823. [PMID: 10584104]

Mallet Finger

- **Essentials of Diagnosis**
  - Mechanism: forced flexion of the distal interphalangeal (DIP) joint in a full extension position (eg, baseball to fingertip)
  - Can occur with distal phalangeal fractures
  - Involves disruption of the extensor mechanism by either avulsion of the terminal slip of the extensor tendon from the dorsal base of the distal phalanx or fracture at the base of the distal phalanx
  - Apparent by resting DIP joint flexion and inability to actively extend the DIP joint
  - Usually clinically obvious and considered an intra-articular injury

- **Differential Diagnosis**
  - Dislocation at the DIP
  - Other phalangeal fracture

- **Treatment**
  - Splint DIP in full extension continuously for 6 weeks; allow functional mobility at the proximal interphalangeal joint
  - Displaced or angulated fractures: often require internal fixation with K-wire; urgent hand surgeon referral

- **Pearl**

Mallet finger is an intra-articular injury, and patients should be referred for prompt hand surgeon follow-up to avoid long-term disability.

Reference

Harrison BP, Hilliard MW: Emergency department evaluation and treatment of hand injuries. Emerg Med Clin North Am 1999;17:793. [PMID: 10584103]

Metacarpal Fracture

- **Essentials of Diagnosis**
  - Mechanism: direct blow, missile, or crush injury
  - Pain, swelling, or ecchymosis overlies injury
  - Axial load of associated finger produces intense pain

- **Differential Diagnosis**
  - Wrist or proximal phalangeal fracture
  - Soft tissue injury

- **Treatment**
  - Metacarpal head fractures: usually intra-articular; splint in "safe position," in which the wrist is immobilized at 20-degrees extension, the metacarpophalangeal (MCP) joint is at 90-degrees flexion, and the proximal interphalangeal (PIP) and distal interphalangeal (DIP) joints are fully extended; hand surgeon referral
  - Metacarpal neck fractures: may allow less than 15-degrees angulation in index and middle metacarpals and up to 35 degrees in ring finger and 45 degrees in little finger; correct any rotational deformity; splint index and middle metacarpal fractures in radial gutter, ring and little fingers in ulnar gutter; splints go from elbow to PIP joint; do not immobilize PIP joint
  - Displaced or angulated index or middle finger metacarpal neck fractures: consult a hand surgeon
  - Metacarpal shaft fractures: no angulation is acceptable in index or middle fingers; may allow 10 and 20 degrees, respectively, in ring and little fingers; no rotational deformity is allowable; appropriate gutter splints are placed to the MCP joint, without immobilizing the joint
  - Metacarpal base fractures: volar splint, hand surgeon referral
  - Thumb metacarpal fractures: thumb spica splint, hand surgeon referral

- **Pearl**

An open fracture of a metacarpal head is suspicious for a "fight bite," and serious infections can develop if diagnosis is delayed or the injury is not treated aggressively.

Reference

Harrison BP, Hilliard MW: Emergency department evaluation and treatment of hand injuries. Emerg Med Clin North Am 1999;17:793. [PMID: 10584103]

Nail Avulsion

- Essentials of Diagnosis
  - May result in total or partial loss of the nailbed, exposing distal phalanx
  - Fragments of nailbed may adhere to the underside of the nail plate
  - Mechanism: catching nail on object or significant direct force to nail plate
  - May be associated with distal phalangeal fracture

- Differential Diagnosis
  - Distal phalangeal fracture
  - Subungual hematoma
  - Nailbed infection

- Treatment
  - In general, repair of associated nailbed laceration is recommended; assess and attempt to repair germinal matrix
  - Clean and place the original nail (secured with sutures) or place either petrolatum or Xeroform gauze at the proximal nail fold to prevent adhesions of the eponychium to the matrix
  - Hand surgeon referral if severe nailbed or germinal matrix damage exists; some cases need split nailbed grafting
  - Notify patient that deformity of the nail may result, especially if the proximal nail plate has been injured

- Pearl

Assess complete nailbed because the germinal matrix and proximal nailbed sometimes are avulsed even though the distal nailbed is intact.

Reference

Harrison BP, Hilliard MW: Emergency department evaluation and treatment of hand injuries. Emerg Med Clin North Am 1999;17:793. [PMID: 10584103]

Paronychia

- **Essentials of Diagnosis**
  - Infection of the nail fold involving collection of pus in the eponychial space
  - Often begins with minor trauma (eg, hangnails or nail biting)
  - Likely pathogen: *Staphylococcus aureus*
  - Chronic, recurrent paronychia usually caused by *Candida albicans*

- **Differential Diagnosis**
  - Cellulitis
  - Felon
  - Lymphangitis
  - Subungual hematoma
  - Underlying fracture

- **Treatment**
  - Incision with 11-blade along nailbed after digital block
  - May require removal of lateral fourth of nail or proximal part of nail plate
  - Packing with petrolatum gauze to allow drainage for 24–48 hours
  - Consider antistaphylococcal antibiotics if significant cellulitis or lymphangitis is present
  - May be able to use antibiotics and warm soaks if no pus apparent
  - Refer to hand specialist for recurrent cases

- **Pearl**

If the patient's hands are exposed to chronic moisture, he or she should discontinue activity and use topical antifungals and steroids.

Reference

Harrison BP, Hilliard MW: Emergency department evaluation and treatment of hand injuries. Emerg Med Clin North Am 1999;17:793. [PMID: 10584103]

Perilunate Dislocation

- ■ Essentials of Diagnosis
  - • Mechanism: forceful hyperextension of wrist (a fall onto an out-stretched hand, or FOOSH)
  - • Not as severe as lunate dislocation
  - • Most common wrist dislocation
  - • Dorsal dislocation of the base of the capitate on the lunate
  - • X-ray evaluation: on lateral wrist view, lunate is palmar flexed and capitate base is dorsally dislocated (interrupts normal vertical alignment on a lateral view of the distal radius, lunate, capitate, and metacarpal bones); on posteroanterior view, loss of normal 2-mm gap between capitate and lunate

- ■ Differential Diagnosis
  - • Lunate dislocation
  - • Scapholunate dissociation
  - • Distal radial or ulnar fracture
  - • Metacarpal fracture
  - • Wrist fracture

- ■ Treatment
  - • Prompt reduction
  - • Urgent hand surgeon consult
  - • Long arm splint for transfer or postreduction
  - • Rest, ice, elevation
  - • Analgesia

- ■ Pearl

For a perilunate dislocation to occur, either a scaphoid fracture or a disruption of the scapholunate ligament must be present.

Reference

Ritchie JV, Munter DW: Emergency department evaluation and treatment of wrist injuries. Emerg Med Clin North Am 1999;17:823. [PMID: 10584104]

Phalangeal Dislocation

- **Essentials of Diagnosis**
  - Typically associated with forced hyperextension or hyperflexion of digit
  - Distal phalanx dislocates dorsally in the majority of cases, often resulting in volar plate disruption or ligamentous injury
  - Need to know patient's dominant hand and occupation, also time of injury
  - Assessment for neurovascular function of the entire hand
  - Restriction in active flexion or extension suggests tendinous or ligamentous rupture or intra-articular osteochondral fragment
  - Test volar plate by passive hyperextension and collateral ligaments by exerting radial and ulnar stress

- **Differential Diagnosis**
  - Phalangeal fracture
  - Soft tissue injury

- **Treatment**
  - Administer digital block 10–15 minutes before reduction
  - Remove patient's rings
  - Grasp finger with gauze, brace hand, and hyperextend digit while gently forcing phalanx into anatomic position
  - Reassess for neurovascular compromise, ligamentous instability
  - Splint for 14–21 days for proximal interphalangeal dislocation, 6 weeks for distal interphalangeal dislocation
  - Buddy tape for 3–6 weeks thereafter
  - Nonsteroidal anti-inflammatory drugs, rest, ice, elevation
  - Follow-up care with a hand surgeon

- **Pearl**

The need for excessive force during a reduction attempt may indicate an intra-articular osteochondral fragment or soft tissue entrapment. Refer the patient to a hand surgeon for urgent follow-up.

Reference

Chinchalkar SJ, Gan BS: Management of proximal interphalangeal joint fractures and dislocations. J Hand Ther 2003;16:117. [PMID: 12755163]

Phalangeal Fracture

- **Essentials of Diagnosis**
  - 15–30% are distal phalangeal fractures (most common phalangeal fracture)
  - Mechanism: crush or shearing forces
  - Consider associated nailbed injuries (ie, open fractures)
  - Be aware of the insertions of the flexor and extensor tendons; tendon avulsions associated with phalangeal fractures significantly affect function of the digit
  - Careful examination of x-rays for displacement of fracture fragments
  - Axial load injuries tend to produce proximal interphalangeal (PIP) joint dislocations and proximal phalangeal fractures

- **Differential Diagnosis**
  - Soft tissue injury
  - Infection
  - Phalangeal dislocation
  - Volar plate injury
  - Sprain

- **Treatment**
  - Patients with closed distal phalangeal fractures with distal interphalangeal (DIP) joint flexion at rest: splint DIP joint in full extension; splint should not cross the PIP joint; refer patient to hand surgeon
  - Patients with closed transverse distal phalangeal fractures with irreducible angulation or displacement: refer patient to hand surgeon for K-wires within 3–5 days
  - Most proximal and middle phalangeal fractures are nondisplaced and stable; buddy splint to adjacent finger; encourage gentle range of motion
  - Displaced or unstable fractures: anatomic reduction and placement in a radial (index and middle finger) or an ulnar (little finger and ring finger) gutter splint for no longer than 3 weeks
  - Hand surgeon follow up within 7–10 days for reevaluation and repeat imaging

- **Pearl**

Consider potential ligamentous injuries and points of attachment when evaluating phalangeal fractures.

Reference

Harrison BP, Hilliard MW: Emergency department evaluation and treatment of hand injuries. Emerg Med Clin North Am 1999;17:793. [PMID: 10584103]

Scapholunate Dissociation

- **Essentials of Diagnosis**
  - Rupture of the scapholunate ligament caused by forced hyperextension of wrist
  - Occurs after a fall onto an outstretched hand (FOOSH)
  - Pain is dorsal, just distal to Lister's tubercle
  - May have clicking with wrist motion
  - Terry Thomas sign on posteroanterior view; diastasis of at least 3 mm between scaphoid and lunate is diagnostic
  - If ligament torn completely, scaphoid may undergo rotary subluxation (produces signet ring sign on posteroanterior view)
  - Injury is suggested if the scapholunate angle is greater than 60 degrees on lateral view

- **Differential Diagnosis**
  - Lunate dislocation
  - Perilunate dislocation
  - Metacarpal fracture
  - Wrist fracture
  - Distal radial or ulnar fracture

- **Treatment**
  - Urgent hand surgeon consult; operative repair required
  - Long arm splint required if patient transferred for specialty care
  - Rest, ice, elevation
  - Analgesia

- **Pearl**

The injury can be subtle and is commonly missed initially. Carefully review wrist films looking for the Terry Thomas sign so as not to miss scapholunate dissociation.

Reference

Ritchie JV, Munter DW: Emergency department evaluation and treatment of wrist injuries. Emerg Med Clin North Am 1999;17:823. [PMID: 10584104]

Subungual Hematoma

- ■ Essentials of Diagnosis
  - • Associated with distal phalangeal blunt trauma, often from getting finger caught in a closing door or under a falling object
  - • May have associated fractures, nail plate injuries, or nailbed injuries
  - • Can cause significant pain
  - • Hematomas larger than 25% of the nail plate area likely require treatment

- ■ Differential Diagnosis
  - • Nailbed or nail plate injury
  - • Open distal phalangeal fracture
  - • Nail bed infection

- ■ Treatment
  - • May require trephination if hematoma causes significant pain and is larger than 25% of the nail plate surface area
  - • Trephination is done with either an 18-gauge needle or electrocautery; usually provides instant relief
  - • Although controversial, traditional treatment of subungual hematomas (involving 50% of the nailbed) consists of removal of the nail plate and repair of nailbed lacerations with 6-0 or 7-0 absorbable suture
  - • Fractures of distal phalanx must be assessed carefully as open or closed with appropriate reduction, irrigation, and repair of open wounds; if an open fracture exists, use cephalexin, 500 mg every 6 hours
  - • Use nail plate as splint by suturing it back on with nonabsorbable suture; if the nail is unavailable, place either petrolatum or Xeroform gauze at the proximal nail fold to prevent adhesions of the eponychium to the matrix
  - • Advise patients that chronic nail deformities may occur with nailbed injury
  - • Hand surgeon referral for early follow-up

- ■ Pearl

With proximal nailbed injuries, the nailbed can become entrapped in bony fragments. This will result in nonunion. Carefully assess all nailbed injuries with associated fractures to prevent this potential complication.

Reference

Harrison BP, Hilliard MW: Emergency department evaluation and treatment of hand injuries. Emerg Med Clin North Am 1999;17:793. [PMID: 10584103]

Tenosynovitis

■ Essentials of Diagnosis

- Flexor tendons are surrounded by sheaths that run from the mid-palmar crease to just distal of the distal interphalangeal joint
- Potential site for inoculation with bacteria after laceration or puncture wounds along their course
- Four cardinal signs: uniform digit swelling ("sausage finger"), semiflexed posture of the finger, tenderness along course of the flexor tendon, significant pain with passive extension of finger
- Spread to deep fascial compartments and flexor tendon scarring can result if treated improperly

■ Differential Diagnosis

- Phalangeal fracture
- Trigger finger
- Sprain
- Cellulitis
- Tendon injury
- Ligamentous injury

■ Treatment

- Emergently consult a hand surgeon for either open debridement or closed irrigation of the tendon sheath
- Start treatment in the emergency department with appropriate intravenous antibiotics (eg, nafcillin, 2 g every 4 hours)
- Obtain wound cultures
- Splint with bulky dressings
- Appropriate analgesia

■ Pearl

Consider disseminated gonorrhea in sexually active patients with flexor tenosynovitis and no history of trauma.

Reference

Harrison BP, Hilliard MW: Emergency department evaluation and treatment of hand injuries. Emerg Med Clin North Am 1999;17:793. [PMID: 10584103]

24

Dermatologic Emergencies

Angioedema

- **Essentials of Diagnosis**
  - Nonpitting edema of skin and mucous membranes in the head and neck areas
  - Causes: hereditary; temperature extremes; trauma; and allergic reaction to foods, food additives, and medications
  - Since mid-1980s angiotensin-converting-enzyme inhibitors have caused at least half the cases; may occur after first dose or after taking the medication for several years
  - May be accompanied by anaphylaxis (with bronchospasm, shock) or with urticaria

- **Differential Diagnosis**
  - Pharyngitis
  - Tetanus
  - Ludwig angina

- **Treatment**
  - Epinephrine, 0.3 cc of a 1:1,000 solution subcutaneously
  - Antihistamines: H_1 and H_2 histamine antagonists should be given intravenously and orally if discharged home
  - Methylprednisolone, 125 mg IV, followed by oral steroids if discharged home
  - Patients with face and oral cavity swelling (not floor of mouth): may be discharged from emergency department with improvement after treatment
  - Patients with massive edema of the tongue and floor of mouth: intubation
  - Patients with potential airway compromise and those with no improvement or worsening symptoms despite aggressive therapy: admission

- **Pearl**

Do not fail to recognize the potential of progression to a compromised airway in all patients with angioedema.

Reference

Chiu AG et al: Angiotensin-converting enzyme inhibitor-induced angioedema: a multicenter review and algorithm for airway management. Ann Otol Rhinol Laryngol 2001;110:834. [PMID: 11558759

Contact Dermatitis

- **Essentials of Diagnosis**
    - Direct contact of exogenous agent (foreign molecule, ultraviolet light, temperature) to the outermost layers of skin
    - Can be in response to allergen (delayed hypersensitivity) or irritant (direct tissue damage)
    - Erythematous, papulovesicular, pruritic rash
    - May have linear streaking; may have soft tissue swelling especially around orbits
    - Rhus (poison ivy, oak, sumac) is common; patients usually present within 8–72 hours of exposure

- **Differential Diagnosis**
    - Eczema
    - Scabies
    - Pediculosis
    - Tinea
    - Phytophotodermatitis
    - Bug bites

- **Treatment**
    - Avoidance of offending cause
    - Cold compresses
    - Over-the-counter lotions
    - Topical steroids for small surface area
    - Oral steroids for facial or orbital dermatitis and if greater than 20% of body surface area
    - Some recommend injectable steroids (eg, triamcinolone, 40 mg IM) as one-time dose; has advantage of lasting for about 3 weeks with autotaper
    - Antihistamines not very effective (reaction is not mediated by mast cells or basophils) but used for pruritus
    - May need to rinse and neutralize irritant
    - Antibiotics for secondary infection

- **Pearl**

Always inform the patient with rhus dermatitis that it will take 2–3 weeks to resolve, despite treatment; and that it may actually worsen for the next few days after treatment is started.

Reference

Tanner TL: Rhus (Toxicodendron) dermatitis. Prim Care 2000;27:493. [PMID: 10815057]

Erythema Multiforme Major (Steven-Johnson syndrome)

- **Essentials of Diagnosis**
  - More severe than erythema multiforme minor (truncal and facial lesions)
  - More extensive and multiple mucosal surfaces involved, typically mouth, vagina, conjunctiva, esophagus, or penile corona
  - Symptoms: fever, arthralgias, myalgias
  - Usually lasts 4–6 weeks, recurrence rare
  - Most common causes: mycoplasma infections and medications including sulfonamides, penicillins, phenytoin, allopurinol, and barbiturates
  - Can evolve to toxic epidermal necrolysis and be life threatening

- **Differential Diagnosis**
  - Pemphigus
  - Pemphigoid
  - DRESS (drug rash with eosinophilia and systemic symptoms)
  - Lupus

- **Treatment**
  - Withdrawal of medications that may be the underlying cause; usually means stopping all that are not life saving
  - Treatment of underlying infection if present
  - Patients with extensive disease, systemic toxicity, or mucous membrane involvement: hospitalization
  - Systemic steroids controversial but usually given
  - Analgesics and antihistamines for symptomatic relief
  - Provision of adequate supportive care

- **Pearl**

The mortality rate of 10% is usually secondary to sepsis.

Reference

Ghislain PD, Roujeau JC: Treatment of severe drug reactions: Stevens-Johnson syndrome, toxic epidermal necrolysis and hypersensitivity syndrome. Dermatol Online J 2002;8:5. [PMID: 12165215]

Erythema Multiforme Minor

- **Essentials of Diagnosis**
  - Erythematous macules on the extensor extremities, which spread to involve flexural surfaces and truncal skin
  - Macules develop into target lesions composed of a dusky center surrounded by a zone of pallor surrounded by an erythematous ring
  - If present, mucosal involvement is limited to oral cavity
  - Prodromal symptoms uncommon
  - Usually self-limited; resolves in 2–4 weeks
  - Thought to be a spectrum from erythema multiforme minor to erythema multiforme major (Stevens-Johnson) to toxic epidermal necrolysis
  - Most common identifiable cause: recurrent herpes simplex infection with or without obvious herpes lesions

- **Differential Diagnosis**
  - Pemphigus
  - Pemphigoid
  - DRESS (drug rash with eosinophilia and systemic symptoms)
  - Lupus
  - Hand-foot-mouth disease

- **Treatment**
  - Frequently no treatment indicated
  - Consider topical steroids, antihistamines, and analgesics
  - Close follow-up advised

- **Pearl**

If the erythema multiforme is secondary to recurrent herpes simplex, consider antiviral therapy.

Reference

Cotell S, Robinson ND, Chan LS: Autoimmune blistering skin diseases. Am J Emerg Med 2000;18:288. [PMID: 10830686]

Herpes Simplex

- **Essentials of Diagnosis**
  - Primary infection: symptomatic, most commonly involves oral mucosa
  - Primary genital herpes: vesicles with ulceration and erosion on the external genitalia or genital mucosa
  - Gingivostomatitis: common primary presentation involving buccal mucosa, palate, tongue, and lips; generally occurs in children
  - Recurrent herpes: appears near site of primary infection as grouped vesicles on an erythematous base; vesicles erode and encrust within 4–5 days and heal within 10–14 days; recurrence is usually less severe and less symptomatic but may be preceded by burning or tingling in the affected area
  - Herpetic whitlow: infection on the fingers, commonly seen in health care workers
  - Viral culture useful if diagnosis is in doubt
  - Tzanck smear will not differentiate between herpes simplex, herpes zoster, and varicella

- **Differential Diagnosis**
  - Contact dermatitis, gonococcus, chancroid
  - Fixed drug eruption, syphilis, impetigo
  - Tinea, pemphigus, pemphigoid
  - Herpes gestationis
  - Aphthous ulcers
  - Hand-foot-mouth disease
  - Behçet disease
  - Erythema multiforme

- **Treatment**
  - Primary infection: oral antivirals (acyclovir, valacyclovir, famciclovir) may be used to shorten course in severe disease and in immunocompromised patients
  - Frequent reoccurrence: may be treated with oral antivirals prophylactically

- **Pearl**

A viral culture is worth obtaining if the patient or the physician has any concern.

Reference

Yeung-Yue KA et al: Herpes simplex viruses 1 and 2. Dermatol Clin 2002;20:249. [PMID: 12120439]

Herpes Zoster (Shingles)

- ■ Essentials of Diagnosis
  - Reactivation of herpes zoster virus in a single dermatome
  - Usually a 3- to 4-day prodrome of sharp, stabbing unilateral pain with headache, fever, malaise; followed by vesicles on an erythematous base
  - Prodrome may mimic colic, appendicitis, pleurisy, or myocardial infarction
  - Trigeminal nerve (ophthalmic branch) with Hutchinson sign indicates eye involvement
  - Ramsay Hunt syndrome: involvement of auditory and facial nerves; may lead to facial paralysis, deafness, tinnitus, and vertigo
  - Immunocompromised patients may develop life-threatening disseminated zoster (presence of more than 20 vesicles outside the primary and adjacent dermatomes)
  - Postherpetic neuralgia: continued dysesthesias and severe pain for many months after the rash resolves

- ■ Differential Diagnosis
  - Zosteriform herpes simplex
  - Burns
  - Insect bites
  - Impetigo

- ■ Treatment
  - Infected patients should be isolated from those without prior infection and from the immunocompromised
  - Goal of antiviral therapy: to suppress severity and duration; most effective if started within 72 hours of skin eruption
  - Oral antivirals (acyclovir, 800 mg orally five times daily for 7–10 days; valacyclovir, 1,000 mg orally three times daily for 7 days; or famciclovir, 500 mg orally three times daily for 7 days)
  - Analgesics required
  - Parenteral antivirals for disseminated zoster and possibly for ophthalmic zoster (ophthalmic involvement should prompt ophthalmologic consult)

- ■ Pearl

Herpes zoster may spread to adjacent dermatomes, and a few scattered lesions (<20) may be in other dermatomes and across the midline.

Reference

Chen TM et al: Clinical manifestations of varicella-zoster virus infection. Dermatol Clin 2000;20:267. [PMID: 12120440]

Impetigo

- **Essentials of Diagnosis**
    - Starts as small, erythematous macules, which progress to fragile blisters that break, releasing a serous discharge that dries to form a honey-colored crust
    - Easily spread with development of satellite lesions
    - Commonly seen on face (especially nose and mouth areas), legs, and feet
    - Immunocompromised patients have involvement more often in the axillary, inguinal, and other intertriginous locations
    - Caused by staphylococci, streptococci, or both

- **Differential Diagnosis**
    - Folliculitis
    - Pseudomonas folliculitis (hot tub folliculitis)
    - Ecthyma
    - Erysipelas
    - Kaposi sarcoma
    - Blistering distal dactylitis (usually in children, distal phalangeal area)

- **Treatment**
    - Topical antibiotics (eg, mupirocin) also may be used intranasally to treat the reservoirs of staphylococci in patients with recurrences and in household contacts
    - Oral antibiotics for highly inflammatory, resistant, or extensive disease (dicloxacillin, 250–500 mg orally four times daily for 5–10 days; clindamycin, 150–300 mg orally four times daily for 5–10 days; or erythromycin, 250–500 mg orally four times daily for 5–10 days)

- **Pearl**

Treatment with antibiotics will not prevent acute poststreptococcal glomerulonephritis because it is caused by the immune response to the infection.

Reference

Hirschmann JV: Impetigo: etiology and therapy. Curr Clin Top Infect Dis 2002;22:42. [PMID: 12520646]

Molluscum Contagiosum

- **Essentials of Diagnosis**
  - Discrete flesh-colored to pink, dome-shaped, umbilicated papules singly or in groups; smooth, shiny, some may have a keratotic plug
  - Mucosal surfaces spared
  - Usually asymptomatic, benign, and self-limited but may last months to a year
  - Infants, sexually active individuals, and HIV patients at risk
  - HIV patients may have larger lesions, both in diameter and height; lesions may coalesce, most commonly on the face
  - Contagious and autoinoculable
  - Cause is a large DNA pox virus

- **Differential Diagnosis**
  - Common wart
  - Genital wart
  - Bullet basal cell carcinoma
  - Keratoacanthoma
  - Pyogenic granuloma, xanthoma
  - Cutaneous cryptococcosis (in HIV patients)
  - Lichen nitidus
  - Milia (usually gone by the second week of life)

- **Treatment**
  - Usually none, particularly in children
  - Adults with genital lesions: cryotherapy, curettage, cantharidin, laser
  - HIV patients: antiretrovirals may help

- **Pearl**

Molluscum contagiosum is occasionally the chief complaint (eg, children with lesions on the face, adults with genital involvement), but frequently a parent will ask about the incidental finding while the clinician is examining the child for another reason.

Reference

Perna AG, Tyring SK: A review of the dermatologic manifestations of poxvirus infections. Dermatol Clin 2002;20:343. [PMID: 12120447]

Pediculosis

- ■ Essentials of Diagnosis
    - • Head lice: most common form; most cases in children (and parents); spread by sharing infected grooming items; pruritus is main complaint; nits (ova of lice) are tiny, whitish oval bodies firmly attached to the hair shaft
    - • Body lice: spread by close contact and infected clothing; pruritus is main complaint; lice live on clothing or bedding and use skin only for feedings; nits may be seen in seams of clothing; predilection for axilla, trunk, and groin
    - • Pubic lice: also very pruritic; predominantly sexually transmitted, affecting genitalia, perineal area, thigh, beard, and eyelashes

- ■ Differential Diagnosis
    - • Scabies
    - • Tinea
    - • Impetigo

- ■ Treatment
    - • Permethrin 5% cream: effective and less toxic than lindane; apply and then wash off after 10 minutes; repeat treatment in 1 week
    - • Lindane 1% shampoo: apply and then wash off after 10 minutes; repeat treatment in 1 week (more toxic, not used for children and pregnant or lactating women)
    - • Permethrin 1% rinse: apply and then wash off after 10 minutes; repeat treatment in 1 week (some resistance, especially head lice)
    - • Petroleum jelly: good for eyelashes; apply to lid margin twice daily for 8 days
    - • After treatment, remove nits with comb or brush
    - • Consider treatment for other family members
    - • For pubic lice, consider treatment for sex partners
    - • Wash clothes, bed linens, bedding, combs, and the like

- ■ Pearl

Because sexual contact is the primary mode of spread for pubic lice, up to one-third of patients may have another sexually transmitted disease.

Reference

Chosidow O: Scabies and pediculosis. Lancet 2000;355:819. [PMID: 10711939]

Pityriasis Rosea

■ Essentials of Diagnosis

- Pruritic brownish to erythematous oval patches with a collarette of scale, classically in a Christmas tree distribution of the trunk
- Long axis of ovals follow the skin lines
- Herald patch precedes eruption by 1 week, similar to other patches but usually larger and commonly located on trunk
- Benign, self-limited disease; resolves in 4–6 weeks
- Cause attributed to human herpes virus-7
- Usually 10–35 years old
- Inverse pityriasis rosea involves extremities rather than the trunk

■ Differential Diagnosis

- Syphilis
- Kaposi sarcoma
- Psoriasis (guttate)
- Tinea corporis

■ Treatment

- Symptomatic treatment with antihistamines, topical antipruritics, and topical steroids
- Short course of oral steroids may cause immediate disappearance

■ Pearl

Testing for syphilis usually indicated.

Reference

Hsu S, Le EH, Khoshevis MR: Differential diagnosis of annular lesions. Am Fam Physician 2001;64:289. [PMID: 11476274]

Psoriasis

- ■ Essentials of Diagnosis
  - • Erythematous plaques with adherent silvery scale usually appearing over the extensor surfaces of the extremities, although variations exist, including lesions on the palms, soles, scalp, umbilicus, and genital areas
  - • Associated symptoms: itching, burning, joint pain, soreness of the lesions
  - • Nail changes: onycholysis, pitting, subungual hyperkeratosis
  - • HIV-related psoriasis: may develop in patients with mild preexisting psoriasis that suddenly undergoes severe exacerbation once AIDS develops, or may develop spontaneously at some point after HIV seroconversion in an individual who has never before had clinical disease

- ■ Differential Diagnosis
  - • Tinea
  - • Pityriasis rosea (guttate psoriasis)
  - • Nummular dermatitis
  - • Cutaneous lupus
  - • Reiter's syndrome

- ■ Treatment
  - • Topical corticosteroids
  - • Emollients
  - • Systemic drugs: etretinate with or without dapsone, psoralen with ultraviolet A therapy and methotrexate

- ■ Pearl

Generalized pustular psoriasis is an emergency; its presentation includes fever, leukocytosis, arthralgias, and malaise, and it can lead to sepsis.

Reference

Prodanovich S, Kirsner RS, Taylor JR: Treatment of patients hospitalized for psoriasis. Dermatol Clin 2000;18:425. [PMID: 10943538]

Scabies

- **Essentials of Diagnosis**
  - Extremely pruritic (constant, pronounced at night) eruption of papules, vesicles, burrows
  - In older children and adults: located in finger webs, flexural areas, belt line, and anogenital area
  - In younger children: located on palms, soles, head, and neck
  - Immunocompromised patients: hyperkeratotic plaques (palms, soles, trunk, extremities) and widespread papulosquamous eruptions
  - Epidemics reported in long-term health care institutions
  - Diagnosis made by scabies prep (intact vesicles or burrows are best used)

- **Differential Diagnosis**
  - Drug-induced eruption
  - Psoriasis
  - Seborrheic dermatitis
  - Impetigo
  - Tinea
  - Bulbous pemphigoid (elderly)
  - Eczema
  - Pediculosis (may coexist)

- **Treatment**
  - Permethrin 5% cream: apply to entire body (except head and eyes) at night and then wash off in the morning; repeat in 1 week
  - Lindane: has possible neurotoxicity in children but is a reasonable alternative; apply 1% cream or lotion from neck down and then wash off after 8 hours; repeat in 1 week
  - Treatment of all household contacts
  - Mites can live 1–2 days off the human body; wash in hot water all clothes and bedding used 2 days before treatment
  - For immunocompromised patients and all resistant cases: ivermectin, 100–200 µg/kg orally each week for 1–3 weeks

- **Pearl**

Posttreatment pruritus may exist for several weeks (hypersensitivity reaction) and may be treated with antihistamines and steroids.

Reference

Chosidown O: Scabies and pediculosis. Lancet 2000;355:819. [PMID: 10711939]

Staphylococcal Scalded Skin Syndrome

- ### Essentials of Diagnosis
  - Diffuse, tender erythema with sandpaper texture (similar to scarlet fever) develops after 1–2 days of fever, malaise, and irritability
  - Strawberry tongue is absent; no mucous membrane involvement
  - Progresses to exfoliative phase with wrinkling and peeling of the skin where minor pressure causes large amounts of skin to peel away (Nikolsky sign)
  - Caused by staphylococcal epidermolytic toxins A and B
  - Usually in children under age 5 years (due to inability to clear toxin thru renal system); most people have antibodies to the toxins by age 10
  - Can occur in adults with renal insufficiency (inability to clear the toxin) or in immunocompromised patients
  - May begin with an unnoticed infection to the throat, nares, umbilicus, or circumcision site

- ### Differential Diagnosis
  - Toxic epidermal necrolysis (biopsy usually done to differentiate)
  - Erythema multiforme major
  - Toxic shock syndrome
  - Streptococcal toxic shock-like syndrome
  - Recalcitrant erythematous desquamating disorder
  - Toxic mediated erythema

- ### Treatment
  - Hydration to replace large fluid loss, especially in neonates
  - Antibiotics (nafcillin, 2 g IV every 4 hours; clindamycin, 600 mg IV every 8 hours; or vancomycin, 1 g IV every 12 hours)
  - Environmental temperature control
  - Steroids thought to be contraindicated

- ### Pearl

Although staphylococcal scalded skin syndrome is rare in adults, the mortality rate is higher than in children because of septicemia.

Reference

Ladhani S: Recent developments in staphylococcal scalded skin syndrome. Clin Microbiol Infect 2001;7:301. [PMID: 11442563]

Tinea

- **Essentials of Diagnosis**
  - Tinea capitis: circumscribed patches of alopecia with varying degrees of scale and erythema; highly inflammatory infection leads to boggy, fluctuant nodules (kerions)
  - Tinea corporis: an annular erythematous patch with leading edge of scale and varying degrees of central clearing on the body, hands, or face
  - Tinea pedis: scale on lateral aspects of feet or maceration between toes
  - Tinea cruris (jock itch): involves the moist areas of groin and buttocks with scrotal sparing
  - Tinea unguium (onychomycosis): causes nails to be dystrophic and yellow, with subungual debris; usually associated with tinea pedis.
  - Diagnosis by KOH prep from active lesion border
  - Patients with peripheral vascular disease, diabetes, impaired immunity, and lymphedema may develop secondary bacterial lymphangitis and cellulitis

- **Differential Diagnosis**
  - Alopecia areata
  - Trichotillomania
  - Seborrheic dermatitis
  - Psoriasis
  - Nummular eczema
  - Scabies
  - Pediculosis
  - Lyme disease (erythema chronicum migrans)

- **Treatment**
  - Topical antifungals for all but tinea capitis and tinea unguium to include miconazole and clotrimazole
  - For tinea capitis: griseofulvin, 500 mg orally every day for 4–6 weeks
  - For tinea unguium: terbinafine, 250 mg orally every day for 6 weeks
  - Kerions appear clinically to have a secondary bacterial infection but antibiotics not usually used; griseofulvin is only FDA-approved treatment

- **Pearl**

Most tinea capitis infections do not demonstrate fluorescence with a Wood lamp.

Reference

Rupke SJ: Fungal skin disorders. Prim Care 2000;27:407. [PMID: 10815051]

Toxic Epidermal Necrolysis

- ■ Essentials of Diagnosis
  - • Most severe of the erythema multiforme spectrum (some authorities consider it a distinct disease)
  - • Usually a prodrome of nonspecific symptoms; disease accompanied by skin pain, fever, asthenia, and anxiety
  - • Initially a macular erythema with vesiculation and ultimately a formation of large bullae that easily spread with pressure to adjacent skin (positive Nikolsky sign)
  - • Widespread purpuric macules
  - • Mucosal involvement is similar to erythema multiforme major and is a prominent finding
  - • Gastrointestinal, renal, liver, and pulmonary involvement possible
  - • Almost always caused by medications; concomitant viral infection may play a role
  - • Paradoxically, high-dose steroids may be a contributory cause

- ■ Differential Diagnosis
  - • Scalded skin syndrome
  - • Erythema multiforme major (Stevens-Johnson syndrome)
  - • DRESS (drug rash with eosinophilia and systemic symptoms)
  - • Paraneoplastic pemphigus
  - • Chemical and thermal burns
  - • Kawasaki disease

- ■ Treatment
  - • Withdrawal of offending drugs; usually means stopping all drugs that are not life saving, particularly those started within the previous month
  - • Massive intravenous fluids with peripheral access in an uninvolved area
  - • Epithelial involvement in tracheobronchial tree may require intubation and ventilation
  - • Aseptic technique because predominant cause of death is sepsis from skin colonization
  - • Initially, antibiotics are pending cultures
  - • Avoid adhesive materials, hypothermia
  - • Do not give steroids

- ■ Pearl

Mortality rate for toxic epidermal necrolysis is high (>30%); these patients are best served with prompt admission or transfer to either a burn unit or the ICU.

Reference

Wolkenstein P, Revuz J: Toxic epidermal necrolysis. Dermatol Clin 2000;18:485. [PMID: 10943543]

Urticaria

- ■ **Essentials of Diagnosis**
  - • Well-demarcated erythematous wheals that are intensely pruritic, usually transient, and resolve in 24–72 hours
  - • May or may not be seen with severe allergic reaction; anaphylaxis
  - • Causes: idiopathic (>50%; particularly in chronic cases, lasting longer than 6 weeks), food, drugs, insect bites, contact, pressure, cholinergic, aquagenic, solar, and cold
  - • Extensive laboratory evaluation not indicated in otherwise healthy patients

- ■ **Differential Diagnosis**
  - • Erythema multiforme
  - • PUPPP (pruritic urticarial papules and plaques of pregnancy)
  - • Early pemphigoid

- ■ **Treatment**
  - • If associated with anaphylaxis (bronchospasm, angioedema, shock), give epinephrine, H_1 and H_2 antagonists, and intravenous steroids
  - • Eliminate exposure if inciting agent identified
  - • Antihistamines (H_1 and H_2 antagonists) are effective
  - • Steroids for symptomatic relief

- ■ **Pearl**

Watch for anaphylaxis in the patient with sudden severe pruritus with or without urticaria, particularly if itching of the scalp, soft palate, palms, or genitalia is present.

Reference

Rusznak C, Peebles RS Jr: Anaphylaxis and anaphylactoid reactions: a guide to prevention, recognition, and emergent treatment. Postgrad Med 2002;111:101. [PMID: 12040857]

25

Psychiatric Emergencies

Alcohol Dependence

- **Essentials of Diagnosis**
  - Continued use of alcohol despite evidence of resultant medical and social problems
  - According to National Institute on Alcohol Abuse and Alcoholism (NIAAA): more than 14 drinks/week for men, 7 for women; more than 4 drinks per occasion for men, 3 for women
  - Frequent absences from school or work
  - Frequent accidents
  - Enlarged or nodular liver on palpation
  - Odor of alcohol on breath
  - Elevated GGT, SGOT, and AST
  - Red cell macrocytosis
  - Elevated carbohydrate-deficient transferrin

- **Differential Diagnosis**
  - Major depressive disorder
  - Bipolar disorder
  - Schizophrenia
  - Anxiety disorder
  - Personality changes due to organic disease
  - Polysubstance abuse

- **Treatment**
  - Patient education about consequences of alcoholism
  - Referral to Alcoholics Anonymous
  - Intervention with family, friends
  - Inpatient rehabilitation

- **Pearl**

Patients with chronic alcoholism may need inpatient detoxification to prevent fatal alcohol withdrawal syndrome.

Reference

Mersy DJ: Recognition of alcohol and substance abuse. Am Fam Physician 2003;67:1529. [PMID: 12722853]

Alcohol Withdrawal

■ **Essentials of Diagnosis**

- History of chronic alcohol use
- Abrupt decrease in blood alcohol concentration
- After 6–12 hours: anxiety, tachycardia, tremor, sleep disturbance, diaphoresis, fever, autonomic symptoms and signs
- After 12–48 hours: alcohol-related seizures, visual hallucinations
- After 48–72 hours: disorientation, agitation, delirium tremens
- Stages may overlap; any symptoms can occur within 7 days
- Alcoholic hallucinosis: hallucinations with otherwise clear sensorium

■ **Differential Diagnosis**

- Hypoglycemia
- Hyponatremia
- Hypercalcemia
- Meningitis
- Encephalitis
- Brain tumor
- Stroke
- Sympathomimetic overdose
- Anticholinergic overdose
- γ-Hydroxybutyrate withdrawal
- Benzodiazepine withdrawal

■ **Treatment**

- Benzodiazepines: treatment of choice; as-needed dosing decreases amount needed compared with scheduled dosing
- Diazepam, lorazepam, and chlordiazepoxide may be used
- Thiamine, magnesium, and folate supplementation
- Phenytoin is ineffective for alcohol-related seizures
- β-Blockers, clonidine may be useful as adjunctive therapy
- Fluid status critical; dehydration often present

■ **Pearl**

Alcohol withdrawal is a potentially life-threatening syndrome.

Reference

Kosten TR, O'Connor PG: Management of drug and alcohol withdrawal. N Engl J Med 2003;348:1786. [PMID: 12724485]

Bipolar Affective Disorder

- **Essentials of Diagnosis**
    - The *Diagnostic and Statistical Manual of Mental Disorders,* 4th edition, divides disorder into bipolar I and bipolar II
    - Bipolar I requires at least 1 week of mania with abnormally elevated, expansive, or irritable mood with three of the following: grandiosity, decreased need for sleep, pressured speech, flights of ideas or racing thoughts, distractibility, increase in goal-directed behavior or psychomotor agitation, reckless involvement in pleasurable activities
    - Bipolar II requires one or more major depressive episodes accompanied by at least one hypomanic episode

- **Differential Diagnosis**
    - Schizophrenia
    - Sympathomimetic, alcohol, or other substance abuse
    - Mixed episodes
    - Response to treatment of major depression
    - Hyperthyroidism
    - Major depressive disorder

- **Treatment**
    - Admit if suicidal, violent, or unable to care for self
    - Consider admission for noncompliance, substance abuse
    - Lithium: drug of choice
    - Valproate: especially useful for rapid-cycling bipolar disorder
    - Carbamazepine
    - Atypical antipsychotics: clozapine, olanzapine
    - Newer anticonvulsants: lamotrigine, gabapentin
    - Combination regimens often necessary
    - Electroconvulsive therapy has been successful

- **Pearl**

Manic patients often lack insight and are referred by their family.

Reference

Moller HJ, Nasrallah MA: Treatment of bipolar disorder. J Clin Psychiatry 2003;64:9. [PMID: 12720475]

Depression

- **Essentials of Diagnosis**
  - Five or more of the following for at least 2 weeks: depressed mood most of the day every day, diminished interest in previously enjoyed activities, significant weight loss or gain, persistent insomnia or hypersomnia, psychomotor retardation or agitation, persistent fatigue or lack of energy, feelings of worthlessness or guilt, decreased concentration or indecisiveness, recurrent thoughts of death
  - Risk factors for suicide: male sex, living alone, alcoholism, access to a firearm, suicidal plan

- **Differential Diagnosis**
  - Organic mood syndrome with major depression
  - Dementia
  - Psychological reaction to physical illness
  - Uncomplicated bereavement
  - Substance abuse, particularly alcohol abuse
  - Schizophrenia
  - Schizoaffective disorder
  - Bipolar affective disorder

- **Treatment**
  - Hospitalization for suicidal ideation, concurrent substance abuse, lack of social support, coexisting psychotic disorder
  - Medication is mainstay of treatment: selective serotonin-reuptake inhibitors, tricyclic antidepressants, atypical antidepressants, monoamine oxidase inhibitors
  - Outpatient treatment for patients with strong social support or vague suicidal ideation
  - Outpatients should form contract with family and physician to return to hospital for strong suicidal feelings
  - Cognitive-behavioral therapy: useful adjunctive treatment
  - Medications prescribed in nonlethal quantities

- **Pearl**

Physicians are required to show a good-faith effort to prevent suicide.

Reference

Schulberg HC et al: Treating major depression in primary care practice. Arch Gen Psychiatry 1998;55:1121. [PMID: 9862556]

Generalized Anxiety Disorder

- ■ Essentials of Diagnosis
    - Unrealistic or excessive anxiety and worry for over 6 months
    - Continued distress over two or more life circumstances
    - Presentation often with predominantly physical symptoms
    - Symptoms of motor tension: twitching, trembling, restlessness
    - Symptoms of autonomic hyperactivity: dyspnea, palpitations, tachycardia, nausea
    - Symptoms of vigilance and scanning
    - Difficulty concentrating, irritability, exaggerated startle response
    - Often associated with depressive or panic disorder

- ■ Differential Diagnosis
    - Hyperthyroidism
    - Sympathomimetic abuse
    - Caffeine intoxication
    - Adjustment disorder with anxious mood
    - Psychotic disorders
    - Eating disorders
    - Depressive disorders
    - Panic disorder
    - Social phobia

- ■ Treatment
    - Benzodiazepines: in emergency department use only for short-term treatment of panic attacks
    - Selective serotonin-reuptake inhibitors: both antidepressant and anxiolytic effects
    - Buspirone: fewer adverse reactions and no withdrawal effects
    - Venlafaxine: effective and well tolerated
    - Tricyclic antidepressants: useful; many cardiovascular side effects; lethal in overdose
    - Monoamine oxidase inhibitors: anxiolytic properties; dangerous interactions with many foods and medicines limit usefulness

- ■ Pearl

Anxiety disorder mimics symptoms of serious disease.

Reference

Arikian SR, Gorman JM: A review of the diagnosis, pharmacologic treatment, and economic aspects of anxiety disorders. Prim Care Companion J Clin Psychiatry 2001;3:110. [PMID: 15014608]

Panic Disorder

- **Essentials of Diagnosis**
  - Brief, recurrent attacks of abnormal apprehension
  - Attacks not in response to normally frightful experience
  - Women affected twice as often as men
  - Four attacks within a month, or fear of another over a month
  - Associated with at least four of the following symptoms: dyspnea, dizziness, palpitations, sweating, choking, nausea, depersonalization, paresthesias, hot flashes or chills, chest pain, fear of dying, fear of "going crazy"
  - Agoraphobia (fear of being in places where escape is difficult or embarrassing) may be present

- **Differential Diagnosis**
  - Hyperthyroidism
  - Hypoglycemia
  - Pheochromocytoma
  - Ménière's disease
  - Sympathomimetic abuse
  - Generalized anxiety disorder
  - Caffeine intoxication
  - Major depression
  - Partial complex seizures
  - Drug or alcohol withdrawal

- **Treatment**
  - Selective serotonin-reuptake inhibitors: becoming treatment of choice; safer in overdose than alternatives
  - Tricyclic antidepressants: effective but with many side effects
  - Benzodiazepines: risk of dependency; duration of action exceeds most panic attacks
  - Clonidine and β-blockers: useful as adjuncts
  - Cognitive-behavioral therapy
  - Community support groups

- **Pearl**

Patients with panic disorder often present to the emergency department with cardiac symptoms.

Reference

Pollak MH et al: WCA recommendations for the long-term treatment of panic disorder. CNS Spectr 2003;8:17. [PMID: 14767395]

Personality Disorders

- **Essentials of Diagnosis**
  - Three clusters of personality disorders: A (paranoid, schizoid, schizotypal), B (borderline, histrionic, narcissistic, antisocial), C (avoidant, dependent, obsessive-compulsive)
  - Maladaptive personality traits causing significant impairment or distress, difficulty with interpersonal relationships
  - Traits pervasive and stable over time
  - Manifest in adolescence; continue through adulthood
  - Diagnosis must reflect both recent and long-term behavior; should not be made during acute illness
  - Structured screening tests available but time consuming: Diagnostic Interview for Personality Disorders, Structured Clinical Interview for *DSM*-III-R Personality Disorders
  - Patient may be unable to modify behavior despite sincere effort

- **Differential Diagnosis**
  - Personality change due to organic illness
  - Substance abuse
  - Major depressive disorder
  - Bipolar disorder
  - Anxiety disorder
  - Schizophrenia
  - Psychotic disorder

- **Treatment**
  - Cognitive-behavioral therapy
  - Highly structured environment required for interactions
  - Setting of clear behavioral limits
  - Consistent, unambiguous role of patient and physician
  - Medications reserved for symptomatic control during periods of decompensation

- **Pearl**

Personality disorders are deeply ingrained and difficult to treat.

Reference

Miller MC: Personality disorders. Med Clin North Am 2001;85:819. [PMID: 11349486]

Psychotic Disorders

■ Essentials of Diagnosis

- Hallmark: delusions or hallucinations
- Delusions: fixed false beliefs; usually persecutory, grandiose, or bizarre
- Hallucinations: false perceptions during clear consciousness; auditory hallucinations most common
- Schizophrenia manifested by over 6 months of psychotic symptoms and impaired functioning
- Symptoms of schizophrenia: loosening of associations, flat or inappropriate affect, loss of volition
- Common diagnosis among homeless
- Onset usually during adolescence but can occur at any age

■ Differential Diagnosis

- Organic mental disorders
- Sympathomimetic abuse
- Mood disorder with psychotic features
- Autistic disorder
- Factitious disorder with psychological symptoms
- Cultural or religious beliefs
- Mental retardation

■ Treatment

- Hospitalization required for decompensation or suicidal ideation
- Risk of suicide is higher in psychotic patients
- Traditional antipsychotics: haloperidol, droperidol, chlorpromazine, fluphenazine
- Older drugs associated with tardive dyskinesia
- Newer atypical agents: ziprasidone, olanzapine, risperidone, quetiapine, clozapine
- Benzodiazepines: may be useful for acute agitation
- Haloperidol, droperidol, and ziprasidone: may be given intramuscularly but all increase the QT interval
- Clozapine: may cause fatal agranulocytosis

■ Pearl

Psychotic disorders inherently affect patient compliance.

Reference

Volavka J et al: Clozapine, olanzapine, risperidone, and haloperidol in the treatment of patients with chronic schizophrenia and schizoaffective disorder. Am J Psychiatry 2002;159:255. [PMID: 11823268]

Somatoform Disorder

- ■ Essentials of Diagnosis
  - • Symptoms for which no medical explanation can be found
  - • Patient not producing symptoms voluntarily
  - • Symptoms not part of a delusion
  - • Symptoms not in context of a depressive or anxiety disorder
  - • Conversion disorder: loss of function (usually neurologic) due to underlying, unresolved psychological stressor
  - • Somatization disorder: "positive review of symptoms"
  - • Frequent unnecessary medical and surgical procedures
  - • Rarely diagnosed in men
  - • Hypochondriasis: preoccupation with serious illness despite adequate medical workup and reassurance
  - • Pain disorder: severe pain without medical explanation

- ■ Differential Diagnosis
  - • Physical disorders
  - • Schizophrenia with multiple somatic delusions
  - • Panic disorder
  - • Depressive disorder
  - • Factitious disorder
  - • Malingering

- ■ Treatment
  - • Rule out medical cause of symptoms
  - • Avoid invasive or potentially harmful procedures
  - • Regular follow-up with primary care provider
  - • Patients often resist psychiatric referral
  - • Cognitive-behavioral therapy

- ■ Pearl

Beware of making this diagnosis in the emergency department.

Reference

De Gucht V, Fischler B: Somatization: a critical review of conceptual and methodologic issues. Psychosomatics 2002;43:1. [PMID: 11927751]

26

Emergencies Due to Physical & Environmental Agents

Acute Mountain Sickness

- **Essentials of Diagnosis**
  - Syndrome caused by rapid exposure to altitudes greater than 6,600 feet without acclimatization; usually occurs in people who live at low altitudes who travel to mountain regions
  - Increased physical activity and preexisting disease conditions account for varying degrees of symptoms
  - Symptoms: headache, lassitude, difficulty concentrating, sleep disturbances, drowsiness, dizziness, insomnia, anorexia, nausea, vomiting, dyspnea on exertion, palpitations
  - Symptoms worse on second and third day of ascent; usually resolve by seventh day
  - Consider blood glucose, CBC, electrolytes, BUN, creatinine, and head CT scan

- **Differential Diagnosis**
  - Viral illness
  - Tension headache
  - Meningitis
  - Intracranial lesion
  - Gastroenteritis
  - High-altitude cerebral edema

- **Treatment**
  - Most effective treatment: descent to lower altitudes
  - Oxygen by mask
  - Antiemetics
  - Opiates may confuse signs of high-altitude cerebral edema
  - For insomnia: acetazolamide, 125 mg orally twice each day
  - Dexamethasone, 4–6 mg orally every 6 hours until improvement

- **Pearl**

Acetazolamide or dexamethasone may be used prophylactically to prevent acute mountain sickness.

Reference

Hacken PH, Roach RC: High altitude illness. N Engl J Med 2001;345:107. [PMID: 11450659]

Arterial Gas Embolism

- ■ Essentials of Diagnosis
  - • Caused by air being forced from the pulmonary alveoli into the venous circulation and forming small bubbles when SCUBA divers ascend to the surface; these air bubbles travel to the heart and then to peripheral arteries where they lodge and cause coronary or cerebrovascular occlusion and ischemia
  - • Occurs when divers hold their breath or when air is trapped in the lungs by bronchospasm on ascent; causes the volume of air in the lungs to expand
  - • Dramatic symptoms within 10 minutes of surfacing
  - • Effects: coma, seizure, blindness, confusion, paralysis, aphasia, chest pain, arrhythmias, collapse, death
  - • Air bubbles may be trapped in interstitial space creating pneumothorax or mediastinal emphysema (non-life-threatening conditions; symptoms appear gradually after ascent)
  - • Untreated, may lead to shock, spinal cord injury, permanent impairment, and death
  - • Blood glucose, CBC, electrolytes, BUN, creatinine, electrocardiogram, head CT scan, chest x-ray

- ■ Differential Diagnosis
  - • Trauma
  - • Myocardial infarction
  - • Cerebrovascular accident
  - • Pulmonary embolism

- ■ Treatment
  - • Only effective treatment: immediate recompression
  - • Rapid transport to nearest hyperbaric chamber
  - • Oxygen by mask
  - • Intravenous fluids for hydration
  - • Transport patient with head down, lying on left side, in Trendelenburg position

- ■ Pearl

Many victims of arterial gas embolism die immediately upon surfacing due to large bubbles in the heart that occlude the large blood vessels.

Reference

Neuman TS: Arterial gas embolism and decompression sickness. News Physiol Soc 2002;17:77. [PMID: 11909997]

Bee & Wasp Stings

■ Essentials of Diagnosis

- Bees, wasps, and ants belong to the order Hymenoptera; females inject venom through a stinger located in posterior abdomen
- Includes honeybees, bumblebees, hornets, yellow jackets, fire ants
- Venom is a complex mixture of enzymes that cause tissue injury
- Most insects sting only when attacked or when their space is invaded (exception is the yellow jacket)
- Major effects: acute severe pain, local inflammatory response, erythema, wheal, vesicle formation, itching
- Anaphylaxis occurs occasionally; urticaria, angioedema, bronchospasm, and shock within 15 minutes of envenomation; death is due to hypotension or asphyxiation
- Multiple stings may produce vomiting, diarrhea, hypotension, syncope, cyanosis, dyspnea, hemolysis, rhabdomyolysis, renal failure, disseminated intravascular coagulation, and death
- Stinger and venom sac may be left in the wound (honeybee) or remain intact so that the insect can sting again (bumblebee)

■ Differential Diagnosis

- Allergic reaction
- Multiple stings

■ Treatment

- Usually pain resolves spontaneously in a few hours
- May apply ice, corticosteroid cream, or antihistamine cream
- Inspect wound carefully for retained stingers, which may be removed by scraping with knife; wash wound with soap and water
- Tetanus prophylaxis if appropriate
- Monitor patient for 1 hour for signs of allergic reaction
- Treatment for anaphylaxis: epinephrine, nebulized β-agonists, intravenous fluids, diphenhydramine, and cimetidine

■ Pearl

More people die from insect bites and stings every year than from injuries caused by any other animal (including dogs, sharks, and snakes).

Reference

Curtis J: Insect sting anaphylaxis. Pediatr Rev 2000;21:256. [PMID: 10922021]

Black Widow Spider Bite

- **Essentials of Diagnosis**
  - Black widow spider (*Lactrodectus mactans*): shiny black spider with red hourglass marking on underside of its abdomen
  - Minute amount of potent venom is injected by hollow fangs long enough to puncture human skin
  - Venom is a neurotoxin that acts at the myoneural junction by releasing excess acetylcholine
  - Bite is often unnoticed at first; erythema or target lesion may be present
  - Effects: severe agonizing pain in bitten extremity, muscle spasm of abdomen and trunk (mimicking a surgical abdomen), muscle fasciculations, piloerection, diaphoresis, headache, dizziness, paresthesias, vomiting, ptosis, severe hypertension, tachycardia; occur within 1 hour
  - Death is rare; occurs in small infants and in the elderly with pre-existing cardiovascular disease
  - Consider blood glucose, CBC, electrolytes, calcium, CPK, electrocardiogram

- **Differential Diagnosis**
  - Acute surgical abdomen
  - Myocardial infarction
  - Peripheral arterial occlusion

- **Treatment**
  - Clean wound with soap and water
  - Apply intermittent ice packs to wound
  - Tetanus prophylaxis if needed
  - Monitor victim for 12 hours; most patients (especially children, elderly or pregnant patients, and those with severe hypertension) require hospitalization for pain control or observation
  - Opiate analgesics
  - For muscle spasms: calcium gluconate, 0.1–0.2 mg/kg slow IV, or methocarbamol, 1 g IV over 10 minutes
  - Equine-derived antivenin is rapidly effective but rarely required; consider it for infants or for seriously ill, elderly, or pregnant patients

- **Pearl**

Symptoms usually peak in 2–3 hours and then resolve in 48 hours.

Reference

Clark RF: The safety and efficacy of antivenin Lactrodectus mactans. J Toxicol Clin Toxicol 2001;39:125. [PMID: 11407497]

Brown Recluse Spider Bite

- **Essentials of Diagnosis**
  - Brown recluse spider (*Loxosceles reclusa*): dark violin-shaped marking on its back
  - Venom contains many digestive enzymes that are hemolytic and cytotoxic (causing local tissue destruction)
  - Bite often unnoticed at first; erythema or target lesion may be present
  - Pain occurs within 4 hours, and an erythematous area with vesicle may be seen; bull's-eye lesion with red blister and pale halo, surrounded by extravasated blood
  - In next 3–4 days, ulcer forms; lymphadenopathy, fever, malaise, arthralgias, and hemolysis (rarely)
  - Lesion may take weeks to heal; most wounds are minor and heal without any specific treatment
  - Death is rare; occurs in children with massive hemolysis, jaundice, hypotension, renal failure, and disseminated intravascular coagulation
  - Diagnosis usually difficult
  - CBC, BUN, creatinine, urinalysis (for free hemoglobin)

- **Differential Diagnosis**
  - Skin infection (bacterial, viral, or fungal)
  - Vasculitis
  - Insect bite
  - Retained foreign body

- **Treatment**
  - Clean wound with soap and water
  - Apply intermittent ice packs to wound
  - Tetanus prophylaxis if needed
  - Dapsone may be helpful if given within 36 hours; do not give to children because of adverse effects
  - Surgical excision, corticosteroids, and prophylactic antibiotics *not* recommended
  - Wounds may become infected and should be treated with antibiotics; it is difficult to discern wound infection from envenomation inflammation

- **Pearl**

Spiders tend to bite only once; insects may cause multiple nearby lesions.

Reference

Forks TP: Brown recluse spider bites. J Am Board Fam Pract 2000;13:415. [PMID: 11117338]

Cat Bite

- **Essentials of Diagnosis**
  - Bites cause deep puncture wounds with little crush injury; claw wounds are infection prone due to cats licking their claws
  - High risk of infection from many different bacteria and viruses (75% due to *Pasteurella multocida*)
  - Routine cultures should not be obtained
  - Extremity x-ray for presence of foreign body or subtle fracture

- **Differential Diagnosis**
  - Puncture wound
  - Dog bite
  - Human bite

- **Treatment**
  - Meticulous wound care is cornerstone of treatment and most important factor to prevent infection
  - Clean wound, debride necrotic tissue and foreign material, and irrigate copiously
  - Immobilize and elevate extremities
  - Tetanus and rabies prophylaxis as appropriate
  - Patients with significant bites: prophylactic antibiotics: amoxicillin/clavulanate, 875/125 mg orally twice each day for 3–5 days
  - Primary closure rarely required; should not be performed except in severe bites to the face
  - Close follow-up to monitor for infection
  - Infections within 24 hours are due to *Pasteurella;* infections occurring after 24 hours are due to streptococci or staphylococci
  - Patients with infections: cefazolin, 1 g IV, then discharge home with amoxicillin/clavulanate, 875/125 mg orally twice each day, or a first-generation cephalosporin for 7–10 days
  - Patients with severe infections or infections of the hand: may require hospitalization

- **Pearl**

Cat bites are more likely than dog bites to become infected.

Reference

Bower MG: Evaluating and managing bite wounds. Adv Skin Wound Care 2002;15:88. [PMID: 11984053]

Ciguatera Toxin Poisoning

- **Essentials of Diagnosis**
    - Caused by ingestion of coral reef fish whose tissues have accumulated toxins from the dinoflagellate *Gambierdiscus toxicus*
    - Most common fish responsible for this poisoning are the large carnivorous fish from endemic regions: barracuda, jack, snapper, and grouper
    - Effects: abdominal pain, vomiting, diarrhea, chills, pruritus, myalgias, fatigue, headache, hypotension, bradycardia; usually occur within 1 hour of ingestion (always within 12 hours)
    - Neurologic effects: paresthesias, dysphagia, athetosis, ataxia, vertigo, seizures, coma, central respiratory arrest
    - Most effects resolve in 24–48 hours; neurologic symptoms may last for weeks; fatality rate is 0.1–12%
    - No laboratory test for the toxin; clinical diagnosis only
    - Consider CBC, electrolytes, BUN, creatinine

- **Differential Diagnosis**
    - Gastroenteritis
    - Paralytic shellfish poisoning
    - Scombroid poisoning
    - Puffer fish poisoning

- **Treatment**
    - Intravenous crystalloid fluids
    - Activated charcoal, 1 g/kg, within 2 hours
    - Mannitol, 1 g/kg IV over 30 minutes; may reverse cardiac depression and severe neurologic symptoms
    - Patients with mild symptoms: monitor for respiratory failure for at least 6 hours
    - Patients with severe symptoms: hospital admission

- **Pearl**

The reversal of the sensation of hot and cold is pathognomonic of ciguatera poisoning.

Reference

Schnorf H, Taurarii M, Cundy T: Ciguatera fish poisoning: a double-blind randomized trial of mannitol therapy. Neurology 2002;58:873. [PMID: 11914401]

Decompression Sickness

- **■ Essentials of Diagnosis**
  - Caused by release of dissolved nitrogen as it bubbles from the body tissues when SCUBA divers ascend to the surface
  - Increased symptoms occur with deeper dives, longer dives, greater physical exertion by diver, and faster ascent
  - Minor symptom: deep, aching pain in the large joints of the extremities (the bends)
  - Major effects: ataxia, paralysis, vertigo, visual or speech disturbance, confusion, chest pain, shortness of breath
  - Untreated, decompression sickness may lead to shock, spinal cord injury, permanent impairment, bladder paralysis, and disseminated intravascular coagulation
  - Consider blood glucose, CBC, electrolytes, creatinine, BUN, chest x-ray, electrocardiogram, and head CT scan

- **■ Differential Diagnosis**
  - Trauma
  - Arterial gas embolism
  - Marine animal envenomation
  - Pneumothorax
  - Cerebrovascular accident
  - Pulmonary embolism

- **■ Treatment**
  - Only effective treatment for minor or major symptoms: immediate recompression
  - Rapid transport to nearest hyperbaric chamber (persistent symptoms may be treated up to 7 days after onset)
  - Oxygen by mask
  - Intravenous fluids for hydration
  - Analgesics during transport

- **■ Pearl**

Never attempt recompression by returning the patient to the water.

Reference

DeGorordo A et al: Diving emergencies. Resuscitation 2003;59:171. [PMID: 14625107]

Dog Bite

■ **Essentials of Diagnosis**

- Causes gaping open wound with necrotic tissue from crush injury
- Risk factors for infection: bites to the hand, puncture wounds, bites older than 6–12 hours
- Routine cultures should not be obtained
- Extremity x-ray for presence of foreign body or subtle fracture

■ **Differential Diagnosis**

- Nonbite wound
- Cat bite
- Human bite

■ **Treatment**

- Meticulous wound care is cornerstone of treatment and most important factor to prevent infection
- Clean wound, debride necrotic tissue and foreign material, and irrigate copiously
- Immobilize and elevate extremities
- Tetanus and rabies prophylaxis as appropriate
- Bites with infection risk factors: do not close after irrigation; prophylactic antibiotics recommended (amoxicillin/clavulanate, 875/125 mg orally twice each day for 3–5 days)
- Bites without infection risk factors: may be sutured; prophylactic antibiotics not required
- Close follow-up to monitor for infection
- Infections are caused from multiple organisms (20–30% due to *Pasteurella multocida*)
- Patients with infections: cefazolin, 1 g IV, then discharge home with amoxicillin/clavulanate, 875/125 mg orally twice each day
- Patients with severe infections or infections of the hand: may require hospitalization

■ **Pearl**

Dog bites account for 89% of all animal bites, 70% of animal-related emergency department visits, and over one-third of all deaths due to animal bites (more than cat bites, snakebites, or shark attacks).

Reference

Goldstein EJ: Current concepts on animal bites: bacteriology and therapy. Curr Clin Top Infect Dis 1999;19:99. [PMID: 10472482]

Electric Shock & Burns

- **Essentials of Diagnosis**
  - Type and amount of current, duration of shock, area of exposure, skin resistance, and pathway through body determine degree of damage
  - Alternating current (house current, 60 Hz) is more dangerous than direct current (battery)
  - Low-voltage current (<200 V) tends to cause minor skin damage but may cause ventricular fibrillation; high-voltage current (>1000 volts) causes severe tissue damage and respiratory arrest
  - Cardiac effects: ventricular fibrillation, sinus tachycardia, bradycardia, atrial fibrillation, asystole
  - Other effects: local pain, burns, seizures, deafness, blindness, aphasia, neuropathy, posterior shoulder dislocations, femoral neck fractures, myoglobinuria, muscular pain, fatigue, headache
  - Flash (arc), flame, or direct tissue burns are possible
  - Entry burn wounds are sharply demarcated, round, and painless; exit wounds are ragged and irregular; after 7 days, ischemia and severe tissue necrosis may become evident
  - Blood glucose, CBC, electrolytes, BUN, creatinine, CPK, electrocardiogram, urinalysis (myoglobinuria)

- **Differential Diagnosis**
  - Trauma, blunt or penetrating
  - Myocardial infarction
  - Pulmonary embolism
  - Seizure disorder

- **Treatment**
  - Monitor for arrhythmias
  - Treat arrhythmias with defibrillation, cardioversion, or antiarrhythmics
  - Intravenous crystalloid fluids for circulatory shock or severe burns
  - Locate entrance and exit wounds
  - Assess need for fasciotomy
  - Hospitalize patients with loss of consciousness, arrhythmias, ischemic chest pain, myoglobinuria, or significant burns

- **Pearl**

High-voltage shock may cause severe muscle damage that has an initial normal or minimal injury appearance.

Reference

Fish RM: Electric injuries, part II: specific injuries. J Emerg Med 2000;18:27. [PMID: 10645833]

Frostbite

- **Essentials of Diagnosis**
  - Injury of the tissues due to freezing; when skin temperature drops to below 25°F (–3.9°C)
  - Difficult to determine degree of frostbite because superficial and severe forms appear similar initially
  - Symptoms: numbness, paresthesias, lack of fine motor control; usually painless until thawing
  - Mild frostbite: white or blue-white, firm and cool to the touch, no sensation
  - Severe frostbite: blisters and swelling
  - Signs and symptoms upon thawing: tenderness, pain, clear blisters, hemorrhagic blisters, ecchymosis, necrosis, gangrene

- **Differential Diagnosis**
  - Trauma
  - Peripheral arterial ischemia
  - Chilblain
  - Immersion syndrome (trench foot)

- **Treatment**
  - Superficial frostbite: rewarming by gentle pressure with warm hand in warm environment
  - Full-thickness frostbite: rewarming by immersion in waterbath at 105°F (40.6°C) in a sterile environment until skin is soft and appears red-purple
  - Intravenous opiates during rewarming
  - Elevation of extremity, left at room temperature; debridement of clear ulcers
  - Apply aloe vera cream every 6 hours
  - Ibuprofen for 3 days
  - Prophylactic antibiotics for severe cases
  - Assess need for fasciotomy
  - Hospitalize patients with blisters or full-thickness frostbite

- **Pearl**

Tissue debridement or amputation should be delayed for days or weeks until tissues are clearly necrotic.

Reference

Murphy JV et al: Frostbite: pathogenesis and treatment. J Trauma 2000;48:171. [PMID: 10647591]

Heat Illness

■ Essentials of Diagnosis

- Risk factors: lack of acclimatization, excessive fatigue, infections, alcohol intoxication, anticholinergics, failure to maintain hydration or salt intake, advanced age, obesity
- Heat edema: swelling of feet and ankles of the elderly due to vasodilatation from prolonged sitting or standing
- Heat syncope: simple fainting from vasodilatation due to volume loss and prolonged standing; skin cool and moist, transient hypotension, core temperature normal
- Heat cramps: due to salt depletion; painful muscle spasms; temperature and serum electrolytes usually normal
- Heat exhaustion: due to sodium depletion and dehydration; core temperature elevated but <104°F (40°C); headache and dizziness, vomiting, muscle cramps, diaphoresis, tachycardia, hypotension, and hyponatremia; may progress to heat stroke
- Heat stroke: altered mental status and temperature >104°F (40°C); effects include those of heat exhaustion plus seizures, delirium, coma, hematuria, hepatic injury, myoglobinuria, thrombocytopenia, concentrated urine; skin usually dry
- Consider blood glucose, CBC, electrolytes, BUN, creatinine, liver enzymes, urinalysis, electrocardiogram, and head CT scan (for heat stroke)

■ Differential Diagnosis

- Viral illness
- Congestive heart failure
- Intracranial lesion
- Hypoglycemia

■ Treatment

- Heat edema: elevation of feet; no diuretics
- Heat syncope: rest; cool place; oral rehydration
- Heat cramps and heat exhaustion: cool place; oral or intravenous salt and fluid replacement; replace glucose and potassium if needed; rest for several days
- Heat stroke: rapidly cool by spraying with water and fanning, cooling blanket; intravenous hydration; monitor urinary output; for myoglobinuria treat with bicarbonate; and hospitalize

■ Pearl

With aggressive treatment, patients with temperatures of 114°F (45.6°C) may recover fully.

Reference

Khosla R, Guntupalli KK: Heat-related illnesses. Crit Care Clin 1999;15:251. [PMID: 10331127]

High-Altitude Cerebral Edema

- **Essentials of Diagnosis**
  - Syndrome related to hypoxemia caused by rapid exposure to altitudes greater than 8,000 feet without acclimatization; usually occurs in people who live at low altitudes who travel to mountain regions
  - Increased physical activity and preexisting disease conditions account for varying degrees of symptoms
  - Early effects: severe headache, ataxia, confusion, incoordination, inability to walk a straight line
  - Later effects: papilledema, retinal hemorrhages, cranial nerve palsy, encephalopathy
  - Death usually due to brain-stem herniation
  - Patients frequently also have high-altitude pulmonary edema
  - Seizures uncommon
  - Blood glucose, CBC, electrolytes, BUN, creatinine, chest x-ray, head CT scan

- **Differential Diagnosis**
  - Acute mountain sickness
  - Tension headache
  - Meningitis
  - Intracranial lesion
  - Drug or alcohol intoxication

- **Treatment**
  - Most effective treatment: descent to lower altitude (5,000 feet)
  - Oxygen by mask; keep patient sitting with head elevated
  - Dexamethasone, 8 mg orally or IM, then 4–6 mg every 6 hours
  - Nifedipine for high-altitude pulmonary edema contraindicated in patients with high-altitude cerebral edema

- **Pearl**

All patients with early acute mountain sickness must be monitored for ataxia, which is an early sign of high-altitude cerebral edema.

Reference

Yarnell PR, Heit J, Hackett PH: High-altitude cerebral edema (HACE): the Denver/Front Range experience. Semin Neurol 2000;20:209. [PMID: 10946741]

High-Altitude Pulmonary Edema

- **Essentials of Diagnosis**
  - Noncardiogenic pulmonary edema caused by rapid exposure to altitudes greater than 8,000 feet without acclimatization
  - Usually occurs in healthy visitors who live at low altitudes who exercise in mountain regions without being acclimatized
  - 60% risk of recurrence
  - Risk factors: congenital absence of one pulmonary artery, valvular disorder, cardiac shunt, pulmonary hypertension
  - Early symptoms (second night at new altitude): dry cough and dyspnea on exertion
  - Later effects: productive cough, pink sputum, dyspnea at rest, weakness, drowsiness, tachycardia, tachypnea, cyanosis, rales, rhonchi, confusion, death
  - Chest x-ray first shows unilateral patchy infiltrates (usually right middle lobe), then later shows bilateral infiltrates with normal heart size and no Kerley lines
  - CBC, electrolytes, BUN, creatinine, electrocardiogram, chest x-ray

- **Differential Diagnosis**
  - Viral illness
  - Pneumonia
  - Congestive heart failure
  - Pulmonary embolism
  - Early acute mountain sickness

- **Treatment**
  - Most effective treatment: descent to lower altitude (below 5,000 feet); oxygen and lower altitude should provide marked improvement in 12–72 hours
  - Oxygen by mask; continuous positive-pressure ventilation relieves symptoms during descent
  - Limited physical activity; may not be able to lie flat
  - Acetazolamide, 250 mg orally every 6 hours, may be useful
  - Nifedipine, 10 mg orally, then 30 mg every 12–24 hours (do not give if patient also has high-altitude cerebral edema)
  - Hospitalization required if symptoms persist for more than a few hours at lower altitude

- **Pearl**

Dry cough and dyspnea in a nonacclimatized person should be considered high-altitude pulmonary edema until proved otherwise.

Reference

Hacken PH, Roach RC: High altitude illness. N Engl J Med 2001;345:107. [PMID: 11450659]

Hydrofluoric Acid Exposure

- ■ Essentials of Diagnosis
  - Hydrofluoric acid is used widely as rust remover, in glass etching, and in semiconductor manufacturing
  - Weak acid that causes severe skin injury (cytotoxic effects of fluoride ion) and severe systemic effects (precipitation of calcium and magnesium)
  - Low concentrations (5–15%) found in household products may cause no initial pain, no initial clinical findings; may cause severe delayed effects after 12–24 hours
  - Intermediate concentrations (20–40%) produce moderate initial pain, slight erythema; may cause severe effects after 1–8 hours
  - High concentrations (50–79%) produce immediate pain, progressive erythema, skin blanching, and increasingly severe pain
  - Systemic hypocalcemia due to small burn (2.5% of total body surface area) with highly concentrated acid or large area of intermediate concentration; vomiting, abdominal pain, seizures, hypotension, arrhythmias, and ventricular fibrillation may occur
  - Electrolytes, magnesium, calcium, BUN, creatinine, electrocardiogram

- ■ Differential Diagnosis
  - Other chemical burns
  - Hypocalcemia

- ■ Treatment
  - Immediately flush burn with copious amount of water
  - Apply gel of calcium gluconate or calcium carbonate tablets in K-Y jelly
  - For hand burns, gel can be placed in a rubber glove that is then placed on the hand
  - If pain is not significantly improved in 1 hour, consider subcutaneous injection
  - Subcutaneous injection of 5–10% calcium gluconate in affected areas (do not use calcium chloride)
  - Intra-arterial injection of calcium for severe burns
  - Opiates may be used; use pain as monitor for calcium effectiveness

- ■ Pearl

Suspect hydrogen fluoride burn when the pain is much more severe than expected based on the appearance of the burn.

Reference

Blodgett DW, Suruda AJ, Crouch BI: Fatal unintentional occupational poisonings by hydrofluoric acid in the US. Am J Ind Med 2001;40:215. [PMID: 11494350]

Immersion Syndrome (Trench Foot)

- **Essentials of Diagnosis**
  - Caused by prolonged immersion in cool or cold water (<60°F [15.6°C]) causing ischemia
  - Initially foot becomes cold, anesthetic, and pulseless
  - Upon rewarming, intense burning, pain, swelling, blistering, redness, ecchymosis, and ulceration result
  - After several weeks, extremity may become cyanotic with increased sensitivity to cold
  - Complications: lymphangitis, cellulitis, thrombophlebitis, gangrene

- **Differential Diagnosis**
  - Trauma
  - Peripheral arterial ischemia
  - Athlete's foot
  - Chilblain
  - Frostbite
  - Cellulitis

- **Treatment**
  - Rewarm extremity gradually by exposing it to warm air
  - Do not massage or soak extremity or apply ice or heat
  - Elevate extremity
  - Treat infection with antibiotics
  - Hospitalization

- **Pearl**

Trench foot was first described in Napoleon's troops in Russia, but the name comes from World War I; it remains a common problem in the military today.

Reference

Ungley CC, Channell GD, Richards RL: The immersion foot syndrome 1946. Wilderness Environ Med 2003;14:135. [PMID: 12825888]

Jellyfish Envenomation

- **Essentials of Diagnosis**
  - Jellyfish use long tentacles with stinging cells called nematocysts to envenomate swimmers
  - Most jellyfish produce only skin reaction of immediate intense pain and local inflammation, paresthesias, pruritus, erythema
  - Portuguese Man-o-War (around North America): sting very painful, nausea, vomiting, muscle cramps; rare deaths
  - Box jellyfish (around Australia): severe incapacitating localized pain with wide erythematous bands; confusion, loss of consciousness, respiratory failure, and cardiac arrest can occur within 5 minutes
  - Irukandji jellyfish (around Australia): sting not felt; severe sacral pain, diaphoresis, headache, nausea, severe hypertension, tachycardia, and pulmonary edema develop 30 minutes later; rare deaths

- **Differential Diagnosis**
  - Scorpion fish envenomation
  - Sea urchin envenomation
  - Stingray envenomation

- **Treatment**
  - Spray or soak affected area with vinegar for 30 minutes to disarm the intact nematocysts; will not relieve pain
  - Effects usually self-limiting; apply cold packs
  - Portuguese Man-o-War: rinse with sea water (not fresh water); intravenous analgesia, supportive care
  - Box jellyfish: compression bandages, antivenom
  - Irukandji jellyfish: intravenous analgesia, control of hypertension, supportive care
  - Monitor patient for 6–8 hours

- **Pearl**

Do not touch affected area and do not wash with fresh water; this can cause intact nematocysts to discharge venom.

Reference

Fenner PJ: Dangers in the ocean: the traveler and marine envenomation. I. jellyfish. J Travel Med 1998;5:135. [PMID: 9772332]

Lightning Injury

- **Essentials of Diagnosis**
  - Lightning attains over 100 million volts and a temperature of 3,000°C (5,432°F); kills over 200 people each year
  - Lightning can strike victims directly, indirectly (splash) from nearby objects, and by step voltage (ground current conducted up through the victim's legs)
  - Burns may be superficial due to "flash over," first or second degree in a branched pattern, starburst pattern, or burns from clothing or metal jewelry; specific skin condition called "feathering" (superficial fern-like pattern)
  - Effects: amnesia, deafness, disorientation, combativeness, loss of consciousness, seizures, coma, paraplegia, respiratory and cardiac arrest
  - Injuries: intracranial hemorrhage, trauma from being thrown or from falls, orthopedic injuries from seizures, myocardial infarction, eye injuries, ruptured tympanic membrane
  - Blood glucose, CBC, electrolytes, BUN, creatinine, CPK, electrocardiogram, urinalysis (myoglobinuria), chest and spine x-rays, head CT scan

- **Differential Diagnosis**
  - Trauma, blunt or penetrating
  - Myocardial infarction or cerebrovascular accident
  - Seizure disorder

- **Treatment**
  - Support respirations and cardiac function
  - Immobilize spine
  - Monitor for arrhythmias and treat with defibrillation, cardioversion, or antiarrhythmics
  - Intravenous crystalloid fluids for circulatory shock or severe burns
  - Locate entrance and exit wounds
  - Assess need for fasciotomy
  - Hospitalization for patients who lose consciousness or who have arrhythmias, myoglobinuria, or significant injuries or burns

- **Pearl**

Lightning victims with cardiopulmonary arrest have been resuscitated after prolonged efforts.

Reference

Fish RM: Electric injuries, part III: cardiac monitoring indications, the pregnant patient, and lightning. J Emerg Med 2000;18:181. [PMID: 10699519]

Near Drowning

- ■ Essentials of Diagnosis
  - Upon submersion, the victim rapidly (over 5–10 minutes) becomes hypoxemic, has laryngospasm, aspirates water into airway and lungs, develops brain injury, and dies
  - Both fresh water and seawater cause pulmonary damage
  - Near drowning victims may quickly regain consciousness when submersion is brief; others respond to artificial ventilation
  - Near drowning causes vomiting (common), loss of consciousness, confusion, cyanosis, trismus, apnea, tachypnea, wheezing, pulmonary edema, metabolic acidosis, tachycardia, arrhythmias, hypotension, anoxic encephalopathy, and cardiac arrest
  - CBC, electrolytes, BUN, creatinine, urinalysis, arterial blood gases, liver enzymes, chest x-ray, pregnancy test, electrocardiogram

- ■ Differential Diagnosis
  - Simple water aspiration
  - Pneumonia
  - Myocardial infarction
  - Head or spinal trauma
  - Venomous animal stings or bites
  - Alcohol or drugs

- ■ Treatment
  - Begin cardiopulmonary resuscitation immediately as required
  - Do not attempt to drain water from victim's lungs
  - Endotracheal intubation as needed
  - Treat hypothermia (hypothermia improves the chances of survival)
  - Monitor patient for 6–12 hours for decline in respiratory function (so-called secondary drowning)

- ■ Pearl

About 10% of near drowning victims have dry drowning and do not aspirate water because of severe laryngospasm after the first gulp.

Reference

Causey AL: Predicting discharge in uncomplicated near-drowning. Am J Emerg Med 2000;18:9. [PMID: 10674523]

Paralytic Shellfish Poisoning

■ Essentials of Diagnosis

- Caused by ingestion of shellfish whose tissues have accumulated saxitoxin from the dinoflagellates *Protogonyaulax* and *Ptychodiscus*
- Most common shellfish responsible for this poisoning: clams, oysters, scallops, mussels
- Shellfish appear and smell normal
- Saxitoxin blocks neuromuscular transmission; lethal dose is 0.1 mg
- Effects: perioral paresthesias, dizziness, incoordination, weakness, incoherence, vomiting, diarrhea, headache, loss of vision, tachycardia, flaccid paralysis, respiratory arrest; usually occur within 1 hour of ingestion
- Fatality rate: 25% within 12 hours
- No laboratory test for the toxin; clinical diagnosis only
- CBC, electrolytes, BUN, creatinine

■ Differential Diagnosis

- Gastroenteritis
- Guillain-Barré syndrome
- Ciguatera poisoning
- Scombroid poisoning
- Puffer fish poisoning

■ Treatment

- Intravenous crystalloid fluids
- Activated charcoal, 1 g/kg, within 2 hours
- Endotracheal intubation and respiratory support
- Patients with mild symptoms: monitoring for respiratory failure for at least 6 hours
- Patients with severe symptoms: hospital admission

■ Pearl

The patient will remain awake and alert but paralyzed.

Reference

Lehane L: Paralytic shellfish poisoning: a potential public health problem. Med J Aust 2001;175:25. [PMID: 11476199]

Puffer Fish (Tetrodotoxin) Poisoning

- ■ Essentials of Diagnosis
  - Caused by ingestion of puffer fish (toadfish, blowfish, balloon fish, porcupine fish) whose tissues have accumulated tetrodotoxin from microbial flora
  - Tetrodotoxin is distributed throughout the fish and is very difficult to remove
  - Tetrodotoxin is a potent toxin that blocks the sodium channel of the nerve cell membrane, causing respiratory depression, intracardiac conduction delays, and skeletal muscle paralysis
  - Effects: paresthesias, hypersalivation, diaphoresis, lethargy, headache, vomiting, ataxia, tremor, paralysis, bradycardia, hypotension, coma, respiratory failure; usually occur within 30 minutes of ingestion, always within 5 hours
  - Most effects resolve in 24–48 hours; fatality rate is 60%, and most die within 6 hours
  - No laboratory test for the toxin; clinical diagnosis only
  - CBC, electrolytes, BUN, creatinine, electrocardiogram

- ■ Differential Diagnosis
  - Gastroenteritis
  - Paralytic shellfish
  - Ciguatera poisoning
  - Guillain-Barré syndrome

- ■ Treatment
  - Intravenous crystalloid fluids
  - Activated charcoal, 1 g/kg, within 2 hours
  - Endotracheal intubation and respiratory support
  - Patients with mild symptoms: monitoring for respiratory failure for at least 8 hours
  - Patients with severe symptoms: hospital admission

- ■ Pearl

Puffer fish ("fugu") are prepared as delicacies in Japan by licensed chefs.

Reference

Field J: Puffer fish poisoning. J Accid Emerg Med 1998;15:334. [PMID: 9785165]

Rabies

- **Essentials of Diagnosis**

  - Caused by an RNA virus and transmitted in saliva; incubation period averages 1–2 months
  - Animals most likely to transmit rabies include carnivorous wild mammals (skunks, bats, raccoons, foxes, coyotes, bobcats)
  - Domesticated cats and dogs less likely to transmit rabies; rabbits, squirrels, hamsters, gerbils, rats, and mice rarely transmit the disease
  - Any penetration of the skin by teeth or any animal saliva on open wound or mucous membrane may transmit rabies
  - Increased risk of animal being infected: unprovoked bite, non-immunized cat or dog, bite in an endemic geographical area
  - Determine if animal is infected; wild mammals should be killed and their brains sent to state laboratory for examination

- **Differential Diagnosis**

  - Nonbite wound
  - Bite from animal with extremely low risk of transmission

- **Treatment**

  - Standard animal bite wound care
  - Rabies immunization not needed for low risk of rabies transmission such as immunized animal, rodent bite, area devoid of rabies, or provoked attack
  - Pet dog or cat bite: observe animal for 10 days; no rabies prophylaxis unless animal becomes ill
  - Wild mammal bite: postexposure immunization recommended
  - Administer rabies immune globulin (RIG) and human diploid cell vaccine (HDCV) as soon as possible; must be within 8 days of bite
  - RIG, 20 IU/kg with one-half of the dose infiltrated in and around the bite and remainder injected intramuscularly at distant site
  - HDCV, 1 ml IM on days 0, 3, 7, 14, and 28 postbite

- **Pearl**

  Rabies is difficult to diagnose, and no effective treatment exists.

Reference

Hemachudha T, Laothamatas J, Rupprecht CE: Human rabies: a disease of complex neuropathogenetic mechanisms and diagnostic challenges. Lancet Neurol 2002;1:101. [PMID: 12849514]

Radiation Injury

- **Essentials of Diagnosis**
    - Amount of injury depends on quantity of radiation, type of radiation, site of exposure, and duration
    - Doses of 400–600 rads will be fatal to most people within 60 days due to hemorrhage, anemia, and infection; 1,000–6,000 rads is always fatal within 2 weeks due to gastrointestinal mucosa and bone marrow destruction; over 3,000 rads will cause death within a few days
    - Radiation causes erythema, skin burns, leukopenia (lymphocytes are most sensitive), anemia, bone marrow depression, pericarditis, sterility, fetal death, pneumonitis, diarrhea, and hepatitis
    - Initial symptom is vomiting followed by latent period; next bone marrow depression and bloody diarrhea; finally, seizures, coma, and death
    - CBC (lymphocyte count indicates amount of radiation), electrolytes, liver enzymes, chest x-ray, pregnancy test, electrocardiogram

- **Differential Diagnosis**
    - Gastroenteritis
    - Cancer
    - Chemical toxin

- **Treatment**
    - Decontaminate patient by removing clothing and washing skin and hair with water
    - If exposed to radioactive iodine, within 1 hour give potassium iodide, 130 mg orally every day for 5 days
    - No specific antidotes; treat symptoms
    - Massive intravenous fluid resuscitation may be needed
    - Consider bone marrow transplantation if patient received more than 300 rads

- **Pearl**

Call REACTS (Radiation Emergency Assistance Center Training Site) at 865-481-1000 for advice regarding specific patients.

Reference

Goans RE et al: Early dose assessment in criticality accidents. Health Phys 2001;81:446. [PMID: 11569639]

Scombroid Poisoning

- **■ Essentials of Diagnosis**
  - Pseudoallergic syndrome caused by ingestion of improperly refrigerated dark-fleshed fish
  - These fish contain bacteria (*Vibrio*) that degrade histidine in muscle causing an increase in histamine; cooking does not prevent the toxic effects of histamine
  - Most common fish responsible for this poisoning: albacore, tuna, mackerel, kingfish, mahi-mahi, bonita, sardine, anchovy, and amberjack
  - Effects: flushing, sensation of warmth, urticaria, pruritus, angioedema, abdominal cramps, vomiting, diarrhea, headache, thirst, tachycardia, palpitations, bronchospasm, and hypotension; usually occur within 1 hour of ingestion
  - Most effects resolve in 12 hours; neurologic symptoms may last for weeks; fatality rate is 0.1–12%
  - No laboratory test for the toxin; clinical diagnosis only
  - CBC, electrolytes, BUN, creatinine

- **■ Differential Diagnosis**
  - Gastroenteritis, viral or bacterial
  - Anaphylaxis
  - Allergic reaction
  - Ciguatera poisoning
  - Puffer fish poisoning

- **■ Treatment**
  - Intravenous crystalloid fluids
  - Activated charcoal, 1 g/kg, within 2 hours
  - Diphenhydramine, cimetidine, nebulized bronchodilators
  - Antiemetics
  - Patients with severe symptoms: hospital admission

- **■ Pearl**

Fish with increased histamine may have a peppery taste.

Reference

Centers for Disease Control and Prevention. Scombroid fish poisoning—Pennsylvania 1998. JAMA 2000;283:2927. [PMID: 10896527]

Scorpion Sting

- **Essentials of Diagnosis**
    - Most scorpions are relatively harmless; these arthropods inject venom with a stinger at the end of their flexible abdomens (resembling a tail); usually produces only local skin reactions
    - Bark scorpion, *Centruroides exilicauda,* is only species in the United States (lives in southwestern states) that produces severe systemic envenomations, usually in small children
    - Venom contains numerous digestive enzymes and neurotoxins
    - Initial sting is painful; usually resolves in 4 hours
    - Bark scorpion stings cause systemic effects within 1 hour: restlessness, jerking movements, nystagmus, diaphoresis, diplopia, incontinence, confusion, seizures, hypertension, hypersalivation, wheezing, respiratory arrest (only in small children)

- **Differential Diagnosis**
    - Venomous snakebite
    - Brown recluse spider bite
    - Bee or wasp sting

- **Treatment**
    - Wash wound with soap and water
    - Tetanus immunization if needed
    - Periodic application of cold packs
    - Immobilize affected extremity
    - For bark scorpion stings causing systemic symptoms: benzodiazepines, atropine (for secretions), monitor for respiratory support, consider antivenom available in Arizona

- **Pearl**

A positive "tap test" (lightly tapping on sting site causes severe pain) indicates a sting from a bark scorpion.

Reference

Suchard JR, Hilder R: Atropine use in Centruroides scorpion envenomation. J Toxicol Clin Toxicol 2001;39:595. [PMID: 11762667]

Sea Snake Envenomation

■ Essentials of Diagnosis

- Family Hydrophiidae; live in all oceans except the Atlantic
- Not aggressive; will bite only when provoked; seldom inject much venom into humans
- Bite usually initially painless, then rapid paralysis, ptosis, ophthalmoplegia, myolysis, and respiratory failure result
- CBC, urinalysis (myoglobin), CPK, BUN, creatinine

■ Differential Diagnosis

- Scorpion fish envenomation
- Jellyfish envenomation
- Sea urchin envenomation

■ Treatment

- Monitor respiratory status and support if necessary
- Sea snake antivenom (or Tiger snake antivenom) for paralysis or myolysis
- Effects should be evident within 6 hours of bite

■ Pearl

Sea snake envenomation does not cause tissue necrosis and rarely causes significant neurologic effects.

Reference

Nimorakiotakis B, Winkle KD: Marine envenomations. Part 2—other marine envenomations. Aust Fam Physician 2003;32:975. [PMID: 14708143]

Smoke Inhalation

- ■ Essentials of Diagnosis
  - • Caused by inhalation of smoke from a burning fire; smoke may cause thermal damage to airway, chemical injury to airway, or systemic chemical injury
  - • Thermal damage to airway usually occurs when victims are trapped in enclosed space breathing hot gases; may have burns to face and neck
  - • Thermal damage to airway causes dysphagia, dyspnea, stridor, drooling; diagnosis made by laryngoscopy
  - • Chemical injury to airway due to toxins produced by combustion such as acrolein, hydrochloric acid, toluene diisocyanate, and nitrogen dioxide
  - • Chemical injury is difficult to diagnose initially; patients may present with wheezing, hypoxia, dyspnea; noncardiogenic pulmonary edema may develop after several hours
  - • Systemic chemical injury caused by carbon monoxide or cyanide commonly produced by fires
  - • Carboxyhemoglobin level, chest x-ray, arterial blood gas, CBC, pregnancy test, electrocardiogram

- ■ Differential Diagnosis
  - • Carbon monoxide poisoning
  - • Cyanide inhalation
  - • Methemoglobinemia
  - • Irritant gas inhalation

- ■ Treatment
  - • Immediate administration of high-flow oxygen by nonrebreathing face mask or endotracheal tube
  - • Treatment of significant carbon monoxide poisoning with hyperbaric oxygen chamber
  - • Inhaled bronchodilators for bronchospasm
  - • Do not administer systemic corticosteroids or antibiotics prophylactically
  - • Continuation of oxygen administration until carboxyhemoglobin level returns to normal

- ■ Pearl

Empiric therapy for cyanide poisoning by inducing methemoglobinemia in a smoke inhalation patient with carbon monoxide intoxication is not recommended.

Reference

Lee-Chiong TL Jr: Smoke inhalation injury. Postgrad Med 1999;105:55. [PMID: 10026703]

Snakebite

■ Essentials of Diagnosis

- Two types of venomous snakes in the United States: pit vipers (rattlesnakes, cottonmouths, copperheads) and coral snakes
- 95% of venomous snakebites are from pit vipers; 20% of these do not involve envenomation (so-called dry bites)
- Pit viper venom contains cytotoxic and hemotoxic enzymes; coral snake venom contains neurotoxic enzymes
- Pit viper envenomation causes immediate pain; over the next few hours, severe swelling, bleeding from puncture site, ecchymosis, and increased pain result; systemic effects include vomiting, paresthesias, dizziness, fasciculations, hemolysis, severe thrombocytopenia, and hypotension
- Coral snake bites produce minimal early signs but systemic effects occur over 6 hours: paresthesias, blurred vision, dysphagia, ptosis, respiratory depression
- CBC, electrolytes, creatinine, BUN, blood type, international normalized ratio, fibrin split products, urinalysis

■ Differential Diagnosis

- Scorpion sting
- Brown recluse spider bite
- Bee or wasp sting

■ Treatment

- Transport patient to hospital with extremity immobilized and patient at rest (do not apply tourniquet, incise wound, suck out venom, or pack in ice)
- Wash wound with soap and water; tetanus immunization if needed
- Assess extremity for progression of signs of envenomation
- Antivenom indicated for progression of pit viper envenomation signs; CroFab antivenom, 4–6 vials IV over 1 hour, may repeat if no improvement
- Surgical treatment not needed in acute management; increased compartment pressure may need fasciotomy
- Antivenom indicated for suspected Eastern or Texas coral snake bites; coral snake antivenom, 3–6 vials IV; monitor for respiratory depression

■ Pearl

Contrary to popular belief, pit viper envenomations are rarely life threatening.

Reference

Dart RC et al: Efficacy, safety, and use of snake antivenoms in the United States. Ann Emerg Med 2001;37:181. [PMID: 11174237]

Stingray Envenomation

■ **Essentials of Diagnosis**

- Most common fish responsible for envenomations
- When disturbed, stingrays strike with tail that contains 1–4 venomous stingers
- Most common injury locations are on legs and arms
- Injuries composed of trauma (from tail strike) and envenomation
- Effects include immediate, severe pain (may be incapacitating), swelling and bleeding; vomiting, weakness, diaphoresis, vertigo, tachycardia, muscle cramps, syncope, paralysis, hypotension, arrhythmias, and cardiac arrest occur within 30 minutes
- Extremity x-ray for presence of foreign body or fracture

■ **Differential Diagnosis**

- Scorpion fish envenomation
- Sea urchin envenomation
- Jellyfish envenomation

■ **Treatment**

- Irrigate wound with fresh water (preferably sterile)
- Remove foreign matter
- Soak wound in hot water (120°F [48.9°C]) for 30–60 minutes to denature venom (do not apply ice)
- Local anesthetic if necessary
- Do not suture wound
- Tetanus immunization if needed
- Prophylactic antibiotics: trimethoprim-sulfamethoxazole, ciprofloxacin, or tetracycline
- Monitor wound for several weeks; may require surgical debridement or intravenous antibiotics

■ **Pearl**

Treat stingray and scorpion fish envenomations with hot water, but treat jellyfish envenomations with cold packs.

Reference

Nimorakiotakis B, Winkle KD: Marine envenomations. Part 2—other marine envenomations. Aust Fam Physician 2003;32:975. [PMID: 14708143]

Tetanus

■ Essentials of Diagnosis

- Frequently fatal illness from the acute infection of a wound by *Clostridium tetani;* incubation period is 1–30 days
- Tetanus-prone wounds are crush wounds, wounds heavily contaminated with soil or feces, puncture wounds, and wounds of individuals who delay medical attention more than 24 hours
- Effects: muscle rigidity, violent muscle contractions, autonomic dysfunction, jaw pain, cranial nerve dysfunction
- Tetanus immunization requires three primary toxoid doses and a booster every 10 years, 5 years if wound is not clean and minor
- Most adults and older children in the United States had primary series of immunization; those over age 50 years, foreign-born, or unable to give immunization history are at risk for not having received the primary series

■ Differential Diagnosis

- Strychnine poisoning
- Neuroleptic malignant syndrome
- Meningitis
- Rabies

■ Treatment

- Usually requires respiratory support, analgesia, tetanus immune globulin (TIG), 3,000–5,000 U IM, and penicillin G, 10 million U IV every 24 hours
- Standard wound care to help prevent other infections
- Tetanus-diphtheria toxoid (Td) and TIG as necessary
- Td, 0.5 cc IM: for those without history of primary series of three injections; for those whose immunization history is uncertain; if wound is clear and minor and last booster was more than 10 years ago; or if wound is not clean and minor and last booster was more than 5 years ago
- TIG, 250 units IM: for those without a history of primary series of three injections and a tetanus-prone wound

■ Pearl

Tetanus frequently begins with pain and stiffness in the jaw.

Reference

Hsu SS, Groleau G: Tetanus in the emergency department: a current review. J Emerg Med 2001;20:357. [PMID: 11348815]

Thermal Burns

■ **Essentials of Diagnosis**

- Burns described as first, second, third, and fourth degree; also classified as partial-thickness or full-thickness (requires skin graft); sometimes difficult to determine depth of burn on initial presentation
- Location of burn determines complications; face (consider smoke inhalation), hands and feet (scarring may produce permanent disability), perineum (susceptible to infection), circumferential burn (may cause obstruction of airway, blood flow, or respirations)
- CBC, carboxyhemoglobin level, electrolytes, BUN, creatinine, urinalysis, blood type, chest x-ray, electrocardiogram

■ **Differential Diagnosis**

- Chemical burn
- Smoke inhalation
- Associated trauma

■ **Treatment**

- Minor burns (second degree <15% total body surface area [TBSA]): tetanus immunization if needed, immerse in cool water, give analgesics, irrigate burn with sterile saline, apply topical antibiotic, elevate extremity (prophylactic antibiotics not indicated)
- Moderate or major burn: crystalloid, 2 ml/kg/% burn IV over 8 hours; adjust intravenous fluids to maintain urine output of 1 ml/kg/hr; analgesia; keep burns sterile
- Patients with major burns and burns in complicated areas: transfer to a burn center

■ **Pearl**

To estimate the percentage of TBSA for smaller burns, use the patient's hand as a guide (1.25% TBSA).

Reference

Sheridian RL: Comprehensive treatment of burns. Curr Probl Surg 2001;38:657. [PMID: 11568825]

27

Poisoning

Acetaminophen

- ■ Essentials of Diagnosis
    - • Found in widely used over-the-counter medications
    - • Acetaminophen (alone or with aspirin) is most common overdose substance in adults; most common cause of fatalities reported to poison centers
    - • Toxic dose: 150–200 mg/kg in children or 6–7 g in adults within a 24-hour period
    - • For acute ingestion, use serum acetaminophen level and the Rumack-Matthew nomogram (4–24 hours postingestion) to determine probability of hepatic toxicity; nomogram may not be accurate for chronic overdose, extended release acetaminophen forms, or overdose involving more than one ingestant
    - • Patients usually asymptomatic for first 24 hours or may have nausea or vomiting
    - • Hepatic injury not seen until 24–48 hours after ingestion

- ■ Differential Diagnosis
    - • Other hepatotoxins
    - • Viral hepatitis

- ■ Treatment
    - • Activated charcoal, 1 g/kg, within 1–2 hours of ingestion
    - • For serum acetaminophen level >140 μg/mL at 4 hours after ingestion or 70 μg/mL at 8 hours after ingestion, begin antidotal treatment with N-acetylcysteine (NAC; Mucomyst): loading dose of NAC at 140 mg/kg orally, then 17 doses of 70 mg/kg every 4 hours
    - • NAC has maximum benefit if given within 8 hours of ingestion
    - • For vomiting, metoclopramide IV, ondansetron IV, or consider giving NAC intravenously

- ■ Pearl

Determine the serum acetaminophen level in all cases of intentional medication overdoses because acetaminophen is widely available and the antidote is very effective when given early.

Reference

Lane JE et al: Chronic acetaminophen toxicity: a case report and review of the Literature. J Emerg Med 2002;23:253. [PMID: 12426016]

Amphetamines & Other Related Stimulants

- ■ Essentials of Diagnosis
  - CNS stimulants that cause sympathetic hyperactivity
  - Include methamphetamine (crank, speed), dextroamphetamine (Dexedrine), methylphenidate (Ritalin), methylenedioxymethamphetamine (MDMA, ecstasy), ephedrine, phenylpropanolamine (PPA), and cocaine (discussed elsewhere in this chapter)
  - Rapid onset of action and short half-life when taken orally or intravenously or when smoked
  - Toxic dose causes euphoria, anxiety, mydriasis, restlessness, sweating, hypertension, tachycardia, hyperthermia, psychosis, seizures, and tachyarrhythmias
  - May cause rhabdomyolysis, myoglobinuria, myocardial infarction, and intracranial hemorrhage
  - Consider serum glucose, electrolytes, BUN, creatinine, CPK, urinalysis, electrocardiogram, and head CT scan
  - Most urine drug screens assess presence of amphetamines; false positives and false negatives possible

- ■ Differential Diagnosis
  - Other sympathomimetics (cocaine, caffeine, PPA)
  - Anticholinergic toxicity (antihistamines, tricyclic antidepressants, atropine)
  - Hallucinogenics (phencyclidine, LSD)
  - Sepsis
  - Sedative-hypnotic withdrawal

- ■ Treatment
  - Activated charcoal, 1 g/kg, within 1–2 hours of ingestion
  - Hyperthermia (>104°F [40°C]) may be lethal; rapid cooling with room-temperature intravenous fluids and removal of clothing, along with evaporative cooling with tepid water and fanning
  - For agitation, seizures, hypertension: benzodiazepines
  - For severe hypertension: nitroprusside or phentolamine
  - For tachyarrhythmias: propranolol or esmolol
  - Dialysis and urine acidification not recommended

- ■ Pearl

Sweating may be used to differentiate anticholinergic and sympathomimetic toxicity.

Reference

Albertson TE et al: Methamphetamine and the expanding complications of amphetamines. West J Med 1999;170:214. [PMID: 10344175]

Anticholinergics

- **Essentials of Diagnosis**
    - Block both central and peripheral cholinergic receptors
    - Include atropine, scopolamine, belladonna, antihistamines, tricyclic antidepressants, antipsychotics, skeletal muscle relaxants, jimsonweed, nightshade, some mushrooms, and many combination medications
    - Toxic dose causes flushed dry skin, dry mouth, mydriasis, restlessness, tachycardia, hyperthermia, ileus, urinary retention, rhabdomyolysis, delirium, hallucinations, psychosis, seizures, coma, and respiratory arrest
    - Consider serum glucose, electrolytes, BUN, creatinine, CPK, urinalysis, electrocardiogram, and head CT scan
    - Most urine drug screens do not assess the presence of most anticholinergics

- **Differential Diagnosis**
    - Sympathomimetics (amphetamines, MDMA, cocaine, phenylpropanolamine)
    - Hallucinogenics (phencyclidine, LSD)
    - Sepsis
    - Sedative-hypnotic withdrawal

- **Treatment**
    - Activated charcoal, 1 g/kg, within 2–4 hours of ingestion (delayed gastrointestinal absorption); no other specific treatment for most patients
    - Intravenous fluids and urinary catheter
    - Hyperthermia (>104°F [40°C]) may be lethal; rapid cooling with room-temperature intravenous fluids and removal of clothing along with evaporative cooling with tepid water and fanning
    - For agitation or seizures: benzodiazepines
    - For wide complex tachycardia: sodium bicarbonate, 1–2 mEq/kg IV
    - For life-threatening seizures or tachycardia: physostigmine, 1 mg slow IV, used with caution; may cause atrioventricular block or asystole, especially with tricyclic antidepressant overdose

- **Pearl**

Always consider anticholinergic toxicity in a patient with unexplained mental status changes.

Reference

Kirages TJ, Sule HP, Mycyk MB: Severe manifestations of Coricidin intoxication. Am J Emerg Med 2003;21:473. [PMID: 14574654]

Arsenic

■ **Essentials of Diagnosis**

- Heavy metal that acts as a cellular toxin through multiple mechanisms
- Used in herbicides, insecticides, rodenticides, wood preservatives, chemical warfare agent, production of semiconductors, and cancer chemotherapy (arsenic trioxide)
- Acute toxic dose causes crampy abdominal pain, vomiting, profuse watery diarrhea, burning sensation in the mucous membranes, hypotension, tachycardia, garlic odor on the breath, and seizures; arsine gas causes intravascular hemolysis and renal failure
- Chronic toxic dose causes stocking-glove sensory and motor neuropathy, malaise, anorexia, alopecia, anemia, and stomatitis
- Consider serum glucose, electrolytes, BUN, creatinine, CBC, liver enzymes, urinalysis, CPK, and abdominal x-rays (may show radiopaque material)
- 24-hour urinary arsenic levels may be misleading; spot urine analysis may be helpful

■ **Differential Diagnosis**

- Gastroenteritis, viral or bacterial
- Iron ingestion
- Lead ingestion
- Mercury ingestion

■ **Treatment**

- Activated charcoal, 1 g/kg, or gastric lavage (for large ingestions) within 1–2 hours of ingestion
- Intravenous fluids
- Chelation therapy: BAL (dimercaprol), 3–5 mg/kg IM, or DMSA (succimer), 10 mg/kg orally
- For arsine inhalation: intravenous fluids, blood transfusions (chelation therapy not useful)

■ **Pearl**

Arsenic (and iron) are heavy metals and may be radiopaque in some poisoned patients.

Reference

Graeme KA, Pollack CV Jr: Heavy metal toxicity, part I: arsenic and mercury. J Emerg Med 1998;16:45. [PMID: 9472760]

β-Adrenergic Blocking Agents

- **Essentials of Diagnosis**
  - Agents block β_1 and β_2 catecholamine receptors
  - Include medications widely used to treat hypertension, arrhythmias, angina pectoris, migraine, and thyrotoxicosis
  - Toxic dose causes hypotension, bradycardia, atrioventricular blocks, hypoglycemia, hyperkalemia, bronchospasm, and pulmonary edema
  - Some agents (propranolol, oxprenolol) cause seizures; others cause wide complex tachycardia
  - Death usually due to severe myocardial depression
  - Obtain electrocardiogram
  - Urine drug screens do not detect the presence of β-blockers

- **Differential Diagnosis**
  - Calcium-channel blockers
  - Antihypertensive medications (clonidine, ACE inhibitors)
  - Antiarrhythmic medications
  - Digitalis
  - Opioids
  - Sedative-hypnotic agents
  - Organophosphates or carbamates

- **Treatment**
  - Activated charcoal, 1 g/kg, within 1–2 hours of ingestion
  - For hypotension: fluid bolus IV; glucagon, 5 mg slow IV bolus (repeat as necessary) and then glucagon, 2–5 mg/h IV infusion; epinephrine, 1–4 μg/min IV
  - For atrioventricular block and bradycardia: atropine, 0.01–0.03 mg/kg IV; isoproterenol, 4 μg/min; glucagon (see above); consider cardiac pacing
  - For seizures: benzodiazepines, phenobarbital, or phenytoin
  - For bronchospasm: may be reversed with nebulized bronchodilators
  - For hypoglycemia: 50% dextrose, 50 mL IV (adults); 25% dextrose, 2 mL/kg IV (children)

- **Pearl**

Glucagon increases cAMP independent of the β-receptors and may improve bradycardia and hypotension.

Reference

Bailey B: Glucagon in beta-blocker and calcium channel blocker overdoses: a systemic review. J Toxicol Clin Toxicol 2003;41:595. [PMID: 14514004]

Calcium-Channel Blocking Agents

- **Essentials of Diagnosis**
  - Agents block slow calcium channels
  - Medications used to treat supraventricular tachycardia, hypertension, atrial fibrillation or flutter, angina pectoris, and vasospasm
  - Toxic dose causes hypotension, bradycardia, and depressed mental function
  - Other effects: nausea, hyperglycemia, atrioventricular block
  - Obtain electrocardiogram
  - Urine drug screens do not detect the presence of calcium-channel blockers

- **Differential Diagnosis**
  - β-Blockers
  - Antihypertensive medications (clonidine, ACE inhibitors)
  - Antiarrhythmic medications
  - Digitalis
  - Opioids
  - Sedative-hypnotic agents
  - Carbamates

- **Treatment**
  - Activated charcoal, 1 g/kg, within 1–2 hours of ingestion; whole-bowel irrigation for sustained-release agents
  - Give 10% calcium chloride, 10 mL for adults (0.1–0.2 mL/kg for children) IV, or 10% calcium gluconate, 30 mL for adults (0.4 mL/kg for children); repeat every 5–10 minutes as needed
  - For hypotension: intravenous fluids; calcium; repeat boluses of glucagon (5 mg slow IV); glucagon infusion at 2–5 mg/h; epinephrine, 1.0 μg/min IV and increase as needed; inamrinone, 0.75 mg/kg slow IV bolus, then infusion at 5–10 μg/kg/min
  - For atrioventricular block and bradycardia: calcium; atropine, 0.01–0.03 mg/kg IV; glucagon (see above); isoproterenol, 4 μg/min and increase; insulin/glucose (HIE therapy: give insulin 1 U/kg IV bolus with 50% dextrose 50 mL IV, then insulin infusion of 1 U/kg/h and additional dextrose to keep serum glucose between 100 and 200 mg/dL); cardiac pacing

- **Pearl**

Calcium-channel blockers do not cause the seizures, hypoglycemia, or hyperkalemia seen in β-blocker overdoses.

Reference

Salhanick SD, Shannon MW: Management of calcium channel antagonist overdose. Drug Saf 2003;26:65. [PMID: 12534324]

Carbon Monoxide

■ Essentials of Diagnosis

- Colorless, odorless gas produced by incomplete combustion of organic materials from fires, gas heaters, motor vehicle engines, and other sources
- Binds to hemoglobin forming carboxyhemoglobin, which cannot transport oxygen; binds to cytochrome A3 and myoglobin
- Pulse oximetry and blood gas measurements may be normal, must order a carboxyhemoglobin concentration; blood may appear cherry-red
- Carboxyhemoglobin levels correlate somewhat with symptoms
- Carboxyhemoglobin level >5% is normal; 5–10% causes slight headache; 10–30% causes severe headache, dyspnea, irritability, fatigue; 30–50% causes tachycardia, confusion, lethargy, collapse; 50–70% causes coma, convulsions, death
- Complications: myocardial infarction, delayed parkinsonism, memory loss, personality changes
- Carboxyhemoglobin level, chest x-ray, arterial blood gas, CBC, pregnancy test, electrocardiogram

■ Differential Diagnosis

- Cyanide inhalation
- Methemoglobinemia
- Other causes of headache

■ Treatment

- Immediately administer high-flow oxygen by nonrebreathing face mask or endotracheal tube (the half-life of carbon monoxide in a patient breathing room air is 5–6 hours; with 100% oxygen, it is 1 hour; and with hyperbaric oxygen, it is only 23 minutes)
- Continue oxygen administration until carboxyhemoglobin level returns to normal
- Consider hyperbaric oxygen treatment for the following: pregnant patients (due to increased sensitivity of fetal hemoglobin); patient with carboxyhemoglobin levels >25%; or patients with loss of consciousness, severe metabolic acidosis, or myocardial ischemia

■ Pearl

Carbon monoxide poisoning is the leading cause of toxic death.

Reference

Weaver LK et al: Hyberbaric oxygen for acute carbon monoxide poisoning. N Engl J Med 2002;347:1057. [PMID: 12362006]

Caustics & Corrosives

- **Essentials of Diagnosis**
    - Substances that cause histologic damage when in contact with body surfaces; cause the most damage when ingested but can damage intact skin
    - Most are acids or alkalis (eg, detergents, toilet bowl cleaners, bleaches, battery acids, drain cleaners)
    - Acid ingestion causes coagulation necrosis that forms an eschar; helps limit damage
    - Alkali ingestion causes liquefaction necrosis with deep penetration into tissues (full-thickness injury)
    - Symptoms: mouth and throat pain, dysphagia, drooling, substernal chest pain, abdominal pain
    - Serum glucose, electrolytes, BUN, creatinine, CBC, chest x-ray (may show free air)

- **Differential Diagnosis**
    - Irritant gas inhalation
    - Endotracheal aspiration

- **Treatment**
    - Skin exposure requires copious irrigation with water
    - For ingestion: do not administer activated charcoal or induce vomiting; dilute with water or milk (4–8 oz)
    - Diagnostic endoscopy for any symptomatic patient within 12–24 hours; results of endoscopy determine management
    - Steroids not indicated before endoscopy
    - For suspected perforation: antibiotics

- **Pearl**

Significant esophageal or gastric injury may be present without oral lesions.

Reference

Ramasamy K, Gumaste VV: Corrosive ingestions in adults. J Clin Gastroenterol 2003;37:119. [PMID: 12869880]

Cocaine & Local Anesthetics

- **Essentials of Diagnosis**
  - Cocaine and the local anesthetics (benzocaine, lidocaine, bupivacaine, mepivacaine, and procaine) block fast sodium channels, producing local anesthesia; stimulate CNS; and cause sympathetic hyperactivity
  - Effects similar to those of amphetamines
  - Cocaine has rapid onset of action and short half-life when taken orally, intravenously, snorted, or smoked
  - Toxic dose causes euphoria, anxiety, mydriasis, restlessness, sweating, chest pain (usually noncardiac), hypertension, hyperthermia, psychosis, seizures, and tachyarrhythmias
  - May cause myocardial infarction, aortic dissection, and intracranial hemorrhage
  - Serum glucose, electrolytes, BUN, creatinine, CPK, urinalysis, electrocardiogram, abdominal x-rays (for body packers), and head CT scan as indicated
  - Most urine drug screens assess presence of cocaine; false positives and false negatives possible

- **Differential Diagnosis**
  - Sympathomimetics (cocaine, caffeine, phenylpropanolamine, amphetamines)
  - Anticholinergics (antihistamines, tricyclic antidepressants, atropine)
  - Hallucinogenics (phencyclidine, LSD)
  - Sepsis
  - Sedative-hypnotic withdrawal

- **Treatment**
  - Activated charcoal, 1 g/kg, within 1–2 hours of ingestion
  - Hyperthermia (>104°F [40°C]) may be lethal; rapid cooling with room-temperature intravenous fluids and removal of clothing along with evaporative cooling with tepid water and fanning
  - For agitation, seizures, hypertension: benzodiazepines
  - For severe hypertension: nitroprusside, nitroglycerin, phentolamine
  - For tachyarrhythmias not responsive to benzodiazepines: consider esmolol or labetalol

- **Pearl**

β-Blockers given to a patient with cocaine intoxication may cause paradoxical hypertension.

Reference

Shanti CM, Lucas CE: Cocaine and the critical care challenge. Crit Care Med 2003;31:1851. [PMID: 12794430]

Cyanide

- **Essentials of Diagnosis**
  - Rapidly absorbed cellular toxin that inhibits the cytochrome oxidase system for oxygen utilization
  - Toxicity from exposure to fumigants, industrial chemicals, amygdalin in fruit pits (Laetrile), burning plastics, artificial nail-removing solution, and sodium nitroprusside
  - May be in solid, liquid, or gas form with the smell of bitter almonds
  - Effects: headache, nausea and vomiting, anxiety, confusion, and collapse; initial hypertension and tachycardia progress to hypotension, bradycardia, severe lactic acidosis, and apnea
  - Death can occur within minutes with a dose of 200 mg
  - Pulse oximetry and blood gas measurements may be normal; venous blood may appear bright red
  - Carboxyhemoglobin level, methemoglobin level, chest x-ray, arterial blood gas, CBC, pregnancy test, electrocardiogram

- **Differential Diagnosis**
  - Carbon monoxide inhalation
  - Cocaine
  - Amphetamines
  - Methemoglobinemia
  - Major vascular catastrophe
  - Myocardial infarction

- **Treatment**
  - Immediately administer high-flow oxygen by nonrebreathing face mask or endotracheal tube
  - For ingestion: activated charcoal, 1 g/kg orally within 1–2 hours of ingestion
  - Nitrates to induce methemoglobinemia, which has a higher affinity for cyanide than cytochrome oxidase
  - Break glass ampule of amyl nitrite under patient's nose every 3 minutes until sodium nitrite given; sodium nitrite, 300 mg IV (6.0 mg/kg in children)
  - Thiosulfate provides sulfur to convert cyanide to thiocyanate
  - Administer 25% sodium thiosulfate 12.5 g IV (1.65 ml/kg in children)

- **Pearl**

For smoke inhalation with both carbon monoxide and cyanide toxicity, inducing methemoglobinemia may be harmful.

Reference

Chin RG, Calderon Y: Acute cyanide poisoning: a case report. J Emerg Med 2000;18:441. [PMID: 10802422]

Digoxin

- **Essentials of Diagnosis**
  - Cardiac glycoside similar to digitalis, digitoxin, and other plant derivatives found in oleander, foxglove, and lily of the valley; inhibits function of sodium-potassium-ATP pump
  - Toxic dose causes blurred vision and color vision disturbance; hyperkalemia; many types of cardiac arrhythmias including third-degree heart block, bradycardia, bidirectional ventricular tachycardia, and paroxysmal atrial tachycardia with atrioventricular block
  - Serum glucose, electrolytes, BUN, creatinine, electrocardiogram, digoxin level, magnesium

- **Differential Diagnosis**
  - Calcium-channel blocker toxicity
  - Antihypertensive medications (clonidine, ACE inhibitors)
  - Antiarrhythmic medication toxicity
  - β-blockers
  - Sedative-hypnotic agents

- **Treatment**
  - Activated charcoal, 1 g/kg, within 1–2 hours of ingestion
  - For hypotension: fluid bolus, pressors
  - For atrioventricular block and bradycardia: atropine, 0.01–0.03 mg/kg IV; isoproterenol, 4 μg/min and increase; cardiac pacing
  - For wide complex tachycardia: lidocaine, 1 mg/kg IV, then infusion; phenytoin, 15–20 mg/kg slow IV (50 mg/min)
  - For hyperkalemia (>5.5 mEq/L): sodium bicarbonate, 1.0 mEq/kg IV; glucose with insulin; and sodium polystyrene sulfonate (Kayexalate); do not use calcium
  - For severe hyperkalemia or symptomatic arrhythmias not responding to other medications: Fab fragments of digoxin-specific antibodies (Digibind); digoxin-Fab dose depends on amount ingested

- **Pearl**

The estimated number of digoxin-Fab vials equals the serum digoxin level (eg, a level of 5.1 ng/mL would require five vials).

Reference

DiDomenico RJ et al: Analysis of the use of digoxin immune Fab for the treatment of non-life threatening digoxin toxicity. J Cardiovasc Pharmacol Ther 2000;5:77. [PMID: 11150387]

Drug-Induced Methemoglobinemia

- **Essentials of Diagnosis**
  - Methemoglobinemia occurs when iron in hemoglobin is oxidized from the ferrous ($2+$) to the ferric ($3+$) state; it can no longer transport oxygen
  - Caused by exposure to nitrites, well water, chloroquine, phenazopyridine, local anesthetics, sulfonamides, aniline dyes, phenacetin, and dapsone
  - Levels correlate with symptoms
  - Methemoglobinemia level >2% is normal; 5–10% causes slight cyanosis; 15% causes chocolate-brown blood; 25% causes marked cyanosis, anxiety, headache, weakness, and lightheadedness; 35% causes confusion, fatigue, and dyspnea; 60% causes coma and death
  - Anemia, acidosis, respiratory illness, and cardiac disease make symptoms more severe
  - Blood gas determination will be normal; pulse oximetry saturations may be normal or decreased
  - Methemoglobin level, chest x-ray, arterial blood gas, CBC, pregnancy test, urinalysis, electrocardiogram

- **Differential Diagnosis**
  - Cyanide inhalation
  - Carbon monoxide inhalation
  - Other causes of cyanosis

- **Treatment**
  - Immediately administer high-flow oxygen by nonrebreathing face mask
  - Usually mild methemoglobinemia (<20%) resolves without treatment when offending agent is removed
  - For symptomatic patients: consider 1% methylene blue, 1–2 mg/kg slow IV; contraindicated in patients with G6PD deficiency
  - Methylene blue reduces ferric iron to ferrous iron

- **Pearl**

A difference between the calculated oxygen saturation on the arterial blood gas and the measured saturation on pulse oximetry (saturation gap) indicates an abnormal type of hemoglobin such as methemoglobin is present.

Reference

Wright RO, Lewander WJ, Woolf AD: Methemoglobinemia: etiology, pharmacology, and clinical management. Ann Emerg Med 1999;34:646. [PMID: 10533013]

Ethanol

- **Essentials of Diagnosis**
  - Found in various concentrations in beer, wine, liquors, colognes, perfumes, mouthwashes, vanilla and lemon extracts, and over-the-counter cold medicines
  - CNS depressant with adverse effects from acute intoxication, chronic use, and withdrawal
  - Acute intoxication causes hypoglycemia, ataxia, nystagmus, impaired judgment, CNS depression (coma usually at levels >300 mg/dL), respiratory depression, hypotension, and pulmonary aspiration
  - Chronic abuse leads to alcoholic hepatitis and cirrhosis, ascites, gastritis, gastrointestinal bleeding, pancreatitis, cardiomyopathy, cerebral atrophy, and nutritional disorders
  - Withdrawal after chronic high-level use first (within 12 hours) causes headache, tremor, anxiety, generalized seizures; then (after 2–3 days) causes delirium tremens with tachycardia, diaphoresis, hyperthermia, and delirium
  - Consider serum glucose, blood alcohol level, electrolytes, magnesium, liver enzymes, international normalized ratio, chest x-ray, and head CT scan

- **Differential Diagnosis**
  - Barbiturates
  - Benzodiazepines
  - Opioids
  - Toxic alcohols (methanol, ethylene glycol, isopropanol)
  - Meningitis or trauma

- **Treatment**
  - Activated charcoal or gastric lavage not useful for acute ethanol ingestions; most patients will recover within 6 hours
  - Intravenous fluids (normal saline)
  - Thiamine, 100 mg (adult) or 50 mg (children) slow IV or IM
  - For hypoglycemia: 50% dextrose 50 mL IV (adults), 25% dextrose 2 mL/kg IV (children)
  - For alcoholic ketoacidosis: intravenous fluid replacement
  - For alcohol-related seizures: benzodiazepines
  - For withdrawal manifestations: benzodiazepines (diazepam, 2–10 mg IV, may repeat)

- **Pearl**

Most patients metabolize ethanol at 20–30 mg/dL/h; a blood level of 300 mg/dL will take about 8 hours to drop to 100 mg/dL.

Reference

Oimedo R, Hoffman RS: Withdrawal syndromes. Emerg Med Clin North Am 2000;18:273. [PMID: 10767884]

Ethylene Glycol & Methanol

- ■ Essentials of Diagnosis
  - • Ethylene glycol: in automobile antifreeze; metabolized by alcohol dehydrogenase to glycolate and oxalate, which precipitates to calcium oxalate crystals
  - • Methanol: in paint stripper, windshield washer fluid, and Sterno; metabolized by alcohol dehydrogenase to formaldehyde and formic acid
  - • Ethylene glycol first causes CNS depression and pulmonary edema; later (4–12 hours after ingestion), severe metabolic acidosis, seizures, and coma; then (24–72 hours after ingestion), renal tubule necrosis, flank pain, hematuria, and renal failure
  - • Methanol first causes CNS depression; later, hyperemia of the optic disk, blurred vision, dizziness, severe metabolic acidosis, blindness, seizures, and coma
  - • Serum glucose, ethanol level, ethylene glycol or methanol level (if possible), electrolytes, BUN, creatinine, urinalysis (for crystals), increased osmolar gap (measured osmolarity minus calculated osmolarity), magnesium, liver enzymes, international normalized ratio, chest x-ray, arterial blood gases, and head CT scan as indicated

- ■ Differential Diagnosis
  - • Other toxic alcohols (ethanol, isopropanol)
  - • Sedative-hypnotic agents
  - • Meningitis or trauma

- ■ Treatment
  - • Activated charcoal or gastric lavage not useful
  - • Fomepizole, 15 mg/kg IV bolus, and ethanol block alcohol dehydrogenase, slowing formation of toxic metabolites
  - • Ethanol may be used if fomepizole is unavailable; give 2 mL/kg of 50% ethanol orally or 7 mL/kg of 10% ethanol IV
  - • For metabolic acidosis: sodium bicarbonate
  - • For methanol: folate, 50 mg IV
  - • For ethylene glycol: thiamine, 100 mg IV; pyridoxine, 50 mg IV
  - • For severe metabolic acidosis or renal failure: hemodialysis

- ■ Pearl

The patient's mouth, clothing, or urine may appear fluorescent under an ultraviolet lamp owing to the fluorescein added to antifreeze.

Reference

Abramson SR, Singh AK: Treatment of the alcohol intoxications: ethylene glycol, methanol and isopropanol. Curr Opin Nephrol Hypertens 2000;9:695. [PMID: 11128434]

Hydrocarbons

■ Essentials of Diagnosis

- Large group of compounds derived from petroleum distillates; used as solvents, degreasers, fuels, and lubricants
- May be ingested, inhaled, or absorbed from skin
- Major complication: aspiration pneumonitis; worse with low-viscosity hydrocarbons (turpentine, pine oil, lighter fluid, furniture polish)
- Severe chemical pneumonitis from aspiration of 1 teaspoon
- Aspiration (from ingestion) causes choking, coughing, or gasping usually immediately; may be delayed up to 6 hours
- Infiltrates on chest x-ray may be delayed
- Inhalation (Freon, trichloroethylene, toluene) causes euphoria, confusion, hallucinations, coma, and cardiac arrhythmias; chronic use leads to myopathy, hypokalemia, renal tubular acidosis, and neuropathy
- Systemic effects from ingestion: vomiting, ataxia, headache, confusion, seizures (camphor), coma, cardiac arrhythmias, respiratory arrest
- Consider serum glucose, electrolytes, BUN, creatinine, CBC, chest x-ray, arterial blood gases, liver enzymes, and electrocardiogram

■ Differential Diagnosis

- Irritant gas inhalation
- Iron ingestion; caustic ingestion

■ Treatment

- For skin exposure: copious irrigation with water
- Aliphatic hydrocarbons (lighter fluid, kerosene, furniture polish, gasoline): usually cause no systemic effects
- *Do not administer activated charcoal;* could precipitate aspiration
- Aromatic and halogenated hydrocarbons (camphor, benzene, toluene, pesticides): may cause systemic effects; consider gastric lavage (only after endotracheal intubation) for large amounts of these hydrocarbons followed by activated charcoal
- For aspiration pneumonitis: oxygen and bronchodilators; steroids and antibiotics not used

■ Pearl

For most hydrocarbon ingestions in children, there is no aspiration and systemic effects do not occur.

Reference

Mickiewicz M, Gomez HF: Hydrocarbon toxicity: general review and management guidelines. Air Med J 2001;20:8. [PMID: 11331818]

Iron

- ■ Essentials of Diagnosis
    - • Widely used for treatment of anemia; found in prenatal vitamins and in daily vitamin combinations
    - • Many different preparations with differing amounts of elemental iron (toxic dose >40 mg/kg elemental iron)
    - • Causes corrosion of gastric and intestinal lining
    - • When iron load exceeds binding capacity, acts as cellular toxin resulting in vasodilatation, lactic acidosis, and death
    - • Acute toxic dose initially (within 4 hours) causes vomiting, diarrhea, abdominal pain, hematemesis, massive fluid loss, shock, metabolic acidosis, coma, leukocytosis, and hyperglycemia
    - • Following acute phase, symptoms improve for 12–24 hours
    - • Third stage consists of return of shock, acidosis, coma, seizures, coagulopathy, renal failure, and sometimes death
    - • Total serum iron, serum glucose, electrolytes, BUN, creatinine, CBC, liver enzymes, urinalysis, coagulation studies, and abdominal x-rays (may show radiopaque material)

- ■ Differential Diagnosis
    - • Gastroenteritis, viral or bacterial
    - • Arsenic ingestion
    - • Lead ingestion
    - • Mercury ingestion

- ■ Treatment
    - • Activated charcoal not useful
    - • Gastric lavage (for large ingestions of liquids or chewed tablets) within 1–2 hours of ingestion
    - • Consider whole-bowel irrigation (GoLYTELY)
    - • Intravenous fluids
    - • For serious symptoms or serum iron level >500 μg/dL: chelation therapy with deferoxamine, 10–15 mg/kg/h (up to 6 g/day); chelation complex is excreted in urine and is pink in color

- ■ Pearl

No serious toxicity results if, after 6 hours, patient did not vomit, WBC is normal, glucose is normal, and no pills are apparent on abdominal x-ray.

Reference

Tran T et al: Intentional iron overdose in pregnancy—management and outcome. J Emerg Med 2000;18:225. [PMID: 10699527]

Isoniazid

- ■ Essentials of Diagnosis
  - • Common medication for treatment of tuberculosis
  - • Reduces the amount of vitamin B6 in the CNS, which lowers the level of the inhibitory neurotransmitter γ-aminobutyric acid (GABA)
  - • Acute ingestion of 80–100 mg/kg causes vomiting, slurred speech, dizziness, lethargy, hyperreflexia, seizures, metabolic acidosis, and cardiorespiratory depression
  - • Seizures usually occur within 2 hours; may not respond to benzodiazepines
  - • Metabolic acidosis may be severe (pH <6.9)
  - • Chronic high dose leads to hepatic toxicity and peripheral neuritis
  - • Serum glucose, electrolytes, BUN, creatinine, CBC, liver enzymes, urinalysis, CPK, liver function tests, arterial blood gases

- ■ Differential Diagnosis
  - • Sympathomimetics
  - • Hypoglycemia
  - • Tricyclic antidepressants
  - • Camphor
  - • Sedative-hypnotic withdrawal

- ■ Treatment
  - • Activated charcoal, 1 g/kg within 1–2 hours of ingestion
  - • For seizures: benzodiazepines and pyridoxine
  - • Pyridoxine usually terminates seizures and improves mental status; if isoniazid dose is known, give identical amount of pyridoxine in grams IV; if dose is unknown, give 5 g IV and repeat as necessary until seizures stop

- ■ Pearl

Hydrazine rocket fuel and Gyromitra mushrooms also deplete vitamin B6 and cause seizures that may require treatment with pyridoxine.

Reference

Ramero JA, Kuczler FJ Jr: Isoniazid overdose: recognition and management. Am Fam Physician 1998;57:749. [PMID: 9490997]

Isopropanol

- ■ Essentials of Diagnosis
  - • Toxic alcohol found in rubbing alcohol (70% isopropanol), antiseptics, and solvents
  - • Metabolized by alcohol dehydrogenase to acetone; does not form organic acids and does not cause severe metabolic acidosis, as do methanol and ethylene glycol
  - • Isopropanol and acetone cause CNS depression
  - • Toxic dose (1 ml/kg) causes vomiting, hematemesis, abdominal pain, isopropanol or acetone smell on the breath, slurred speech, ataxia, stupor, coma, hypotension, and respiratory arrest
  - • Abnormal laboratory values: increased osmolar gap, ketonemia, ketonuria, slight metabolic acidosis, and isopropanol serum level (>150 mg/dL usually causes coma)
  - • Serum glucose, ethanol level, electrolytes, BUN, creatinine, measured osmolarity (large difference from calculated osmolarity indicates presence of toxic alcohol), magnesium, liver enzymes, international normalized ratio, chest x-ray, arterial blood gases, and head CT scan

- ■ Differential Diagnosis
  - • Other toxic alcohols (ethanol, methanol, ethylene glycol)
  - • Sedative-hypnotic agents
  - • Meningitis
  - • Trauma

- ■ Treatment
  - • Activated charcoal or gastric lavage not useful
  - • Usually supportive care only; treat as for ethanol intoxication
  - • Fomepizole and ethanol not indicated
  - • For isopropanol levels >400–500 mg/dL with coma or hypotension: hemodialysis

- ■ Pearl

Alcoholics may ingest isopropanol as a substitute for ethanol.

Reference

Stemski E, Hennes H: Accidental isopropanol ingestion in children. Pediatr Emerg Care 2000;16:238. [PMID: 10966340]

Lead

- ## Essentials of Diagnosis
  - Inorganic lead: found in paint in older homes; foreign pottery glazes; and fumes from welding, smelting, and battery production
  - Organic lead (tetraethyl lead): may be found in gasoline
  - Widespread cellular enzyme toxin with multiple mechanisms affecting multiple organ systems; more than 70% of lead burden is stored in bone
  - Acute large ingestions may cause abdominal pain, hemolytic anemia, hepatitis, and encephalopathy
  - Chronic exposure (more common) causes fatigue, irritability, anorexia, arthralgias, hypertension, abdominal pain, nausea, constipation, headache, tremor, wrist drop, normochromic or microcytic anemia (with basophilic stippling), encephalopathy, and seizures
  - Whole-blood lead level, CBC, serum glucose, electrolytes, BUN, creatinine, liver enzymes, urinalysis, coagulation studies, abdominal x-rays (may show radiopaque material), and head CT scan

- ## Differential Diagnosis
  - Gastroenteritis, viral or bacterial
  - Viral respiratory infection
  - Arsenic ingestion
  - Mercury ingestion

- ## Treatment
  - Activated charcoal probably not useful
  - Blood level <25 μg/dL is normal; 25–45 μg/dL requires no emergency treatment
  - For blood level 45–70 μg/dL: oral DMSA (succimer) if no encephalopathy is present; calcium EDTA or BAL parenterally if encephalopathic
  - For blood level >70 μg/dL: medical emergency; calcium EDTA or BAL parenterally
  - Consider whole-bowel irrigation (GoLYTELY) if radiopaque material seen on x-ray

- ## Pearl

Retained lead bullets do not usually cause elevation of blood lead levels unless they are in or near a synovial space.

Reference

Graeme KA, Pollack CV Jr: Heavy metal toxicity, part II: lead and metal fume fever. J Emerg Med 1998;16:171. [PMID: 9543397]

Lithium

- ■ **Essentials of Diagnosis**
  - Used to treat bipolar disorder and other psychiatric illnesses
  - Acute toxic ingestion causes nausea, vomiting, diarrhea, and delayed neurologic symptoms
  - Chronic intoxication (more common) usually due to regular dosing with a sudden change in hydration or kidney function such as acute gastroenteritis; dehydration; hyponatremia; nephrogenic diabetes insipidus; or initial therapy with diuretics, nonsteroidal anti-inflammatory drugs, or ACE inhibitors
  - Chronic intoxication causes lethargy, weakness, slurred speech, ataxia, tremor, extrapyramidal side effects, delirium, coma, seizures, hyperthermia, and death
  - Abnormal findings: leukocytosis, electrocardiogram with T-wave inversion and bradycardia, very high early lithium levels with acute ingestions (before equilibrium)
  - Lithium level (>2 mEq/L usually very toxic for chronic intoxication), CBC, serum glucose, electrolytes, BUN, creatinine, electrocardiogram, urinalysis, and head CT scan

- ■ **Differential Diagnosis**
  - Gastroenteritis, viral or bacterial
  - Sedative-hypnotic agents
  - Tricyclic antidepressants
  - Arsenic ingestion

- ■ **Treatment**
  - Activated charcoal not useful
  - Consider gastric lavage if recent, large ingestion
  - Consider whole-bowel irrigation for sustained-released products
  - Intravenous normal saline bolus; correct serum sodium
  - Oral sodium polystyrene sulfonate (Kayexalate) may decrease lithium level
  - For severe symptoms (seizures or coma): hemodialysis

- ■ **Pearl**

Chronic lithium therapy may cause nephrogenic diabetes insipidus.

Reference

Nagappan R, Parkin WG, Holdsworth SR: Acute lithium intoxication. Anaesth Intensive Care 2002;30:90. [PMID: 11939450]

Mercury

- **Essentials of Diagnosis**
    - Reacts with sulfhydryl groups causing enzyme inhibition and damage to cellular membranes
    - Elemental mercury: used in thermometers, electrical equipment, dental amalgam, and paints; not toxic when ingested; inhaled heated vapor may cause encephalopathy and pneumonitis
    - Inorganic salts (mercuric chloride): used in disinfectants; may cause hemorrhagic gastroenteritis, abdominal pain, acute tubular necrosis, shock, and death when ingested; chronic exposure leads to CNS toxicity
    - Organic substances (methylmercury, ethylmercury): used in fungicides; cause tremor, neuropsychiatric symptoms, paresthesias, loss of hearing, smell, sight, or taste, incoordination, choreoathetosis, stupor, incontinence, and birth defects when ingested
    - Whole-blood mercury level, 24-hour urine collection, CBC, serum glucose, electrolytes, BUN, creatinine, liver enzymes, urinalysis, coagulation studies, abdominal x-rays (may show radiopaque material), and head CT scan

- **Differential Diagnosis**
    - Gastroenteritis, viral or bacterial
    - Viral respiratory infection
    - Arsenic ingestion

- **Treatment**
    - For inorganic mercury salt ingestion: initiate gastric lavage, activated charcoal, intravenous fluids, hemodialysis if renal failure develops, oral succimer (DMSA), or intramuscular BAL chelation early
    - Organic mercury ingestion: initiate gastric lavage, activated charcoal, DMSA, or oral *N*-acetylcysteine may be effective (BAL should not be used)

- **Pearl**

The symptoms of classic chronic mercury poisoning (erethism) consist of tremor, anxiety, incapacitating shyness, and irritability.

Reference

Graeme KA Pollack CV: Heavy metal toxicity, part I: arsenic and mercury. J Emerg Med 1998;16:45. [PMID: 9472760]

Neuroleptic Malignant Syndrome

- ■ Essentials of Diagnosis
  - • An uncommon and potentially fatal reaction to high-potency antipsychotic medications; not dose related
  - • May develop after years of antipsychotic therapy
  - • Effects: hypertension, tachycardia, severe hyperthermia, muscle rigidity, altered mental status, diaphoresis, lactic acidosis, rhabdomyolysis
  - • Lactate level, hepatic enzymes, chest x-ray, arterial blood gas, CBC, electrolytes, BUN, creatinine, CPK, serum glucose, urinalysis, electrocardiogram, and head CT scan

- ■ Differential Diagnosis
  - • Hallucinogenics (phencyclidine, LSD)
  - • Cocaine
  - • Lithium
  - • Anticholinergics
  - • Salicylates
  - • Malignant hyperthermia
  - • Serotonin syndrome
  - • Sedative-hypnotic withdrawal

- ■ Treatment
  - • Immediate discontinuation of antipsychotic
  - • For hyperthermia: rapid cooling with tepid water and fanning
  - • Aggressive intravenous hydration
  - • Intravenous benzodiazepines
  - • Bromocriptine, 5 mg every 8 hours orally
  - • Neuromuscular paralysis may be necessary for cooling
  - • Dantrolene, 1 mg/kg, may be helpful

- ■ Pearl

Consider neuroleptic malignant syndrome in any patient who is taking antipsychotic medications and who has hyperthermia and altered mentation.

Reference

Khan M, Farver D: Recognition, assessment and management of neuroleptic malignant syndrome. S D J Med 2000;53:395. [PMID: 11016275]

Opiates

- **Essentials of Diagnosis**
  - Large number of naturally occurring and synthetic compounds that stimulate specific opiate receptors in the CNS; cause sedation, analgesia, and respiratory depression
  - Include opium, morphine, heroin, codeine, hydrocodone, fentanyl, butorphanol, meperidine, methadone, dextromethorphan, tramadol, propoxyphene, and oxycodone
  - Mild overdose symptoms: lethargy, pinpoint pupils, diminished bowel sound, flaccid muscles
  - Severe overdose symptoms: coma, respiratory depression, sudden death
  - Diagnosis is certain if comatose patient awakens rapidly after naloxone
  - Opiate withdrawal occurs rapidly in addicted patients; although not life threatening, the anxiety, piloerection, abdominal cramps, diarrhea, and insomnia are extremely uncomfortable
  - Serum glucose, electrolytes, BUN, creatinine, electrocardiogram, head CT scan, chest x-ray, KUB radiograph (for body packers)
  - Urine drug screens may not detect some synthetic opioids such as fentanyl or tramadol

- **Differential Diagnosis**
  - Sedative-hypnotic agents
  - Toxic alcohols
  - Meningitis
  - Intracranial lesion

- **Treatment**
  - Activated charcoal, 1 g/kg, within 2–4 hours of ingestion (delayed gastrointestinal absorption), if airway is protected
  - Naloxone, 0.4–2.0 mg IV (may repeat); propoxyphene overdose may require 20 mg to reverse
  - Naloxone may precipitate opiate withdrawal symptoms; although not life threatening, these symptoms may be prevented by careful titration of naloxone

- **Pearl**

Naloxone reversal effects will last only 1–3 hours, but the effects of most opiates last much longer; these patients will relapse and require more naloxone.

Reference

Watson WA et al: Opioid toxicity recurrence after an initial response to naloxone. J Toxicol Clin Toxicol 1998;36:11. [PMID: 9541035]

Organophosphates & Other Cholinesterase Inhibitors

- ■ Essentials of Diagnosis
  - Organophosphates (insecticides), carbamates (flea collars), and some chemical warfare agents (nerve agents) inhibit acetylcholinesterase, allowing accumulation of acetylcholine at muscarinic and nicotinic receptors
  - Organophosphates irreversibly bind to acetylcholinesterase; carbamates are reversible
  - Rapidly absorbed from skin, gastrointestinal tract, and respiratory tract
  - Toxic dose causes miosis, salivation, bronchospasm, hyperactive bowel sounds, garlic odor, lacrimation, lethargy, bradycardia or tachycardia, diarrhea, urination, muscle fasciculation, anxiety, and seizures; death occurs from bronchospasm and bronchorrhea
  - Plasma or RBC cholinesterase levels confirm diagnosis
  - Consider serum glucose, electrolytes, BUN, creatinine, CPK, urinalysis, electrocardiogram, and head CT scan
  - Most urine drug screens do not assess the presence of cholinesterase inhibitors

- ■ Differential Diagnosis
  - Opiates
  - Sepsis
  - Sedative-hypnotic agents
  - Congestive heart failure
  - Pneumonia

- ■ Treatment
  - Activated charcoal, 1 g/kg, within 1–2 hours of ingestion
  - Airway management, oxygen, suction, endotracheal intubation as needed
  - Removal of patient's contaminated clothing
  - Atropine, 1–2 mg IV; repeat many times until bronchorrhea has resolved; large doses may be required
  - For significant organophosphate toxicity: pralidoxime (2-PAM), 1–2 g slow IV
  - For seizures: benzodiazepines

- ■ Pearl

Pesticides usually contain both organophosphates and hydrocarbons; ingestions may cause hydrocarbon aspirations.

Reference

Kwong TC: Organophosphate pesticides: biochemistry and clinical toxicology. Ther Drug Monit 2002;24:144. [PMID: 11805735]

Phencyclidine

- ■ Essentials of Diagnosis
  - • Phencyclidine (PCP, angel dust, crystal, supergrass, ozone, crack, rocket fuel, peace pill) may be smoked, snorted, ingested, or injected; common drug of abuse
  - • Sympathomimetic, hallucinogenic, dissociative agent that has rapid onset of action and long half-life
  - • Severe intoxication causes CNS fluctuations (severe agitation to quiet stupor), bizarre behavior, extreme violence, vertical and horizontal nystagmus, hypertension, tachycardia, muscle rigidity, hyperthermia, seizures, rhabdomyolysis, and renal failure
  - • Consider serum glucose, electrolytes, BUN, creatinine, CPK, urinalysis, electrocardiogram, and head CT scan
  - • Most urine drug screens assess presence of phencyclidine; false positives and false negatives possible

- ■ Differential Diagnosis
  - • Other sympathomimetics (cocaine, caffeine, phenylpropanolamine)
  - • Anticholinergics (antihistamines, tricyclic antidepressants, atropine)
  - • Amphetamines
  - • Hallucinogenics (LSD)
  - • Sepsis
  - • Sedative-hypnotic withdrawal

- ■ Treatment
  - • Activated charcoal, 1 g/kg, within 1–2 hours of ingestion; no other specific treatment for most patients because usual symptoms resolve in a few hours
  - • Hyperthermia (>104°F [40°C]) may be lethal; rapid cooling with room-temperature intravenous fluids and removal of clothing along with evaporative cooling with tepid water and fanning
  - • For agitation, seizures, hypertension: benzodiazepines
  - • For psychosis: may require haloperidol

- ■ Pearl

Phencyclidine and ketamine have similar pharmacologic and clinical characteristics, and both are drugs of abuse.

Reference

Brust JC: Acute neurological complications of drug and alcohol abuse. Neurol Clin 1998;16:503-19. [PMID: 9537972]

Phenothiazines & Other Antipsychotics

- **Essentials of Diagnosis**
  - Include phenothiazines (chlorpromazine, prochlorperazine, promethazine), butyrophenones (haloperidol), and others
  - Complex effects: anticholinergic, α-adrenergic-receptor blocking, quinidine-like cardiac activity, CNS depression, and extrapyramidal dystonic reactions due to dopamine receptor blockade
  - Toxic dose causes sedation, miosis, orthostatic hypotension, dry mouth, dry skin, agitation, tachycardia, and urinary retention seizures; severe toxicity causes hypothermia or hyperthermia, coma, seizures, and death
  - Cardiac effects: widening QRS complex and prolonged QT
  - Consider serum glucose, electrolytes, BUN, creatinine, CBC, CPK, urinalysis, electrocardiogram, abdominal KUB (for radiopaque material), and chest x-ray
  - Urine drug screens do not detect all antipsychotics

- **Differential Diagnosis**
  - Sympathomimetics (amphetamines, MDMA, cocaine, phenylpropanolamine)
  - Hallucinogenics (phencyclidine, LSD)
  - Tricyclic antidepressants
  - Sepsis
  - Sedative-hypnotic withdrawal

- **Treatment**
  - Activated charcoal, 1 g/kg, within 2–4 hours of ingestion (delayed gastrointestinal absorption)
  - Monitor electrocardiogram for QRS widening (>100 msec)
  - For hypotension: intravenous fluids; norepinephrine may be more effective than other pressors
  - For agitation or seizures: benzodiazepines
  - For ventricular dysrhythmias: lidocaine, 1–2 mg/kg IV bolus
  - For dystonic reactions: diphenhydramine, 0.5–1 mg/kg IM or IV, or benztropine, 1–2 mg IV or IM

- **Pearl**

Overdoses with antipsychotic medication without other ingestants seldom cause death.

Reference

James LP et al: Phenothiazine, butyrophenone, and other psychotropic medication poisonings in children and adolescents. J Toxicol Clin Toxicol 2000;38:615. [PMID: 11185968]

Poisonous Mushrooms

- **Essentials of Diagnosis**
    - Of the thousands of varieties of mushrooms, only about 100 are toxic; most of the poisonous mushrooms are in six categories
    - Identification of specific mushrooms can be difficult; may require an experienced mycologist
    - Acute gastrointestinal symptoms (<2 hours): vomiting, diarrhea due to gastrointestinal irritant; no critical toxicity
    - Delayed gastrointestinal symptoms (>6 hours): vomiting, diarrhea, and abdominal pain, followed in 2–3 days by hepatic or renal failure; *Amanita phalloides* (amatoxin), *Gyromitra esculenta* (monomethylhydrazine)
    - Cholinergic symptoms (<1 hour): vomiting, diarrhea, diaphoresis, bronchospasm, bradycardia, salivation, lacrimation, miosis; *Inocybe, Clitocybe*
    - Anticholinergic symptoms (<1 hour): vomiting, drowsiness, tachycardia, seizures, dry skin, mydriasis, hallucinations, delirium, psychosis; *Amanita muscaria*
    - Visual hallucinations (<1 hour), tachycardia, mydriasis, ataxia; *Psilocybe cubensis*
    - Disulfiram symptoms within 1 hour of drinking alcohol, headache, flushing, tachycardia, hyperventilation, palpitations; *Coprinus*
    - Serum glucose, electrolytes, BUN, creatinine, CBC, chest x-ray, arterial blood gases, liver enzymes, international normalized ratio, and electrocardiogram

- **Differential Diagnosis**
    - Gastroenteritis, viral or bacterial
    - Iron ingestion
    - Hallucinogenics
    - Anticholinergics

- **Treatment**
    - Activated charcoal, 1 g/kg within 1–2 hours of ingestion
    - Intravenous hydration and antiemetics
    - For cholinergic symptoms: atropine, 0.01 mg/kg as needed
    - For hallucinations or agitation: benzodiazepines

- **Pearl**

If vomiting occurs within 2 hours of ingestion, a critical poisoning is very unlikely.

Reference

Broussand CN et al: Mushroom poisoning—from diarrhea to liver transplantation. Am J Gastroenterol 2001;96:3195. [PMID: 11721773]

Salicylates

■ **Essentials of Diagnosis**

- Found in many medications (Pepto-Bismol, aspirin, oil of wintergreen); one teaspoon of oil of wintergreen contains 5,000 mg of methyl salicylate
- Toxicity results in metabolic acidosis and pulmonary and cerebral edema
- Acute toxicity (>150 mg/kg): vomiting, hyperventilation, tinnitus, lethargy, mixed respiratory alkalosis and metabolic acidosis, seizures, coma, hypoglycemia, hyperthermia, and pulmonary edema; death caused by CNS failure and cardiovascular collapse
- Chronic toxicity (>100 mg/kg/d): nonspecific symptoms (confusion, dehydration, and metabolic acidosis); death more common than in acute toxicity and occurs at lower serum salicylate levels
- Serum levels >100 mg/dL following acute ingestions and >60 mg/dL following chronic ingestions are associated with severe toxicity; Done nomogram no longer used
- Salicylate level and repeat salicylate level (4 hours later), serum glucose, electrolytes, BUN, creatinine, CBC, liver enzymes, urinalysis, coagulation studies

■ **Differential Diagnosis**

- Gastroenteritis, viral or bacterial
- Arsenic ingestion
- Lead ingestion
- Sepsis
- Pneumonia

■ **Treatment**

- Activated charcoal, 1 g/kg every 4 hours
- Treatment of hypoglycemia, metabolic acidosis, and hypokalemia
- Urine alkalinization by adding 1–2 mEq/kg of sodium bicarbonate followed by an infusion of 3 amps in 1 L of 5% dextrose in water running at 1.5–2 times maintenance
- If serum level >100 mg/dL and severe symptoms present: consider dialysis

■ **Pearl**

The Phenistix test of urine may be positive (purple) with salicylate toxicity.

Reference

Dargan PI, Wallace CI, Jones AL: An evidence-based flowchart to guide the management of acute salicylate (aspirin) overdose. Emerg Med J 2002;19:206. [PMID: 11971828]

Sedative-Hypnotics

■ Essentials of Diagnosis

- Broad range of medications used to treat anxiety or insomnia
- May induce tolerance and may cause withdrawal syndrome similar to ethanol withdrawal
- Include benzodiazepines, barbiturates, γ-hydroxybutyrate (GHB), chloral hydrate, meprobamate, and methaqualone
- Acute intoxication causes nystagmus, ataxia, diplopia, dysarthria, lethargy, respiratory depression, hypotension, hypothermia, and coma with nonreactive pupils
- Withdrawal after chronic high-level use causes headache, tremor, anxiety, generalized seizures, tachycardia, diaphoresis, and delirium
- Consider serum glucose, blood alcohol level, electrolytes, liver enzymes, international normalized ratio, chest x-ray, and head CT scan
- Urine drug screens detect many but not all sedative-hypnotics

■ Differential Diagnosis

- Opioids
- Toxic alcohols (ethanol, methanol, ethylene glycol, isopropanol)
- Meningitis
- Trauma
- Anticholinergics
- Antidepressants

■ Treatment

- Activated charcoal, 1 g/kg, within 1–2 hours of ingestion
- Intravenous fluids (normal saline) for hypotension
- Treatment of hypothermia
- Flumazenil should not be used for most overdosed patients; may cause seizures
- Dialysis may be clinically efficacious for phenobarbital and meprobamate poisoning
- For withdrawal: benzodiazepines (diazepam, 2–10 mg IV; may repeat)

■ Pearl

Contraindications to flumazenil are known seizure disorder, benzodiazepine addiction, or tricyclic antidepressant overdose.

Reference

Mason PE, Kerns WP 2nd: Gamma hydroxybutyric acid (GHB) intoxication. Acad Emerg Med 2002;9:730. [PMID: 12093716]

Serotonin Antagonists

- ■ Essentials of Diagnosis
  - • Selective serotonin reuptake inhibitors (SSRIs) are used for treatment of depression and other psychiatric illnesses
  - • Include citalopram, fluoxetine, fluvoxamine, paroxetine, and sertraline
  - • Unlike tricyclic antidepressants, overdoses with SSRIs are rarely life threatening
  - • SSRI overdose causes nausea, vomiting, dizziness, blurred vision, mild tachycardia, and CNS depression; rarely, hyponatremia, seizures, and QRS widening; citalopram causes widening of QT complex and seizures
  - • SSRIs when used in combination or with other serotonergic agents or in overdose may cause serotonin syndrome
  - • Consider serum glucose, acetaminophen level, pregnancy test, electrolytes, BUN, creatinine, CPK, urinalysis, and electrocardiogram
  - • Most urine drug screens do not assess the presence of SSRIs

- ■ Differential Diagnosis
  - • Sepsis
  - • Sedative-hypnotic agents
  - • Toxic alcohols (ethanol, methanol, ethylene glycol, isopropanol)

- ■ Treatment
  - • Activated charcoal, 1 g/kg, within 1–2 hours of ingestion
  - • Supportive care

- ■ Pearl

Most patients with SSRI overdose require no specific treatment; however, the presence of other more toxic ingestants or other illnesses must be determined.

Reference

Borys DJ et al: Acute fluoxetine overdose: report of 234 cases. Am J Emerg Med 1992;10:115. [PMID: 08285970]

Serotonin Syndrome

■ Essentials of Diagnosis

- Reaction seen when a selective serotonin reuptake inhibitor (SSRI) is taken with a monoamine oxidase inhibitor, when SSRIs are combined, or in the case of SSRI overdose; other medications implicated include dextromethorphan, meperidine, trazodone, lithium, MDMA, and clomipramine
- Because of the long half-lives of these medications, one drug may be discontinued and another one initiated leading to the presence of both drugs and causing serotonin syndrome
- Mechanism is not well understood but involves stimulation of serotonin receptors
- Patients with serotonin syndrome have at least three of the following: altered mental status, agitation, myoclonus, hyperreflexia, diaphoresis, tremor, diarrhea, incoordination
- Serotonin syndrome may progress to lactic acidosis, rhabdomyolysis, myoglobinuria, renal and hepatic dysfunction, disseminated intravascular coagulation, and adult respiratory distress syndrome
- Serum glucose, acetaminophen level, pregnancy test, electrolytes, BUN, creatinine, CPK, urinalysis, and electrocardiogram

■ Differential Diagnosis

- Neuroleptic malignant syndrome
- Meningitis
- Sympathomimetics
- Sedative-hypnotic withdrawal

■ Treatment

- For hyperthermia: rapid cooling
- For muscle rigidity and hyperthermia: benzodiazepines
- For severe muscle rigidity not responding to benzodiazepines: neuromuscular blockade
- Cyproheptadine, 4 mg orally, may help

■ Pearl

Serotonin syndrome usually resolves within 24 hours after the offending agent is removed.

Reference

Gillman PK: The serotonin syndrome and its treatment. J Psychopharmacol 1999;13:100. [PMID: 10221364]

Theophylline

- **Essentials of Diagnosis**
  - A methylxanthine used to treat asthma and chronic obstructive pulmonary disease; intravenous form (aminophylline) is used to treat bronchospasm and neonatal apnea
  - Antagonizes adenosine receptors, releases endogenous catecholamines, and inhibits phosphodiesterase causing increase of intracellular cAMP
  - Sustained-release preparations; minimum toxic dose: 10 mg/kg
  - Acute ingestion causes vomiting, tremor, anxiety, tachycardia, hypokalemia, hyperglycemia, and metabolic acidosis; with severe overdose (serum level >80 mg/L): hypotension, ventricular arrhythmias, and seizures (resistant to treatment)
  - Chronic intoxication causes less vomiting; causes tachycardia, arrhythmias, and seizures at lower serum levels
  - Serum theophylline level and repeat level, serum glucose, electrolytes, BUN, creatinine, CPK, electrocardiogram

- **Differential Diagnosis**
  - Amphetamines
  - Other sympathomimetics (cocaine, caffeine, phenylpropanolamine)
  - Anticholinergics (antihistamines, tricyclic antidepressants, atropine)
  - Sedative-hypnotic withdrawal
  - Diabetic ketoacidosis

- **Treatment**
  - Activated charcoal, 1 g/kg, within 1–2 hours of ingestion; may repeat every 4 hours
  - Consider whole-bowel irrigation if sustained-release preparation is ingested
  - For seizures: benzodiazepines, phenobarbital, phenytoin
  - Hypokalemia usually resolves spontaneously without aggressive treatment
  - For tachyarrhythmias: propranolol or esmolol
  - For severe toxicity: charcoal hemoperfusion

- **Pearl**

Theophylline is one of the few toxins that is effectively removed by multiple doses of activated charcoal, dialysis, or charcoal hemoperfusion.

Reference

Shannon M: Life-threatening events after theophylline overdose. Arch Intern Med 1999;159:989. [PMID: 10326941]

Tricyclic Antidepressants

- **Essentials of Diagnosis**
  - Complex effects: anticholinergic, α-adrenergic-receptor blocking, and quinidine-like cardiac activity
  - Includes amitriptyline (Elavil), imipramine (Tofranil), doxepin (Sinequan), amoxapine, desipramine, and nortriptyline
  - Common cause of toxic deaths
  - Toxic dose causes dry mouth, mydriasis, agitation, tachycardia, seizures, and hallucinations; onset of coma may be precipitous
  - Cardiac effects: widening QRS complex, prolonged QT and PR intervals, atrioventricular block, ventricular tachycardia, profound hypotension
  - Consider serum glucose, electrolytes, BUN, creatinine, CPK, urinalysis, electrocardiogram, and head CT scan
  - Serum level not helpful for acute overdose

- **Differential Diagnosis**
  - Sympathomimetics (amphetamines, MDMA, cocaine, phenylpropanolamine)
  - Hallucinogenics (phencyclidine, LSD)
  - Sepsis
  - Sedative-hypnotic withdrawal

- **Treatment**
  - Activated charcoal, 1 g/kg, within 2–4 hours of ingestion (delayed gastrointestinal absorption)
  - Consider gastric lavage if <1 hour postingestion and lethal dose
  - Monitor electrocardiogram for QRS widening (>100 msec)
  - For agitation or seizures: benzodiazepines
  - For wide complex tachycardia: sodium bicarbonate, 1–2 mEq/kg IV bolus; lidocaine, 1–2 mg/kg IV bolus
  - For hypotension: 1–2 L crystalloid fluids; norepinephrine or epinephrine may be more effective than dopamine

- **Pearl**

Tricyclic antidepressant overdose patients go quickly from being awake and talking to coma, seizure, or pulselessness.

Reference

Kerr GW, McGuffie AC, Wilkie S: Tricyclic antidepressant overdose: a review. Emerg Med J 2001;18:236. [PMID: 11435353]

Warfarin & Other Anticoagulants

- ■ Essentials of Diagnosis
  - • Warfarin (Coumadin) used as therapeutic anticoagulant; other long-acting anticoagulants (super-warfarins) used as rodenticides
  - • Inhibit blood clotting by interfering with the synthesis of vitamin K–dependent clotting factors (II, VII, IX, X)
  - • Effects usually not seen until 1–2 days after ingestion due to long-half lives of clotting factors
  - • Multiple drug and food interactions increase or decrease antico-agulation effects
  - • Single overdose of warfarin does not usually cause significant bleeding because the half-life of warfarin is shorter than the half-lives of clotting factors; however, single overdose of super-warfarin may produce effects for months
  - • Chronic warfarin toxicity is more likely to produce serious bleeding
  - • Toxic dose causes ecchymosis, hematuria, uterine bleeding, melena, epistaxis, gingival bleeding, hematemesis, hematomas, cardiac tamponade, and intracranial hemorrhage
  - • CBC, international normalized ratio, liver enzymes, blood type

- ■ Differential Diagnosis
  - • Trauma
  - • Cirrhosis

- ■ Treatment
  - • Activated charcoal, 1 g/kg, within 1–2 hours of ingestion
  - • For major bleeding: fluid resuscitation; vitamin K, 5–10 mg IV; and fresh-frozen plasma, 15 mL/kg
  - • For asymptomatic abnormal international normalized ratio: vitamin K, 2–5 mg orally

- ■ Pearl

Accidental ingestion of super-warfarins by children does not usually cause serious bleeding.

Reference

Cruickshank, Ragg M, Eddey D: Warfarin toxicity in the emergency department: recommendations for management. Emerg Med (Freemantle) 2001;13: 91. [PMID: 11476421]

28

Pediatric Emergencies

Apnea

- **Essentials of Diagnosis**
    - Cessation of respiration for 20 seconds or more, *or* for any duration if pallor, cyanosis, or bradycardia is present
    - Apparent life-threatening event (ALTE): an apneic event that has associated change in color (pallor or cyanosis), muscle tone, or mental status
    - For stable patients, history is crucial to determine if a potentially significant event took place
    - History: where the event happened, who was with the infant and what they observed, when the infant was last fed, how long the episode lasted and was there associated color change or loss of muscle tone, what resuscitative measures were taken

- **Differential Diagnosis**
    - Sepsis
    - Meningitis
    - Respiratory syncytial virus: apnea may occur in up to 25% of infants <2 months; increased risk if baby was premature
    - Child abuse
    - Periodic breathing
    - Seizure
    - Infection
    - Airway obstruction
    - Ingestion
    - Breath-holding spell

- **Treatment**
    - For unstable patients: address ABCs emergently
    - For stable patients: testing and treatment guided by history and physical exam findings; admit for observation

- **Pearl**

Admit any infant with an ALTE, no matter how good he or she looks at the time of examination.

Reference

Farrell PA, Weiner GM, Lemons JA: SIDS, ALTE, apnea, and the use of home monitors. Pediatr Rev 2002;23:3. [PMID: 11773587]

Appendicitis

- ### Essentials of Diagnosis
  - Difficult and frequently delayed diagnosis in children <2 years due to nonspecific symptoms: vomiting, diarrhea, pain, fever, irritability, grunting
  - Most children <2 years have a perforated appendix (84%), due to an average of >4 days from symptom onset to diagnosis and subsequent surgical removal
  - Important part of differential diagnosis of abdominal pain in children >2 years
  - Classic progression is anorexia followed by vague periumbilical pain, with progression to vomiting and pain localization to the right lower quadrant
  - WBC frequently 11,000–15,000; neither sensitive nor specific for diagnostic purposes
  - Urinalysis may demonstrate WBCs, which may represent sterile pyuria associated with appendicitis and not a urinary tract infection
  - Abdominal x-rays: frequently nonspecific, unless a calcified appendicolith is present (<10% of all patients)
  - Imaging modalities of choice: ultrasound or CT (sensitivity and specificity >90% for both)

- ### Differential Diagnosis
  - Gastroenteritis
  - Constipation
  - Urinary tract infection
  - Pneumonia

- ### Treatment
  - Strong consideration or confirmation of appendicitis dictates prompt surgical referral
  - Intravenous fluids; nothing-by-mouth status
  - For patients who are septic or who have a suspected perforated appendix: antibiotics

- ### Pearl
Rely on the history, physical exam, and your clinical suspicion to enlist surgical consultation, because no test or combination of tests and exam findings is 100% reliable for diagnosis.

Reference

Rothrock SG, Pagane J: Acute appendicitis in children: emergency department diagnosis and management. Ann Emerg Med 2000;36:39. [PMID: 10874234]

Asthma

- **Essentials of Diagnosis**
  - Increased work of breathing (increased respiratory rate, nasal flaring, retractions, abdominal breathing)
  - Decreased or differential breath sounds
  - Prolonged expiratory phase
  - Wheezing
  - Chest x-ray for patients with first-time wheezing; not needed routinely for those with known asthma
  - Peak flow (PEFR) is a simple, inexpensive, objective measure of airway obstruction; can be used in school-aged children
  - Patients with prior ICU admission or intubation are high risk

- **Differential Diagnosis**
  - Bronchopulmonary dysplasia
  - Cystic fibrosis
  - Bronchiolitis
  - Bronchiectasis
  - Pneumonia
  - Aspiration
  - Foreign body
  - Tracheomalacia
  - Bronchial stenosis
  - Congestive heart failure
  - Vocal cord dysfunction

- **Treatment**
  - Avoid intubation, if at all possible
  - Mainstay of therapy: inhaled β-agonists
  - Nebulized albuterol, 2.5–5.0 mg every 20 minutes; goal of three treatments in the first hour or continuous treatments at 10–20 mg/h
  - Glucocorticoids (prednisone/prednisolone) early in treatment: initial dose, 2 mg/kg orally or IV, followed by 5- to 7-day course of 2 mg/kg/d divided twice daily (daily max = 80 mg)
  - For severe cases of respiratory distress, poor air movement, or rapid decompensation: epinephrine or terbutaline subcutaneously or IV

- **Pearl**

Put down your stethoscope and look at the child, because observation of work of breathing frequently reveals more than auscultation.

Reference

Baren JM, Zorc JJ: Contemporary approach to the emergency department management of pediatric asthma. Emerg Med Clin North Am 2002;20:115. [PMID: 11831222]

Bronchiolitis

- **Essentials of Diagnosis**
    - Usually caused by respiratory syncytial virus (RSV)
    - Occurs in annual epidemics from winter to early spring
    - Symptoms: cough, coryza, fever, wheezing, increased work of breathing, difficulty feeding
    - Symptoms vary significantly between patients; frequently peak between third and fifth days of illness
    - Risk factors for severe disease: age <3 months, prematurity, immunocompromised state, underlying pulmonary or cardiac disease
    - Diagnosis established on clinical grounds or by means of rapid diagnostic testing for RSV
    - Chest x-ray findings: usually include hyperexpansion or atelectasis

- **Differential Diagnosis**
    - Sepsis
    - Pneumonia
    - Asthma
    - Gastroesophageal reflux disease with aspiration

- **Treatment**
    - For infants with respiratory failure or apnea: emergently evaluate patient and address ABCs; may require nasal CPAP or intubation and mechanical ventilation
    - For bronchiolitis: general supportive measures are mainstay of treatment; oxygen and fluids as needed
    - Most infants and young children with bronchiolitis have a benign course; may be treated as outpatients
    - Primary reasons for hospital admission: hypoxemia, severe tachypnea, difficulty feeding, dehydration
    - Albuterol and racemic epinephrine have limited therapeutic roles; glucocorticoids have no proven benefit

- **Pearl**

Children with underlying cardiopulmonary disease, congenital heart disease, bronchopulmonary dysplasia, prematurity, or age less than 6 weeks and infants with congenital or acquired immune disorders are at high risk for severe RSV infection.

Reference

Steiner RW: Treating acute bronchiolitis associated with RSV. Am Fam Physician 2004;69:325. [PMID: 14765771]

Colic

- ■ **Essentials of Diagnosis**
  - • Daily paroxysms of crying and irritability, with onset in first few weeks of life, lasting several hours per day and usually occurring during evening hours
  - • Crying episodes not relieved by routine parental interventions such as feeding, burping, holding, rocking, or giving a pacifier
  - • Spontaneous improvement or resolution by age 3–4 months

- ■ **Differential Diagnosis**
  - • Gastroesophageal reflux
  - • Esophagitis
  - • Sandifer syndrome
  - • Urinary tract infection
  - • Corneal abrasion
  - • Ocular foreign body
  - • Hair tourniquet
  - • Septic joint
  - • Supraventricular tachycardia
  - • Intussusception
  - • Midgut volvulus
  - • Anal fissure
  - • Child abuse

- ■ **Treatment**
  - • No effective treatments
  - • Counsel parents as to natural history of this disorder and give reassurance
  - • Avoid formula changes
  - • Avoid medications with potentially toxic effects such as paregoric, hyoscyamine, or dicyclomine

- ■ **Pearl**

Perform a good history and physical examination that is sufficient to make the diagnosis of colic. It is a diagnosis of exclusion.

Reference

Hofer MA: Unexplained infant crying: an evolutionary perspective. Acta Paediatr 2002;91:491. [PMID: 12113311]

Congestive Heart Failure

- **Essentials of Diagnosis**
  - Primary cause in infancy and childhood: congenital heart disease
  - Clinical presentation in childhood are highly variable and may include any of the following: feeding difficulties or diaphoresis while feeding; growth failure or failure to thrive; tachycardia, often with a gallop rhythm; weak, thready pulses; cool, moist extremities and pallor; tachypnea, increased work of breathing or wheezing; hepatomegaly; jugular venous distention; peripheral edema (rare in infants)
  - Ancillary testing: chest x-ray, electrocardiogram, echocardiography

- **Differential Diagnosis**
  - Primary pulmonary disease
  - Anemia
  - Cardiac arrhythmias
  - Intrathoracic mass lesion

- **Treatment**
  - Determine underlying cause and initiate appropriate treatment
  - Ensure adequate oxygenation and ventilation
  - For severe pulmonary edema: morphine
  - For diuresis: furosemide, initial dose of 1 mg/kg
  - Inotropic support: digitalis is mainstay of therapy, but other inotropic agents (isoproterenol, dopamine, dobutamine) may be used in certain instances
  - Afterload and preload reduction agents: nitroprusside, nitroglycerin most commonly used

- **Pearl**

Have a high index of suspicion for this relatively uncommon pediatric disorder in the infant with tachycardia, respiratory distress, difficulty feeding, and hepatomegaly.

Reference

Kay JD, Colan SD, Graham TP Jr: Congestive heart failure in pediatric patients. Am Heart J 2001;142:923. [PMID: 11685182]

Dehydration

- **Essentials of Diagnosis**
  - Most commonly due to extensive vomiting or diarrhea
  - History will provide clues that infant or child should be dehydrated: decreased oral intake, decreased urine output, numerous episodes of vomiting or diarrhea
  - Estimation of dehydration is divided into three categories: mild (5%), moderate (10%), severe (15%)
  - Clinical signs and symptoms used to assess the degree of dehydration: acute weight loss (may be several kg), mental status (normal to hyperirritable or comatose), heart rate (normal to extremely tachycardic), delayed capillary refill time (normal <2 seconds), mucous membranes (moist to very dry), eyes (normal to very sunken), tears (normal/present to absent), blood pressure (normal to hypotensive)
  - Hypotension is a late finding in infants and children; reflects uncompensated shock (estimate 15% dehydration)
  - Electrolytes, BUN, creatinine, and urine specific gravity are helpful

- **Differential Diagnosis**
  - Shock

- **Treatment**
  - For mild dehydration: consider oral rehydration
  - For moderate to severe dehydration: initial 20 ml/kg bolus of isotonic fluids (normal saline or lactated Ringer's); reassess and repeat boluses until perfusion has improved
  - To calculate fluid losses, 1 gm of body wt = 1 cc of water; therefore, 1 kg = 1,000 cc; translate extent of dehydration into amount of fluid lost (deficit), ie, for a 10-kg child who is 10% dehydrated: $10 \text{ kg} \times 0.1 = 1\text{-kg}$ deficit (would require 1 L of intravenous fluids to replace the calculated deficit)
  - Calculate fluid deficit plus maintenance fluid requirements and replace over 24 hours for isotonic dehydration or over 48 hours for significant hypotonic or hypertonic dehydration

- **Pearl**

The degree of dehydration in infants is frequently underestimated; make sure the history and exam findings match.

Reference

Roberts KB: Fluid and electrolytes: parenteral fluid therapy. Pediatr Rev 2001;22:380. [PMID: 11691948]

Esophageal Foreign Body

- **Essentials of Diagnosis**
  - Have an index of suspicion for this diagnosis; caregivers will not always observe the child swallowing a foreign body
  - Most common esophageal foreign bodies are coins; pennies are the most commonly swallowed coins
  - Patients usually asymptomatic; can present with chest discomfort, drooling, or inability to swallow
  - Esophageal foreign bodies typically become lodged at one of three areas: at the cricopharyngeus muscle (the thoracic inlet), at the level of the aortic arch, or at the lower esophageal sphincter
  - Chest x-ray is gold standard for diagnosis; be sure that the film gets enough of the cervical area to see a "high" foreign body

- **Differential Diagnosis**
  - Airway foreign body
  - Retropharyngeal abscess (dysphagia)
  - Stomatitis (drooling and refusal to swallow)

- **Treatment**
  - Patients with coins impacted for less than 1 day may be observed as outpatients and have a follow-up chest x-ray to determine if passage has occurred
  - Esophageal disc batteries may produce electrical current and subsequent tissue injury; remove promptly
  - Removal of esophageal foreign bodies can be performed by several techniques (usually operator dependent): esophagoscopy (widely used, patient must undergo deep sedation or general anesthesia, use for all sharp objects), Bougienage (used to gently "push" items into the stomach), Foley catheter (insert past object, inflate balloon, and pull out the object through the oral cavity)
  - Don't use Foley catheter or Bougienage technique if object lodged 1–2 days or more

- **Pearl**

Be patient. Amazing things pass uneventfully.

Reference

McGahren ED: Esophageal foreign bodies. Pediatr Rev 1999;20:129. [PMID: 10208086]

Exanthems

- **Essentials of Diagnosis**
  - Illnesses that have exanthems often follow seasonal patterns; frequently have characteristic age group distributions
  - Historical clues to the cause include exposure to affected individuals, current medications, associated symptoms, and progression of the rash
  - Physical exam should focus on how ill the child appears, rash distribution and morphology, involvement of mucous membranes, and presence of lymphadenopathy or hepatosplenomegaly
  - Diagnosis usually made on clinical grounds; ancillary tests frequently unnecessary
  - Laboratory testing may require serology or cultures to determine offending agent

- **Differential Diagnosis**
  - Measles (rubeola virus)
  - Rubella
  - Erythema infectiosum
  - Enteroviruses (coxsackie, echovirus, and other enteroviruses)
  - Adenovirus
  - Chicken pox
  - Roseola
  - Lyme disease
  - Rocky Mountain spotted fever
  - Kawasaki disease
  - Gianotti-Crosti syndrome
  - Scarlet fever

- **Treatment**
  - For most viral agents: supportive treatment
  - For rickettsial and bacterial agents: appropriate antibiotics

- **Pearl**

Become proficient in the diagnosis of exanthems, to avoid making rash decisions.

Reference

Gable EK, Liu G, Morrell DS: Pediatric exanthems. Prim Care 2000;27:353. [PMID: 10815048]

Febrile Seizure

- **Essentials of Diagnosis**
  - Common; incidence of 2–5% in children aged 6 months to 5 years
  - Either simple or complex (atypical)
  - Simple febrile seizure: brief period of generalized, tonic-clonic activity associated with a febrile illness; onset within first 24 hours of fever
  - Complex or atypical febrile seizures (have any of the following features): occurrence more than 24 hours after onset of fever, duration >15 minutes, focal seizure, more than one discrete seizure event occurring during the illness, abnormal neurologic findings
  - Consider workup as dictated by exam; if child has an atypical seizure, consider head CT, lumbar puncture, and electrolytes
  - Risk of recurrence of febrile seizures is 30% after the first febrile seizure and increases to 50% with the second febrile seizure; risk is higher in infants <1 year of age (50%) or if family history of seizures is present
  - Risk of developing epilepsy (recurrent seizures not associated with fever) is 1% in the general population; risk increases to 2% with known febrile seizures

- **Differential Diagnosis**
  - Epilepsy
  - Breath-holding episodes
  - Infantile spasms
  - Benign paroxysmal vertigo
  - Sandifer syndrome

- **Treatment**
  - For simple febrile seizures: antiepileptic drugs not indicated
  - For prolonged atypical febrile seizures: lorazepam, phosphenytoin or phenobarbital may be needed

- **Pearl**

Seizures are extremely frightening events for parents to witness. Being able to provide information and reassurance to parents is crucial in this situation.

Reference

Warden CR et al: Evaluation and management of febrile seizures in the out-of-hospital and emergency department settings. Ann Emerg Med 2003;41:215. [PMID: 12548271]

Fever in Children Aged <3 Months

- **Essentials of Diagnosis**
  - Fever (≥100.4°F [38°C]) in infancy dictates thorough evaluation based on age and risk for serious bacterial illness
  - Infants ≤30 days old are at high risk for serious illness with pathogens reflecting maternal flora including group B *Streptococcus, Streptococcus pneumoniae, Escherichia coli, Klebsiella* sp., *Listeria monocytogenes, Haemophilus influenzae,* enterococci, and herpes simplex virus
  - Infants presenting with fever at ≤30 days old should have a complete evaluation: CBC, blood culture, urinalysis with culture, lumbar puncture with CSF analysis and culture, and chest x-ray if indicated
  - Infants 30–90 days of age may need limited or no workup if they meet low-risk criteria (Rochester, Philadelphia, or Boston criteria) or if a viral source is proved; if not, consider workup as for infants ≤30 days old

- **Differential Diagnosis**
  - Bacteremia
  - Sepsis
  - Meningitis
  - Urinary tract infection
  - Pneumonia
  - Omphalitis
  - Acute otitis media
  - Cellulitis
  - Viral illness (eg, respiratory syncytial virus, influenza, herpes virus, cytomegalovirus)

- **Treatment**
  - For infants ≤30 days old: intravenous antibiotics (ampicillin and gentamicin or ampicillin and cefotaxime), hospitalization
  - For infants >30 days old: treatment based on risk stratification and potential diagnosis; low-risk criteria are met, may withhold antibiotics and arrange for close follow-up; consider ampicillin plus either ceftriaxone or cefotaxime

- **Pearl**

Fever may be conspicuously absent in septic infants because they are frequently hypothermic.

Reference

King C: Evaluation and management of febrile infants in the emergency department. Emerg Med Clin North Am 2003;21:89. [PMID: 12630733]

Fever in Children Aged 3–36 Months

- **■ Essentials of Diagnosis**
  - Fever (≥100.4°F [38°C]) is one of the most common presenting complaints in pediatric emergency medicine
  - Myriad of commonly recognized conditions cause fever in this age group
  - For children with fever without a source, assess for serious bacterial illness
  - In post–Hib vaccine era, rates of occult bacteremia have dropped to less than 2% and will probably decline even further with introduction of universal pneumococcal immunization
  - Rates of urinary tract infection in girls <2 years of age reach 8% and peak for males <1 year of age at 3.3%
  - Rate of radiographic pneumonia is 7% with fever and tachypnea for age; occult pneumonia is present in 26% of patients with a WBC >20,000 and a temperature of >102.2°F (39°C)
  - Choose tests according to risk and clinical suspicion

- **■ Differential Diagnosis**
  - Acute otitis media
  - Upper and lower respiratory tract infections
  - Viral illness
  - Sepsis
  - Bacteremia
  - Meningitis
  - Urinary tract infection
  - Pneumonia

- **■ Treatment**
  - For children with an identifiable source of fever: treat illness according to standard of care
  - Recognize viral syndromes and avoid treatment with antibiotics
  - For the well-appearing child with fever and no identifiable source of fever: consider empiric antibiotics when WBC >15,000 and temperature >102.2°F (39°C)

- **■ Pearl**

Being able to recognize the myriad common viral illnesses that affect this age group will enable you to avoid unnecessary testing and overtreatment of viral illness with antibiotics.

Reference

Steere M, Sharieff GQ, Stenklyft PH: Fever in children less than 36 months of age—questions and strategies for management in the emergency department. J Emerg Med 2003;25:149. [PMID: 12902000]

Hemolytic Uremic Syndrome

■ Essentials of Diagnosis

- Caused by infection with a toxin-producing agent, most commonly *Escherichia coli* 0157:H7; others implicated include *Shigella, Salmonella, Yersinia, S. pneumoniae, Campylobacter,* varicella, echovirus, and coxsackievirus
- Peak incidence occurs between 6 months and 4 years of age
- Prodrome of abdominal pain and diarrhea, followed by bloody diarrhea with or without fever
- After 5–7 days, abrupt onset of pallor, petechiae, listlessness to obtundation, oliguria, hypertension, and hepatomegaly
- Diagnosis based on typical clinical picture of hemolytic anemia, thrombocytopenia, and acute renal failure
- Specific laboratory findings: anemia (hemoglobin may be as low as 5–9 g/dL); platelet count as low as 20,000/mm^3; urinalysis with hematuria, proteinuria, and WBCs; azotemia, metabolic acidosis, hyperbilirubinemia, and elevated LDH
- Routine stool culture will not yield *E coli* 0157:H7; detection is by use of specialized antiserum to identify *E coli* 0157:H7 antigen

■ Differential Diagnosis

- Sepsis
- Autoimmune hemolytic anemia
- Idiopathic thrombocytopenia purpura
- Thrombotic thrombocytopenia purpura

■ Treatment

- Primarily supportive; control hypertension; transfusions as needed
- Dialysis if BUN >100, congestive heart failure, encephalopathy, or hyperkalemia
- Use of antimicrobial therapy is controversial; no scientific evidence currently supports antibiotic use

■ Pearl

The hemolytic uremic syndrome triad consists of hemolytic anemia, thrombocytopenia, and renal failure.

Reference

Corrigan JJ Jr, Boineau FG: Hemolytic-uremic syndrome. Pediatr Rev 2001;22:365. Erratum in Pediatr Rev 2002;23:1. [PMID: 11691946]

Henoch-Schönlein Purpura

- ■ Essentials of Diagnosis
  - A vasculitis characterized by rash, joint swelling, abdominal pain, renal involvement, and occasionally scrotal involvement
  - Rash is purpuric and symmetric and usually involves legs, buttocks, and less commonly arms; in infants the face may be affected
  - Arthritis and subsequent arthralgias affect the larger joints and are migratory
  - Abdominal pain occurs in many affected individuals; may be colicky and severe; submucosal hemorrhage may occur and can serve as a lead point for intussusception
  - Renal involvement is variable; usually consists of asymptomatic microscopic hematuria (80%); transient azotemia may be present
  - Scrotal involvement may occur in approximately 30% of patients; usually follows onset of rash and joint and abdominal pain by several days; may last for a week or more
  - Laboratory studies: CBC, chemistries, serum proteins, and C3 complement; all generally normal
  - Urinalysis frequently demonstrates microscopic hematuria
  - Platelet count and coagulation tests normal

- ■ Differential Diagnosis
  - Meningococcemia (purpura fulminans)
  - Appendicitis
  - Intussusception

- ■ Treatment
  - Usually symptomatic treatment, unless patient is having severe joint or abdominal pain, in which case corticosteroids are beneficial

- ■ Pearl
  The rash of Henoch-Schönlein purpura generally looks bad, but the patient feels well; this is an important distinguishing characteristic between Henoch-Schönlein purpura and meningococcemia.

Reference

Ballinger S: Henoch-Schonlein purpura. Curr Opin Rheumatol 2003;15:591. [PMID: 12960486]

Intussusception

- **Essentials of Diagnosis**
  - Occurs when proximal portion of bowel telescopes into distal segment of intestine; most common location is ileocolic (90%)
  - Most cases are idiopathic, although lymphoid hyperplasia is present in approximately 90% of all cases and usually occurs in children <2 years
  - Children >2 years often have pathologic lead point (10% of cases), such as a Meckel diverticulum, polyps, cystic fibrosis, neoplasm, Henoch-Schönlein purpura, or Peutz-Jeghers syndrome
  - Most common cause of intestinal obstruction in children between 3 and 12 months of age
  - Classic triad: intermittent abdominal pain, vomiting, and bloody (currant jelly) stools; present as a triad in 10–20% of patients
  - 80–95% have intermittent abdominal pain; child often appears normal between episodes
  - 70% present with vomiting; may become bilious
  - 75–80% have grossly bloody or hemoccult-positive stools
  - 60–85% have a palpable right upper quadrant mass
  - Profound, isolated lethargy: unclear mechanism, may be due to endogenous opioid release triggered by ischemic bowel
  - Plain x-rays may show soft tissue mass in right upper quadrant, absence of gas and stool, and loss of visualization of tip of liver
  - Ultrasound: sensitive and specific means of diagnosis
  - CT helpful in older children; may identify a lead point
  - Barium or air contrast enema is diagnostic and curative

- **Differential Diagnosis**
  - Incarcerated hernia
  - Malrotation
  - Volvulus
  - Gastroenteritis

- **Treatment**
  - Stabilize patient; give intravenous fluids
  - Barium and air contrast enemas usually curative; success rate is 80% for barium and 95% for air
  - Surgical consult for perforation or if irreducible

- **Pearl**

Consider intussusception in the differential of lethargy.

Reference

D'Agostino J: Common abdominal emergencies in children. Emerg Med Clin North Am 2002;20:139. [PMID: 11826631]

Meckel Diverticulum

- ■ Essentials of Diagnosis
  - A remnant of the omphalomesenteric duct located in the small intestine; may contain ectopic gastric mucosa; usually located within 50–75 cm of the ileocecal valve
  - 2% of the population is born with a Meckel diverticulum, although only 2% of patients with a Meckel diverticulum ever manifest a clinical problem
  - Most common clinical presentation: rectal bleeding, which may or may not be painful
  - Bleeding is due to gastric acid secretion from the ectopic gastric mucosa, which leads to a bleeding ulcer
  - Bleeding may be minimal or severe; may cause bright red to tarry stools
  - Average age at presentation is 2 years old; rare in children over age 5 years
  - Index of suspicion needed for this diagnosis; routine radiographic tests not diagnostic
  - Radiographic test of choice is nuclear scintigraphy; will demonstrate a well-defined area of uptake of the 99m-technetium pertechnetate in the distal small bowel that will correspond with the uptake seen in the stomach; diagnostic for an area of ectopic gastric mucosa
  - Routine lab tests not beneficial for diagnostic purposes, although with extensive bleeding, anemia may be present

- ■ Differential Diagnosis
  - Intestinal duplication containing gastric mucosa
  - Diverticulitis
  - Intestinal perforation with peritonitis
  - Intussusception with the Meckel diverticulum as a lead point

- ■ Treatment
  - Surgical resection of the affected area is curative

- ■ Pearl

Remember the "rule of twos" for Meckel diverticulum: it occurs in 2% of the population, is 2 inches in length (or less), and typically is located within 2 feet of the ileocecal valve.

Reference

McCollough M, Sharieff GQ: Abdominal surgical emergencies in infants and young children. Emerg Med Clin North Am 2003;21:909. [PMID: 14708813]

Meningitis

- **Essentials of Diagnosis**
  - Most common causes: bacteria and viruses
  - Aseptic meningitis: meningitis caused by any agent not demonstrated on Gram stain
  - Most common viral pathogens: enteroviruses
  - Most common bacterial pathogens: 0–3 months, group B *Streptococcus, Escherichia coli* and other gram-negative enteric organisms, *Listeria monocytogenes;* ≥3 months, *Streptococcus pneumoniae, Neisseria meningitidis, Haemophilus influenzae* (if unimmunized)
  - Clinical signs and symptoms vary among age groups: 0–3 months, paradoxical irritability, altered sleep, vomiting, lethargy, bulging fontanelle, shock; 4–24 months, irritability, altered sleep, lethargy, fever, nuchal rigidity (some will argue difficult to tell even up to 1 year), coma, shock; >24 months, headache, neck pain, lethargy, photophobia, fever, nuchal rigidity, irritability, coma, shock
  - Diagnosis made by lumbar puncture to obtain CSF for WBC count and differential, glucose, protein, Gram stain, and culture
  - Always obtain a culture, but result takes several days

- **Differential Diagnosis**
  - Retropharyngeal abscess
  - Pharyngitis
  - Cervical adenitis
  - Osteomyelitis of the spine
  - Intracranial hemorrhage

- **Treatment**
  - Rapid administration (within 30 minutes) of presentation of broad-spectrum intravenous antibiotics: <1 month of age, ampicillin and cefotaxime, 50 mg/kg each or ampicillin and gentamicin 2.5 mg/kg; >1 month of age, vancomycin, 15 mg/kg, and either cefotaxime, 75 mg/kg, or ceftriaxone, 50 mg/kg
  - Consider dexamethasone, 0.15 mg/kg, prior to initial antibiotics; studies have shown a reduction in hearing loss and neurologic sequelae

- **Pearl**

If meningitis is in the differential, do the lumbar puncture.

Reference

Bonthius DJ, Karacay B: Meningitis and encephalitis in children. An update. Neurol Clin 2002;20:1013. [PMID: 12616679]

Osteomyelitis

- **Essentials of Diagnosis**
  - An inflammation of the bone, usually with an infectious cause
  - More common in boys; higher incidence in infants and preschool children
  - Routes of infection: hematogenous spread, direct spread, or inoculation via a penetrating wound
  - Fever in up to 90% of affected children
  - Other findings are age dependent and related to pain: infants may demonstrate paradoxical irritability or refuse to move the affected limb; toddlers may manifest irritability or simply present with a limp, refusal to walk, or refusal to move an arm; older children may be able to localize pain
  - Decreased range of motion and pain with movement occur in all age groups
  - Laboratory findings: WBC elevated in approximately 33%, ESR and CRP elevated in more than 90% of cases
  - Obtain blood cultures and consider bone aspirate for culture prior to starting antibiotics
  - Plain x-rays show soft-tissue swelling 3–4 days after symptoms, lytic bone at 7–10 days
  - Triple-phase technetium bone scan: sensitivity and specificity >90% within 24–48 hours of symptom onset

- **Differential Diagnosis**
  - Septic arthritis
  - Transient synovitis
  - Neoplasm
  - Vertebral discitis
  - Fracture

- **Treatment**
  - Consult an orthopedic surgeon prior to initiating therapy
  - Obtain cultures and admit for intravenous antibiotics; oxacillin or nafcillin, consider vancomycin if high likelihood of methicillin-resistant *Staphylococcus aureus,* and consider addition of gentamicin for neonates

- **Pearl**

Fever, bone pain, and elevated ESR or CRP equals osteomyelitis until proven otherwise.

Reference

Vazquez M: Osteomyelitis in children. Curr Opin Pediatr 2002;14:112. [PMID: 11880745]

Otitis Media, Acute

- **Essentials of Diagnosis**
  - Most common bacterial pathogens: *Streptococcus pneumoniae, Haemophilus influenzae, Moraxella catarrhalis*
  - Viral pathogens: account for approximately 50% of infections
  - Young children often present with nonspecific symptoms: poor sleeping, fussiness, poor feeding, vomiting or diarrhea
  - In older children, ear pain is most frequent complaint
  - At any age, child may be afebrile or have low-grade fever
  - High fever (>40°C or 104°F) should prompt search for another source for the fever (eg, bacteremia, pneumonia)
  - Tympanic membrane may rupture, causing pus to exude from ear canal
  - Pneumatic otoscopy demonstrating decreased mobility of the tympanic membrane is both sensitive and specific for diagnosis
  - Other findings: loss of landmarks, decreased or absent light reflex, bulging tympanic membrane
  - Erythema or hyperemia of tympanic membrane not very specific; may be due to fever or may be seen in a child who is screaming or crying

- **Differential Diagnosis**
  - Otogenic causes: otitis externa, foreign body, cerumen impaction, tympanic perforation, hemotympanum, cholesteatoma
  - Nonotogenic causes: stomatitis, dental caries or abscess, parotitis, temporomandibular joint dysfunction, mastoiditis, lymphadenitis

- **Treatment**
  - Infants <30 days old: evaluation to rule out sepsis; hospitalize for initial intravenous antibiotic therapy
  - First-line therapy: amoxicillin, 60–90 mg/kg/d divided twice daily
  - Second-line therapy: amoxicillin/clavulanate, 80 mg/kg/d divided twice daily, cefdinir; cefuroxime axetil; or ceftriaxone
  - Children <2 years: oral antibiotics for 10 days; children >2 years with uncomplicated cases: may be treated for 5 days
  - For recurrent or refractory cases: tympanostomy tubes

- **Pearl**

Proficiency in pneumatic otoscopy reduces overdiagnosis of otitis media.

Reference

Takata GS et al: Evidence assessment of management of acute otitis media: I. the role of antibiotics in treatment of uncomplicated acute otitis media. Pediatrics 2001;108:239. [PMID: 11483783]

Periorbital Cellulitis

- **Essentials of Diagnosis**
  - Periorbital or preseptal cellulitis is an infection of the eyelids that does not extend into the posterior orbit
  - Periorbital cellulitis must be differentiated from orbital cellulitis, which may be a potentially vision- or life-threatening condition
  - Periorbital cellulitis is usually unilateral and presents with a swollen, erythematous, and tender eyelid with normal visual acuity and eye movements
  - In cases with severe eyelid swelling where ocular motility cannot be evaluated, a CT scan of the orbits will distinguish between periorbital and orbital cellulitis
  - Laboratory evaluation generally not helpful in diagnosis

- **Differential Diagnosis**
  - Orbital cellulitis
  - Insect bite or sting
  - Allergic reaction
  - Sinusitis
  - Conjunctivitis
  - Trauma to the eye or eyelids

- **Treatment**
  - For children who do not appear systemically ill: outpatient treatment
  - Mainstay of therapy: oral antibiotics effective against *Staphylococcus* and *Streptococcus*
  - Follow-up within 24–48 hours; patients not improving or who are getting worse should be hospitalized for intravenous antibiotic therapy

- **Pearl**

Perform a CT scan to rule out orbital cellulitis for all children in whom age makes a reliable eye examination difficult.

Reference

Givner LB: Periorbital versus orbital cellulitis. Pediatr Infect Dis J 2002;21:1157. [PMID: 12488668]

Pharyngitis

■ Essentials of Diagnosis

- Respiratory viruses account for majority of infectious cases of pharyngitis (70–80%): adenovirus, coxsackievirus, Epstein-Barr virus (EBV), cytomegalovirus (CMV), rhinoviruses, parainfluenza, and influenza
- Group A β-hemolytic *Streptococcus* (GABHS) is the most common bacteria causing pharyngitis in children (20–30%)
- Diagnostic clues may provide key to diagnosis: age <3 years, almost exclusively viral pathogens; pharyngitis with conjunctivitis is likely due to adenovirus; erythematous ulcers on posterior palate are due to coxsackievirus A (herpangina); significant cervical adenopathy, "kissing tonsils," and hepatosplenomegaly are most likely due to EBV and less commonly due to CMV
- No absolute diagnostic criteria for GABHS; suggestive features include fever, tender cervical adenopathy, palatal petechiae, and absence of upper respiratory symptoms; other associations include scarlatiniform rash, headache, abdominal pain, nausea, and vomiting.
- Diagnosis of GABHS is made with rapid antigen testing or throat culture

■ Differential Diagnosis

- Cervical lymphadenitis
- Peritonsillar abscess or cellulitis
- Retropharyngeal abscess

■ Treatment

- For viral pharyngitis: supportive care
- For GABHS: treatment required to prevent rheumatic heart disease; oral penicillin V or amoxicillin for 10 days
- If compliance is an issue, long-acting benzathine penicillin may be given as a one-time intramuscular dose
- Penicillin-allergic patients may take erythromycin, cephalosporins, or clindamycin

■ Pearl

Use rapid diagnostic testing for diagnosis and to guide therapy because it is more accurate than clinical signs or symptoms.

Reference

Attia MW, Bennett JE: Pediatric pharyngitis. Pediatr Case Rev 2003;3:203. [PMID: 14520082]

Physical Abuse

- ■ **Essentials of Diagnosis**
  - Bruising is most common abusive injury; look at location, pattern, and marks (eg, cord, belt, buckle)
  - Fractures in any child <1 year old should raise possibility of abuse; special concerns: rib fractures (<2 years), femur fractures (<3 years), and any metaphyseal chip fracture (virtually diagnostic of abuse)
  - Head injury results in highest morbidity and mortality in abused children; injuries due to direct impact or shaking and resulting in axonal injury or CNS hemorrhage; look for associated retinal hemorrhages
  - Burns: evaluate based on history and burn distribution; immersion in hot water may be used as a means of discipline and frequently causes burns to the feet and buttocks
  - Diagnosis can be made only if clinician suspects abuse
  - Ancillary tests: skeletal series, head CT, MRI, coagulation tests, amylase, lipase, liver enzymes, urinalysis

- ■ **Differential Diagnosis**
  - Mongolian spots
  - Idiopathic thrombocytopenia purpura
  - Ehlers-Danlos syndrome
  - Henoch-Schönlein purpura
  - Metabolic bone disease
  - Osteogenesis imperfecta
  - Acute abdomen

- ■ **Treatment**
  - Acute management dictated by specific type of injury
  - Make sure the infant or child is not discharged into an unsafe environment; enlist social services assistance

- ■ **Pearl**

Have a high index of suspicion for child abuse when the child has traumatic injuries that do not match the history.

Reference

Listman DA, Bechtel K: Accidental and abusive head injury in young children. Curr Opin Pediatr 2003;15:299. [PMID: 12806261]

Pneumonia

- **Essentials of Diagnosis**
  - Signs and symptoms suggestive of viral cause: nontoxic appearance, preceding upper respiratory infection symptoms, gradual onset, diffuse findings on auscultation (wheezing)
  - Signs and symptoms suggestive of bacterial cause: acute onset of high fever, grunting respirations, inspiratory rales, decreased breath sounds
  - Tachypnea common in both viral and bacterial pneumonia
  - Respiratory viruses predominate in infants and younger children with pneumonia and commonly include respiratory syncytial virus, influenza, parainfluenza, and adenovirus
  - Bacterial pathogens vary by age group and include group B *Streptococcus, Escherichia coli,* and *Listeria monocytogenes* in neonates; *Chlamydia trachomatis* in infants aged 1–3 months; *Streptococcus pneumoniae* in children aged 3 months to 5 years; and *Mycoplasma pneumoniae, Chlamydia pneumoniae,* and *S pneumoniae* in school-aged children
  - Diagnosis of both viral and bacterial pneumonia is made by combination of exam findings and chest radiography
  - Chest x-ray findings: viral pneumonia (normal to hyperinflation, atelectasis, or patchy infiltrates), bacterial pneumonia (lobar consolidation is classic; pleural effusion may be present)
  - Laboratory findings: WBC is frequently >15,000 with bacterial pneumonia

- **Differential Diagnosis**
  - Bronchiolitis
  - Asthma
  - Foreign body
  - Empyema
  - Pertussis

- **Treatment**
  - For viral pneumonia: supportive care
  - For bacterial pneumonia: supportive care and antibiotics (amoxicillin or ceftriaxone) or macrolide antibiotics for atypical agents (*Mycoplasma* or *C pneumoniae*)

- **Pearl**

Atelectasis is frequently misdiagnosed as lobar consolidation in differentiating viral versus bacterial pneumonia on chest x-ray.

Reference

Lichenstein R, Suggs AH, Campbell J: Pediatric pneumonia. Emerg Med Clin North Am 2003;21:437. [PMID: 12793623]

Pyloric Stenosis

- ■ Essentials of Diagnosis
    - • Caused by hypertrophy of the pyloric musculature, resulting in a gastric outflow obstruction
    - • Male-to-female ratio is 5:1; usual presentation between 2 and 6 weeks of age
    - • Projectile vomiting but without blood or bile
    - • Infants hungry all of the time
    - • Infants with a prolonged course before diagnosis may present with weight loss and significant electrolyte abnormalities secondary to gastric losses
    - • Firm, elongated mass, known as an "olive" palpated in the right upper quadrant
    - • Significant gastric peristaltic waves that move from left to right in an attempt to empty the stomach can be seen
    - • Laboratory finding: hypochloremic, hypokalemic, metabolic alkalosis secondary to gastric losses
    - • Ultrasound of the pylorus is test of choice to confirm diagnosis

- ■ Differential Diagnosis
    - • Gastroesophageal reflux
    - • Esophageal or intestinal webs
    - • Hirschsprung disease
    - • Increased intracranial pressure

- ■ Treatment
    - • Intravenous fluids to correct fluid and electrolyte status
    - • When the infant is well hydrated and the electrolytes are corrected, surgical pyloromyotomy should be performed

- ■ Pearl
    Classic findings are an "olive" in the right upper quadrant and a hypochloremic, hypokalemic, metabolic alkalosis.

Reference

Letton RW Jr: Pyloric stenosis. Pediatr Ann 2001;30:745. [PMID: 11766203]

Septic Arthritis

- **Essentials of Diagnosis**
  - Presence of bacterial pathogens within the articular capsule
  - Delay in diagnosis or treatment can result in severe and permanent disability
  - Routes of infection: hematogenous spread, direct spread, or inoculation via a penetrating wound
  - 80–90% of cases occur in lower extremities; knee and hip affected most commonly
  - 90% of cases involve single joints; multiple infected joints more common in infants
  - Pain is most common presenting complaint: infants exhibit paradoxical irritability or refusal to move a limb; toddlers limp or refuse to bear weight; older children more likely to accurately localize pain
  - Range of motion is restricted and causes significant distress
  - Laboratory tests: WBC >15,000 in less than 50% of cases, ESR and/or CRP elevated in more than 90–95% of cases
  - Plain x-rays may demonstrate blurring or widening of joint space
  - Ultrasound useful in diagnosis of a septic hip but does not distinguish infected versus sterile fluid
  - Diagnosis confirmed by arthrocentesis with presence of purulent fluid in joint space

- **Differential Diagnosis**
  - Osteomyelitis
  - Transient synovitis
  - Neoplasm
  - Fracture

- **Treatment**
  - Emergent orthopedic consult
  - Intravenous antibiotics: oxacillin or nafcillin; consider vancomycin if high likelihood of methicillin-resistant *Staphylococcus aureus;* add gentamicin for neonates

- **Pearl**

The sun should never rise or set on an untreated septic hip.

Reference

Shetty AK, Gedalia A: Septic arthritis in children. Rheum Dis Clin North Am 1998;24:287. [PMID: 9606760]

Sexual Abuse

- ■ Essentials of Diagnosis
  - Involvement of children or adolescents in sexual activities beyond their developmental level, activities for which they are unable to give consent, or activities that violate social norms
  - Most victims are female; mean age 7–8 years
  - Younger children most commonly molested by males who are well known to them; unlikely to disclose the event
  - Adolescents more frequently molested by strangers
  - Children who have been sexually assaulted within 72 hours of presentation should be evaluated immediately and have evidence collection performed by a knowledgeable health care professional
  - If the reported sexual assault occurred more than 72 hours prior to seeking medical care, examination should be deferred and child should be referred to a center that provides specialized services to child victims of sexual abuse
  - Symptoms of sexual abuse are varied; may range from behavioral problems to physical evidence of genital injury
  - Most common finding is a normal genital exam
  - Genital injuries: contusions, lacerations, abrasions, hymenal injury
  - Perform age-appropriate exam and collect evidence; consider Gram stain, wet prep, cultures, hepatitis B and HIV serology
  - *Neisseria gonorrhoeae* and syphilis are virtually diagnostic of sexual abuse in prepubertal children beyond infancy; other sexually transmitted diseases are less diagnostic because they may be transmitted by nonsexual routes

- ■ Differential Diagnosis
  - Urethral prolapse
  - Perianal streptococcal disease
  - Lichen sclerosis

- ■ Treatment
  - Treat physical injuries and sexually transmitted diseases
  - Offer pregnancy prophylaxis and consider HIV prophylaxis for high-risk encounters

- ■ Pearl

Do not perform sexual abuse evaluations in children unless you have developed expertise in this area.

Reference

Atabaki S, Paradise JE: The medical evaluation of the sexually abused child: lessons learned from a decade of research. Pediatrics 1999;104:178. [PMID: 10390286]

Upper Airway Obstruction

- **Essentials of Diagnosis**
  - Hallmark is stridor
  - Laryngotracheobronchitis (croup): usually due to parainfluenza virus; consists of brief upper respiratory infection prodrome followed by acute stridor, a "seal-barking" cough, and hoarseness
  - Epiglottitis: rare in post-Hib era; now seen more in adults; due to staphylococci or streptococci; manifested by acute onset of drooling and varying amounts of respiratory distress
  - Retropharyngeal abscess: due to mixed bacterial flora (oral); insidious onset over several days; presentation often with drooling or dysphagia
  - Bacterial tracheitis: due to *Staphylococcus aureus;* high fever, painful cough, and toxic appearance
  - X-ray findings: "steeple" sign in croup; "thumb" sign in epiglottitis; widened prevertebral soft tissues in retropharyngeal abscess; shaggy trachea in bacterial tracheitis

- **Differential Diagnosis**
  - Croup
  - Epiglottitis
  - Retropharyngeal abscess
  - Bacterial tracheitis
  - Laryngomalacia
  - Tracheal compression or foreign body
  - Laryngeal or tracheal polyps

- **Treatment**
  - For croup: cool mist; oxygen; nebulized racemic epinephrine; dexamethasone, 0.6 mg/kg; heliox
  - Epiglottitis: airway stabilization; emergency ENT consult; cefuroxime, 50 mg/kg, or cefotaxime, 50 mg/kg
  - Retropharyngeal abscess: airway stabilization; ampicillin/sulbactam, 200 mg/kg/d divided every 6 hours, or clindamycin, 40 mg/kg IV every 6 hours; ENT consult for incision and drainage
  - Bacterial tracheitis: airway stabilization; vancomycin, 15 mg/kg, and ceftriaxone, 100 mg/kg

- **Pearl**

Inspiratory stridor usually indicates extrathoracic pathology, whereas expiratory stridor is usually associated with an intrathoracic compression of the trachea.

Reference

Baines PB, Sarginson RE: Upper airway obstruction. Hosp Med 2004;65:108. [PMID: 14997779]

Urinary Tract Infection

- ■ **Essentials of Diagnosis**
    - *Escherichia coli* responsible for majority of urinary tract infections
    - Clinical manifestations are variable and age dependent: neonates have fever or sepsis; infants present with fever, vomiting, diarrhea, irritability; children >2 years of age have symptoms more consistent with urinary tract (dysuria, suprapubic pain, flank pain)
    - For practical purposes, febrile (>101.2°F [38.4°C]) children should be presumed to have pyelonephritis
    - Diagnosis made by urinalysis and urine culture
    - Collect urine by catheterization or suprapubic aspiration (for males <6 months of age and females <2 years of age)
    - Toilet-trained children may provide clean-catch specimens
    - Absence of leukocyte esterase (LE) or nitrite on the urine dipstick is not sensitive enough to rule out infection
    - Negative LE and nitrite, in combination with absence of pyuria on microscopy, makes infection highly unlikely (applies to males >6 months and females >2 years)

- ■ **Differential Diagnosis**
    - Bubble bath or chemical vaginitis
    - Pinworms

- ■ **Treatment**
    - Intravenous antibiotics: if <3 months of age, or for any toxicity, vomiting, abnormal urinary tract anatomy, or resistant infections
    - Oral antibiotics such as trimethoprim-sulfamethoxazole (TMP-SMZ), cefixime, or amoxicillin
    - Treat pyelonephritis for 10–14 days; cystitis for 7 days

- ■ **Pearl**

Urinary tract infection is the most common bacterial illness in febrile infants and toddlers who present with fever and no source of infection.

Reference

Santen SA, Altieri MF: Pediatric urinary tract infection. Emerg Med Clin North Am 2001;19:675. [PMID: 11554281]

Volvulus

- ■ Essentials of Diagnosis
  - Malrotation: due to an incomplete or reverse rotation of the embryonic midgut about the superior mesenteric artery, which results in an abnormal fixation of the mesentery of the bowel
  - Volvulus: occurs when midgut twists around the mesenteric stalk, causing vascular compromise and small bowel obstruction
  - Malrotation with volvulus most commonly occurs in utero or during the neonatal period
  - Clinical presentation: sudden onset of abdominal pain and bilious emesis in an infant or child who was previously well; sudden onset of small bowel obstruction in an infant who has had previous feeding difficulties with transient episodes of bilious emesis; children with failure to thrive and chronic vomiting
  - Physical findings: abdominal distention; distended loops of bowel on abdominal palpation; tenderness to palpation, progressing to peritoneal signs; gross blood in the stool or on rectal examination
  - Diagnosis based on radiographic findings: flat and upright films with duodenal obstruction (double bubble sign); upper GI series shows displacement of the duodenal-jejunal junction to the right of the spine and displacement of the jejunum and cecum to the right upper quadrant

- ■ Differential Diagnosis
  - Sepsis
  - Intussusception
  - Meckel diverticulum
  - Necrotizing enterocolitis

- ■ Treatment
  - Intravenous fluids to correct shock, nasogastric tube, blood type, and cross-match
  - Immediate surgical correction (Ladd procedure)

- ■ Pearl

Strongly consider malrotation with volvulus in any infant or child who presents with bilious emesis and abdominal pain.

Reference

McCollough M, Sharieff GQ: Abdominal surgical emergencies in infants and young children. Emerg Med Clin North Am 2003;21:909. [PMID: 14708813]

29

Nuclear, Biologic, & Chemical Agents of Terrorism

Anthrax

- **Essentials of Diagnosis**
  - Disease forms: inhalational, gastrointestinal, cutaneous
  - Biologic attack would likely involve the aerosol release of anthrax spores causing inhalational disease: initial symptoms of fatigue, malaise, minimal or nonproductive cough, then fever, nausea, vomiting, and drenching sweats, followed by chest pain and dyspnea; average time from onset of symptoms to death is 3 days with overall mortality once initial symptoms develop of 95%
  - Gastrointestinal anthrax: (1) oral or esophageal ulcers followed by regional lymphadenopathy and sepsis or (2) abdominal anthrax with lower abdominal symptoms of nausea, vomiting, bloody diarrhea, acute abdomen, and sepsis; mortality over 50%
  - Cutaneous anthrax: causes pruritic papule that develops into ulcer, vesicle, and painless eschar; regional lymphadenopathy and occasional sepsis may develop 1–2 weeks after onset; without treatment, mortality is 20%, with treatment 1% (most common natural form of disease)
  - Organisms can be seen on routine Gram stain; chest x-ray may show widened mediastinum

- **Differential Diagnosis**
  - Pulmonary disease: tuberculosis, fungal infection, sarcoidosis, lymphoma with mediastinal adenopathy, plague
  - Skin lesions: staphylococcal or streptococcal infection

- **Treatment**
  - Prophylaxis with oral ciprofloxacin or doxycycline
  - Treatment with intravenous followed by oral doxycycline or ciprofloxacin for 60 days or 30 days with use of vaccine

- **Pearl**

A cluster of patients with atypical upper respiratory infection and mediastinal widening might be the earliest clue to a terrorist attack. Person-to-person transmission does not occur.

Reference

Inglesby TV et al: Anthrax as a biological weapon, 2002: updated recommendations for management. JAMA 2002;287:2236. [PMID: 11980524]

Botulinum Toxin

- **Essentials of Diagnosis**
  - Ptosis, diplopia, dysphagia, dysarthria, dysphonia, and possibly dilated, poorly reactive pupils (common)
  - Anticholinergic symptoms: xerostomia, intestinal ileus
  - Eventually paralysis moves to lower muscle groups leading to paralysis and respiratory compromise
  - Does *not* cause altered sensorium, sensory changes, or fever
  - Botulism is caused by protein toxin produced by *Clostridium botulinum,* a gram-positive, spore-forming, obligate anaerobe found naturally in soil
  - Toxin binds to cholinergic and motor neurons and prevents release of acetylcholine
  - Incubation period of 12–80 hours followed by flaccid symmetric descending muscle paralysis
  - Obtain electrolytes and arterial blood gas
  - Mouse bioassay is definitive test for botulism though not widely available

- **Differential Diagnosis**
  - Poliomyelitis
  - Myasthenia gravis (edrophonium test can be falsely positive in botulism; electromyography will differentiate the cause)
  - Tick paralysis (ascending paralysis)
  - Guillain Barré syndrome (ascending paralysis)
  - Periodic paralysis
  - Multiple sclerosis

- **Treatment**
  - Botulinum antitoxin binds free toxin but will not restore nerve terminals that have already been compromised
  - May require airway management and ventilatory support
  - Avoid clindamycin and aminoglycosides; may worsen neurologic blockade
  - Person-to-person transmission of botulism does not occur

- **Pearl**

Obtain an early negative inspiratory force (NIF) and tidal volume (weaning criteria) to determine need for airway support; these criteria are more sensitive than waiting for hypoxemia.

Reference

Arnon SS et al: Botulinum toxin as a biological weapon: medical and public health management. JAMA 2001;285:1059. [PMID: 11209178]

Cyanide Agents

- **Essentials of Diagnosis**
  - Cyanide gas has characteristic scent of bitter almonds
  - Tachycardia, hypertension, tachypnea followed by anxiety, mental status changes, coma, seizures, cardiac arrest, and death within 6–8 minutes
  - Cyanide distributes rapidly throughout body and bonds with a high affinity to the cytochrome a3 complex within the mitochondria, blocking aerobic cellular respiration
  - Anaerobic metabolism leads to lactic acidosis
  - Cyanosis does not develop; skin appears cherry-red
  - Laboratory studies show elevated venous oxygen saturation and increased lactic acid level

- **Differential Diagnosis**
  - Other causes of a high anion gap metabolic acidosis: lactic acidosis, diabetic ketoacidosis, uremia, salicylates, methanol, iron, isoniazid

- **Treatment**
  - Cyanide antidote kit (Taylor): amyl nitrate, sodium nitrite, sodium thiosulfate
  - Nitrites: amyl nitrate via inhalation or intravenous sodium nitrite will cause formation of methemoglobin, which will preferentially bind cyanide; sodium nitrite dose is adjusted for weight and hemoglobin concentration in children; fatal methemoglobinemia has occurred from overzealous use of nitrites
  - Sodium thiosulfate interacts with cyanide to form thiocyanate, which is secreted in urine; sodium thiosulfate is much safer than nitrites; may be considered as a sole therapy when carbon monoxide is present
  - Persistent symptoms may require repeat dosing at half the initial dose

- **Pearl**

Think cyanide or carbon monoxide when venous blood looks "arterial."

Reference

Chin RG, Calderon Y: Acute cyanide poisoning: a case report. J Emerg Med 2000;18:441. [PMID: 10802422]

G Agents & VX

- ### Essentials of Diagnosis
  - Nerve agents classified as organophosphates; usually rapid onset of action, absorbed via cutaneous or inhalation exposure
  - No significant latent period with vapor exposure; latent periods up to 18 hours after skin contamination
  - G agents more volatile than VX and will form a vapor more readily
  - Initial symptoms with lower vapor concentrations: miosis, rhinorrhea, and chest tightness; severe intoxication: salivation, involuntary defecation and urination, sweating, lacrimation, bradycardia or hypotension, respiratory depression, collapse, convulsions, and death (usually from respiratory failure)
  - Peripheral nicotinic effects: muscle fasciculations and weakness may progress to paralysis

- ### Differential Diagnosis
  - Other causes of a cholinergic toxidrome: organophosphates, carbamates

- ### Treatment
  - Patients *must* be decontaminated to prevent downstream contamination to the emergency department
  - Atropine, 1–2 mg IV or IM, and repeat every 3–5 minutes until patient reaches end point of drying of secretions (large doses may be required)
  - Pralidoxime chloride (2-PAM), 1–2 g IV, counteracts nicotinic activity if given before enzyme is irreversibly bound
  - For seizure activity: benzodiazepines
  - Supportive care, careful attention to ABCs, including rapid intubation for ventilatory support

- ### Pearl
  Failure to respond to a trial dose of atropine at routine doses supports the diagnosis of organophosphate or nerve gas exposure, especially if multiple patients are involved.

Reference
Reutter S: Hazards of chemical weapons released during war: new perspectives. Environ Health Perspect 1999;107:985. [PMID: 10585902]

Hemorrhagic Fever

- **Essentials of Diagnosis**
  - After an incubation period of 3–8 days, alterations in the vascular bed and increased vascular permeability lead to marked fever, conjunctival injection, mild hypotension, prostration, flushing, vomiting, diarrhea, and petechial hemorrhaging
  - Eventual shock and mucous membrane hemorrhage possible as well as hepatic, pulmonary, and neurologic involvement
  - Leukopenia, thrombocytopenia, proteinuria, hematuria, elevated liver enzymes may be seen
  - Definitive diagnosis possible with rapid enzyme immunoassays and with viral culture from the Centers for Disease Control and Prevention
  - Consider diagnosis in ill travelers with fever or in any patient with a severe febrile illness and evidence of vascular involvement

- **Differential Diagnosis**
  - Disseminated intravascular coagulation
  - Meningococcemia
  - Sepsis syndrome

- **Treatment**
  - Treatment is supportive
  - Ribavirin may improve mortality in some forms of hemorrhagic fever; can be initiated as prophylaxis for close contacts of patients
  - Limit intravenous lines and invasive procedures; use caution with fluid resuscitation
  - Consider heparin therapy for frank disseminated intravascular coagulopathy
  - Vaccine for yellow fever available (others exist though not available to the general public)
  - Strict body fluid precautions, airborne precautions; double-seal all laboratory specimens in airtight containers

- **Pearl**

Person-to-person transmission is a real danger to those caring for patients with hemorrhagic fever. HEPA filter masks and full infection control measures such as a negative-flow room are necessary.

Reference

Darling RG et al: Threats in bioterrorism. I: CDC category A agents. Emerg Med Clin North Am 2002;20:273. [PMID: 12120480]

Plague

■ **Essentials of Diagnosis**

- *Yersinia pestis* is a nonmotile, gram-negative bacillus with a "safety-pin" morphology causing bubonic, septicemic, and pneumonic plague
- Bubonic: bite of contaminated flea may cause fevers, chills, and weakness followed by regional lymph node swelling and tenderness (bubo)
- Septicemic: fever, dyspnea, hypotension, purpuric skin lesions, gangrene of extremities and nose (black death)
- Pneumonic: form most likely to occur from terrorist attack with dissemination of an aerosolized bacteria; latent period of 1–6 days followed by fever, productive cough, blood-tinged sputum, dyspnea, hypoxia, and possible gastrointestinal symptoms
- Organism seen on routine Gram stain or with characteristic bipolar staining pattern on special stains; routine cultures may be helpful; fluorescent antibody staining of capsular antigen
- Chest x-ray shows patchy or confluent lobar infiltrate

■ **Differential Diagnosis**

- Adenopathy, abscess, lymphogranuloma venereum (bubonic form)
- Pneumonia, influenza, chancroid, tuberculosis, scrub typhus, meningitis, encephalitis

■ **Treatment**

- Historically streptomycin, 15 mg/kg IM, has been treatment; gentamicin or gentamicin-chloramphenicol combinations, doxycycline, or ciprofloxacin are also described
- For meningitis or hemodynamically unstable patients: chloramphenicol
- Treatment duration is for a minimum of 10 days or at least 4 days after clinical recovery
- Intensive supportive care
- Respiratory and droplet isolation
- Unprotected direct contacts should receive postexposure prophylaxis for 6 days with tetracycline, 15–30 mg/kg/d, or doxycycline, 100 mg twice a day

■ **Pearl**

Primary pneumonic plague from an aerosolized terrorist attack does not typically cause the bubo adenopathy seen with naturally occurring disease.

Reference

Inglesby TV et al: Plague as a biological weapon: medical and public health management. Working Group on Civilian Biodefense. JAMA 2000;283:2281. [PMID: 10807389]

Q Fever

■ Essentials of Diagnosis

- Caused by sporelike form of the rickettsial organism *Coxiella burnetii*
- Incubation period 5–30 days followed by nonspecific symptoms of fever, chills, malaise, myalgias, headache, anorexia, nausea, vomiting, diarrhea, and maculopapular rash
- Presentation much like an atypical pneumonia; when cough is present, it is usually nonproductive
- Cardiac manifestations: endocarditis, myocarditis, pericarditis
- Elevated liver enzymes common, mainstay of diagnosis is by complement fixation, indirect fluorescent antibody testing, or enzyme-linked immunosorbent assay
- Debilitating disease; mortality typically less than 2.5%
- Routine tests and cultures not helpful; specialized testing may be available in specialized reference laboratories
- Chest x-ray may show multiple round opacities and, in up to one-third of cases, a pleural effusion

■ Differential Diagnosis

- Atypical pneumonia
- Influenza

■ Treatment

- Most cases resolve without antibiotic therapy, but a 7-day course of tetracycline is used most commonly; other drugs include macrolides, quinolones, chloramphenicol, rifampin, or trimethoprim-sulfamethoxazole
- Person-to-person spread of disease is unlikely
- Prophylactic course of antibiotics should be started 8–12 days after exposure

■ Pearl

Q fever is the only rickettsial infection spread via inhalation rather than tick vector; therefore, it has potential to be used as a terrorist weapon.

Reference

Marrie TJ: Q fever pneumonia. Curr Opin Infect Dis 2004;17:137. [PMID: 15021054]

Smallpox

- **Essentials of Diagnosis**
  - Caused by the *variola* virus of the genus *Orthopoxvirus*
  - Spread via inhalation, direct contact, and fomites such as clothes and sheets
  - Inhalation of virus is followed by 7- to 17-day incubation period as virus replicates in lymph nodes, bone marrow, and spleen
  - Secondary viremia causes high fever, malaise, headache, backache, and sometimes delirium; 2 days later, the characteristic rash begins: initially in the mouth and then on the hands and forearms followed by the legs and trunk; the rash does not spare the palms or soles; progression from macules to papules to pustules, eventually forming scabs that separate to leave scars; all lesions will be in similar stages of development; patient is extremely contagious until all scabs have fallen off
  - A fatal hemorrhagic form of the rash may occur
  - Virus particles in pustular fluid easily recognized via electron microscopy; analysis by special cultures, polymerase chain reaction, and biologic assays
  - Humans are only natural host; no carrier state

- **Differential Diagnosis**
  - Varicella: in contrast to smallpox, lesions are at different stages of development

- **Treatment**
  - No specific therapy exists (cidofovir promising in animal studies)
  - Treatment is supportive
  - Strict isolation or quarantine
  - Vaccine available for prophylaxis; may lessen illness if given within 4 days after exposure
  - Early involvement of appropriate government public health agencies is essential for rapid containment

- **Pearl**

Varicella (chicken pox) rash appears in crops at multiple stages usually concentrated on the extremities although sparing the hands and feet.

Reference

Henderson DA: Smallpox as a biological weapon: medical and public health management. Working Group on Civilian Biodefense. JAMA 1999;281:2127. [PMID: 10367824]

Sulfur Mustard

- **Essentials of Diagnosis**
  - Vesicant readily absorbed through intact skin
  - May exist as vapor or liquid; characteristic odor of garlic or mustard
  - Initial exposure is asymptomatic; patients may not decontaminate
  - After latent period of 2–48 hours, patients may display effects that range from mild dermal injury to rapid death
  - Skin: erythema, burning, blisters with straw-colored fluid
  - Eyes: ocular pain, photophobia, conjunctivitis, blepharospasm, possible denuding of superficial cornea
  - Respiratory: oronasal burning, rhinorrhea, epistaxis, cough, dyspnea, mucous membrane necrosis, pulmonary edema, respiratory failure
  - Gastrointestinal: nausea and vomiting, diarrhea, constipation
  - CNS (with severe exposures): mental status changes, seizure activity
  - Bone marrow suppression may occur; leukocytosis early followed by pancytopenia
  - The metabolite thiodiglycol may be detected in urine
  - Chest x-ray may reveal focal or diffuse pneumonitis or pulmonary edema

- **Differential Diagnosis**
  - Corrosive exposure; other vesicants

- **Treatment**
  - Decontamination with soapy water or 0.5% hypochlorite solution; leave small blisters intact, unroof large blisters
  - Topical antibiotics for skin and eyes
  - For bronchospasm: systemic steroids and inhaled bronchodilators
  - For gastrointestinal symptoms: antispasmodics
  - Supplemental oxygen, airway management, and ventilation may be required
  - Bone marrow transplant or factor replacement may be necessary

- **Pearl**

Decontamination to prevent downstream contamination is critical.

Reference

Rice P: Sulphur mustard injuries of the skin. Pathophysiology and management. Toxicol Rev 2003;22:111. [PMID: 15071821]

Index

A

ABCs
  in chest trauma, 277
  in children, 461, 464
Abdomen, occult injuries to, 338
Abdominal aortic aneurysm, 111
Abdominal pain, 116, 127, 152, 161, 166
  in children, 462, 475, 489
  in endocrine disorders, 159, 160,
    163, 165
  in GI emergency, 52, 56, 57, 59, 65, 69,
    70, 75, 76
  in gynecologic emergency, 198, 199,
    204, 207
Abortion
  septic, 208
  spontaneous, 202
Abscess
  amebic, 65
  Bartholin, 193
  brain, 79
  breast, 201
  "collar button," 353
  deep space, 351
  of distal phalanx, 354
  hepatic, 65
  hordeolum, 222
  parapharyngeal, 247
  pelvic, 204, 208
  peritonsillar, 245
  pyogenic, 65
  retropharyngeal, 247, 487
  "shooter's," 142
  on side of nose, 221
  tuboovarian, 210
Accelerated idioventricular rhythm
  (AIVR), 18
Acetamonphen poisoning, 427
Achilles tendonitis, 191
Achilles tendon rupture, 312
Acid ingestion, 434
Acidosis, 438
  lactic, 161
  metabolic, 160, 161, 176
  respiratory, 178
Acoustic neuroma, 78
Acromioclavicular (AC) joint injury, 314
Acute mountain sickness, 396, 408
Acute respiratory distress syndrome
  (ARDS), 37

Adenopathy, 48, 124. *See also*
  Lymphadenopathy
Adenovirus, 481
Adnexal torsion, 192
Adolescents. *See also* Children
  gonococcal infection in, 137
  patella dislocation in, 332
Adrenal insufficiency, 153, 164
Affective disorders, bipolar, 389
Agoraphobia, 392
AIDS, 136. *See also*
  Immunocrompromised patients
Airway management, 178, 242, 245, 247,
  491. *See also* Intubation
  in angioedema, 371
  in children, 487
  in facial trauma, 266, 267, 275
  in nasal fracture, 268
  in neck trauma, 262, 271
  in neurologic emergency, 88,
    89, 90
  in poisoning, 450
  in tonsillary enlargement, 124
Alcohol
  and ketoacidosis, 159
  in neurologic disorders, 97
  rubbing, 444
Alcohol dependence, 387
Alcoholic hepatitis, 439
Alcoholics Anonymous, 387
Alcoholism, 67, 74, 89, 186, 387, 444
Alcohol withdrawal, 387, 388
Alkali ingestion, 434
Alkalosis, 172
  metabolic, 177, 484
  respiratory, 179
Altitude
  and acute mountain sickness, 396
  and cerebral edema, 408
  and pulmonary edema, 409
  and retinal hemorrhages, 231
Alveolar infiltrates, in pneumonia, 45
Amebiasis, 57
Amebic abscess, 65
Amiodarone, 36, 43
Amphetamine poisoning, 428, 435
Amputation, 406
  fingertip, 355
  traumatic, 347
Amygdalin, exposure to, 436